Nursing: Clinical Research and Practice

Volume II

Nursing: Clinical Research and Practice
Volume II

Edited by **Cynthia Wison**

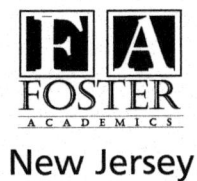

FOSTER
ACADEMICS

New Jersey

Published by Foster Academics,
61 Van Reypen Street,
Jersey City, NJ 07306, USA
www.fosteracademics.com

Nursing: Clinical Research and Practice
Volume II
Edited by Cynthia Wison

International Standard Book Number: 978-1-63242-295-8 (Hardback)

Contents

              Making Independent Decisions over Time**   **163**
              Agneta Breitholtz, Ingrid Snellman and Ingegerd Fagerberg

Chapter 21   **Epigenetic Mechanisms Shape the Biological Response to
              Trauma and Risk for PTSD: A Critical Review**   **171**
              Morgan Heinzelmann and Jessica Gill

Chapter 22   **Toothbrush Contamination: A Review of the Literature**   **181**
              Michelle R. Frazelle and Cindy L. Munro

Chapter 23   **Primary Health Care: Comparing Public Health
              Nursing Models in Ireland and Norway**   **187**
              Anne Clancy, Patricia Leahy-Warren,
              Mary Rose Day and Helen Mulcahy

Chapter 24   **Planning for Serious Illness amongst
              Community-Dwelling Older Adults**   **196**
              Donna Goodridge

              Permissions

              List of Contributors

Preface

Nursing research is most commonly the research that provides evidence which can be used to support nursing practices. Nursing is an evidence-based area of practice. It has been developing since the 19th century and in this age many nurses now work as researchers based in universities as well as in the health care field. It is a field of study that places stress upon the use of evidence from research and practice in order to explain and justify nursing interventions. Nursing research can be broadly branched off into two methodologies- Quantitative Research where the dominant method is randomised controlled trial and Qualitative Research where the methods focus on are interviews, case studies, focus groups and ethnography. Advances in science of nursing through research have broadened our knowledge and understanding of health and illness in man. Research is used by nurses to provide evidence-based care that encourages quality health solutions for individuals, families, communities and health care systems. Research is also useful in the shaping of global and national health policies in or within an organization, at local, state and federal levels. Nurses therefore conduct research projects, practice research or rather apply research in practical situations and teach about research. Nursing research can thus build foundations for clinical practise, prevent disease and disability as well as manage symptoms and also provide and enhanced palliative care.

This book attempts to collate research and data on nursing under a common aegis. I am grateful to those who put in their hard work and efforts in this endeavour. I am also thankful to those who supported this undertaking. I especially wish to thank my friends and family. I would not have been able to complete this vast project without their support and understanding.

Editor

A Comparison of a Traditional Clinical Experience to a Precepted Clinical Experience for Baccalaureate-Seeking Nursing Students in Their Second Semester

Kristin Ownby, Renae Schumann, Linda Dune, and David Kohne

The University of Texas Health Science Center School of Nursing at Houston, 6901 Bertner Avenue, Room 691, Houston, TX 77030, USA

Correspondence should be addressed to Kristin Ownby, kristin.k.ownby@uth.tmc.edu

Academic Editor: Florence Myrick

The shortage of nursing faculty has contributed greatly to the nursing workforce shortage, with many schools turning away qualified applicants because there are not enough faculty to teach. Despite the faculty shortage, schools are required to admit more students to alleviate the nursing shortage. Clinical groups in which preceptors are responsible for student learning extend faculty resources. *Purpose.* To determine the effectiveness of an alternative clinical experience (preceptorship). *Methods.* quasi-experimental, randomized, longitudinal design. Students were randomized to either the traditional or precepted clinical group. The clinical experience was a total of 12 weeks. Groups were compared according to several variables including second semester exam scores, HESI scores, and quality and timeliness of clinical paperwork. *Sample.* Over a two-year period, seventy-one undergraduate nursing students in the second semester medical-surgical nursing course participated. 36 were randomized to the experimental group. The preceptors were baccalaureate-prepared nurses who have been practicing for at least one year. *Setting.* Two hospitals located in the Texas Medical Center. *Statistical Analysis.* Descriptive statistics and independent *t*-test. *Results.* There was no difference between the groups on the variables of interest. *Conclusion.* Students in the precepted clinical group perform as well as those in a traditional clinical group.

1. Introduction

A recent report published by the American Association of Colleges of Nursing (AACN) noted that over 67,000 qualified applicants were not accepted into baccalaureate and graduate nursing programs in the USA in 2010. The report also noted that almost two-thirds of the nursing schools participating in the survey noted that faculty shortage is the primary reason for not accepting all qualified applicants into baccalaureate programs [1]. The consequence of a nursing shortage is nurses work longer hours under stressful conditions, which leads to nurses being more prone to making mistakes and medical errors. Subsequently, patient care suffers.

Schools of nursing are increasingly using hospital-based nurses to precept students during clinical rotations. These nurse preceptors extend the faculty at a time when a shortage of nursing faculty limits nursing school enrollment. Combined with initiatives already in place, such as using master's prepared nurses at the hospital as loaned faculty, compressing students' clinical rotations and assigning clinical rotations to off-shifts or, in less popular nursing units, using nurse preceptors as clinical faculty helps in two ways: it increases the number of available clinical nursing slots and it provides qualified clinical instructors. As little quantitative research on the effectiveness of using preceptors as clinical instructors early in a nursing program has been reported, this study looks at the question "Given baccalaureate students in their second medical-surgical class, do precepted students perform as academically well as traditionally prepared students?"

Clinical groups in Texas traditionally have a ratio of one master's prepared instructor to 10 students. The instructor's role is to monitor students in the clinical setting and instruct them in meeting their educational learning objectives. When class size is extended to increase enrollment, procuring a sufficient number of qualified clinical instructors is often difficult. That nurses qualified for teaching can make higher salaries working as a nurse in a hospital than as faculty in a university exacerbates the faculty shortage problem. Additionally, as the number of clinical slots dedicated to nursing students is limited, schools in the region compete with each other.

Nursing students today differ from students of past generations [2]. Students often demand accessible and timely information, and they want flexibility to meet their needs of working, studying, and raising a family. The younger students rely heavily on technology for learning, entertainment, and life scheduling. Learning experiences must be not only timely, but also relevant [3]. Students precepted one-on-one with registered nurses (RN) in hospital settings are more likely to find their needs met than is possible under a traditional group model, which permits less interaction between faculty and student, limits student opportunities for learning and skills practice, and provides an inaccurate view of the profession [4, 5].

According to the Texas Board of Nurse Examiners [6], master's prepared faculty can oversee the teaching activities of 12 RN preceptors, each of whom can supervise two undergraduate students. Using preceptors as clinical faculty alternatives more than doubles the number of students ($N = 12 \times 2 = 24$) than can be placed in traditional clinical rotations ($N = 10$). The policy established by the Texas Board of Nursing states that a precepted student must be visited by a faculty member at least once a month. Faculty conducting the study rounded on precepted students at least twice a month since the students were early in their nursing program.

Hospital-based clinical preceptors, as alternatives to clinical faculty, expect adequate support to function within the educator role [7]. According to Yonge and Myrick [8], preparation of preceptors includes teaching educational principles that help prepare the preceptors beyond their usual staff nurse orientation. Wilkes et al. [9] identified that continued support materials, beyond orientation, were essential to success. This support can be online and extended to faculty and students [10]. Using hand-held computers allows preceptors to obtain support at the bedside when time is at a premium and desktop services are not available [11]. The use of hand-held computers with internet access is an effective way for preceptors to obtain information, such as faculty contact information, school policies, and student clinical schedules, prepare anecdotal notes, and search for useful clinical information [12, 13].

Use of the precepting alternative also frees up additional nurses and hospital units for clinical training; nurses on smaller units not able to support a traditional group of 10 students could precept one-on-one and nurses working off-shifts can serve as preceptors [14]. Students participating in precepted groups find that they have more scheduling flexibility, greater opportunities for learning and practicing skills, and more relevant learning experiences [15].

TABLE 1: Online Modules Available to Nurse Preceptors.

Module No.	Module title
1	Nurses and the educational process
2	Preceptorship and nursing education
3	Applying learning theories to teaching
4	Assessing learning styles
5	Learning contracts
6	Motivation to learn
7	Critical thinking
8	Communicating with students
9	The impact of technology on education
10	Ethical and legal issues in clinical nursing education
11	Clinical evaluation of students
12	Evidence-based practice
13	Cultural competency and health care
14	Educating students with special needs

To prepare the nurses for the preceptor role, the researchers developed a 14-module online preceptor education course. The module units, listed in Table 1, were designed to provide direction on teaching students as adult learners and to promote critical thinking in nursing students. The online training was offered through Blackboard. The project team, including faculty and hospital educators, attended the preceptors' presentations to offer technical training and support. Upon completion of the preceptor training, nurses received 9.6 continuing education units.

Having Blackboard access also gave the RN preceptors access to the students' course materials, including syllabi and lecture notes, which permitted the RN preceptors to provide clinical experiences that met the learning objectives and to keep pace with the students learning progression. As nurses traditionally work with new hire graduates and not students in their second semester of nursing education, it was important that preceptors knew that these students would not perform at the same level as a new graduate nurse.

Technology assisted in permitting continuous availability of faculty and in forming a communication net for students, preceptors, and faculty. Communication was via a dedicated web page, E-mail, cellular phones, traditional pagers, and handheld computers. Preceptors working at the bedside could communicate with nursing faculty in the office. Using the handheld computers, preceptors had a rapid means of access to relevant nursing and drug information while they were working with the students.

In addition, the research faculty and project staff developed a project-specific website to provide quick access to contact information, school policies, performance issue information, tips and topics, and links for emergencies and needle sticks. The website was a resource for preceptors and students whether the students were precepted during school hours or on off-shifts. Both preceptors and students could rapidly locate faculty contact information or receive technical support 24 hours a day. This was necessary as

A Comparison of a Traditional Clinical Experience to a Precepted Clinical Experience for Baccalaureate-Seeking Nursing Students in Their Second Semester

3

the precepted students worked the schedule their preceptor worked, whether this was a day, night, or weekend shift. E-mail group links permitted communication to the project staff and the control and experimental student groups. The availability of student performance information and school policies assisted preceptors to take appropriate action in addressing student attendance, dress and appearance, safety, and professionalism issues.

Using Blackboard to deliver the education course online permitted the RN preceptors to complete the training at their convenience; it also gave them access to additional learning resources. Since the students worked all shifts, discussion boards were set up to support communication and submission of assignments. Nursing faculty moderated the discussion postings and responded accordingly. Additionally, faculty and hospital educators periodically made rounds when students were scheduled to be with their preceptors to stay in contact, answer questions, and provide support. This also permitted faculty to assess student progress and preceptor effectiveness. The use of technology helped to decrease preceptor resistance in precepting students without the instructor being present and increased faculty assurance in the quality and relevance of the preceptors teaching.

The students had to complete a total of 96 hours in the clinical setting and were permitted to work between 8 and 24 hours per week. For faculty to keep track of student schedule and hours, students posted their clinical schedule at least 48 hours prior to working with their preceptor. Faculty held weekly post-clinical conferences with students at the school to answer questions and reinforce learning objectives. However, faculty were available to the students and preceptors by cellular phone twenty-four hours a day.

2. Methodology

The study used a quasi-experimental design where students ($N = 69$) were randomly assigned to a control group (traditional clinical group) or experimental group (precepted group). The subjects were in the second semester of their nursing education, and instruction that semester included pharmacology, gerontology, pathophysiology, and the second medical-surgical nursing course. Both experimental and control students volunteering to participate in the study submitted an informed consent form in accordance with the university's Institutional Review Board policy.

For experimental and control groups, the student's accumulative numerical course grade in medical-surgical course 1 (taken in the first semester) was used as an independent variable. The dependent variables were students' numerical grades on unit examinations given throughout the semester, comprehensive final examination grades, and accumulative numerical course grades in both the medical-surgical course 2 and the corequisite pharmacology course. Both experimental and control students took a standardized medical-surgical exam. Although scores earned on exams administered to measure what the student learned in the classroom does not have established reliability and validity for measuring clinical performance, issues surrounding clinical evaluation exist.

Some of the identified issues pertinent to this study include the subjectivity of the evaluation especially when using "novice" clinical faculty. Novice faculty (bedside nurses serving as preceptors) may have limited formal education and experience in evaluation of students and often lack confidence in their ability to fairly evaluate students [16, 17].

Using a grading rubric, two faculty members on the research team reviewed the precepted student's nursing process papers at weeks 4, 8, and 12 and recorded these grades. To increase interrater reliability, the two researchers critiqued one student's paper prior to week 4 to standardize scoring.

A clinical evaluation form was developed for preceptor use (Table 1 in supplementary material available online at doi:10.1155/2012/276506). After each 12-hour shift, the preceptor evaluated the student's clinical performance and faxed the form to the research team. Content covering the process of clinical evaluation was included within the online preceptor course. Faculty reviewed clinical evaluations after each shift worked by the student. If a student is consistently scoring 2 or less on the evaluation, the faculty meets with the preceptor to discuss the weaknesses of the student. Faculty would meet with the student as well to discuss strategies for improving their clinical performance. The final clinical evaluation was completed by the faculty and was based on data from the preceptor evaluations, the nursing process paper grades, and the faculty's impressions when rounding on the student in the hospital.

2.1. Sample and Setting. The students were randomized into two groups, experimental or precepted group ($N = 37$) and control or traditional group ($N = 32$). The sample consisted of 6 male and 63 female students. The precepted students were assigned clinical rotations at two tertiary-level hospitals, where they worked one-on-one with a baccalaureate-prepared registered nurse (RN) on a medical or surgical unit or a surgical intermediate care unit. As per the request of the two hospitals, precepted students could not work on the days other school of nursing held their traditional clinical. This meant that there was one day a week in which the precepted students could not schedule a clinical day. Precepted students were not exposed to the traditional students or their faculty when working. The control students were mixed within the traditional training groups of 10 students, and these groups were assigned to medical-surgical floors at various local hospitals.

Hospital educators recruited the preceptors. The criteria for eligibility were that the RNs (1) have at least one year experience as a registered nurse; (2) have a recent satisfactory annual evaluation by their nurse manager; (3) have a current BCLS and nursing license; (4) completed the online preceptor education course; (5) graduated from a baccalaureate nursing program. Inclusion criteria for students were that they were in their second semester of nursing school and had not previously withdrawn from or failed a class.

2.2. Data Analysis. The students' final numerical course grade from the first semester medical-surgical course was analyzed using an independent sample *t*-test to determine whether the first semester grade needed to be used as a co-variant. However, this test showed no significant difference between the experimental and control designated groups. Student 2nd semester medical-surgical examination scores (4 units and 1 comprehensive final) were analyzed using a mixed model approach for repeated measures ANOVA. Final numerical grades from their pharmacology course and a standardized specialty medical-surgical examination (HESI) were analyzed using independent sample t-tests.

3. Results

No significant differences between the experimental and control groups on any measurement were found. For discussion purposes, an implication is that precepted students did as academically well as students in the control group. Likewise, this could be stated, as precepted students do no better than traditional students academically despite the one-on-one clinical treatment. Given this, the study supports using hospital-based RN nurses as clinical preceptors. Using RNs as preceptors not only provides much needed clinical faculty but also frees up clinical slots that previously have not been available.

3.1. Analysis of the Medical-Surgical Course Grades. The four unit examination grades and the final examination grade were analyzed using a mix model approach for repeated measures ANOVA. There was no statistically significant difference between the precepted and control groups ($F = .936$, df = 63, $P = .449$). Mean grade scores for the examinations are presented in Table 2.

An independent sample t test was computed to determine if there was a significant difference between precepted and control groups in academic performance as demonstrated by the final course grade students received in their second semester medical-surgical course. Students in the traditional clinical group had a mean of 83.7 (SD = 5.9), and the precepted students had a mean of 83.5 (SD = 4.6). There was no statistical difference between the two groups ($t = .118$, df = 67, $P = .906$).

3.2. HESI Medical-Surgical Specialty Exam. As second semester students take the Health Education Services Inc. (HESI, now owned by Elsevier) medical-surgical specialty exam at the end of the semester, this mean score was considered in the analysis. The mean standard score for the traditional students was 784.19 (SD = 182.5) as compared to a mean standard score of 807.76 (SD = 136.7) for the precepted students. However, there was no statistical difference between the two groups ($t = -.612$, df = 67, $P = .543$).

3.3. Pharmacology Final Course Grade. Students in the traditional clinical groups usually prepared medication cards the day before each clinical session. As students in the precepted group did not know which patients their preceptor would have until report, they had to take a different approach. They reviewed each medication and presented the information to their preceptor before administering the medication. In

TABLE 2: Mean Scores for 2nd semester BSN student medical-surgical course.

Examination	Group	Mean	SD
1	Control	88.7	6.3
	Experimental	88.4	5.5
2	Control	87.3	7.9
	Experimental	87.6	7.3
3	Control	84.9	5.5
	Experimental	86.1	5.5
4	Control	83.0	8.5
	Experimental	81.1	9.0
Comprehensive	Control	78.1	8.1
	Experimental	77.9	6.8

analyzing pharmacology final course grades, there was no statistical difference between the two groups ($t = -.786$, df = 67, $P = 434$). The students in the control group had a mean grade of 89.1 (SD = 3.8), and the precepted group had a mean of 88.3 (SD = 4.8).

3.4. Clinical Evaluations. On average, the students in the precepted group received ratings of 3–5 for the clinical competencies listed on the clinical evaluation form. As expected, some preceptors were more confident in their role as clinical evaluator. Confident preceptors not only rated the clinical performance, but also provided anecdotal information to justify the given ratings. Preceptors did note that the clinical evaluation process was an added responsibility to their busy clinical day.

3.5. Nursing Process Papers. Unlike students in the traditional group, precepted students arrived for their shift with no preparatory work in place. The student and their preceptor selected one patient as the student's primary patient for that shift. Although the precepted student was responsible for obtaining the same information as that of a traditional student, the precepted students did this on shift and completed the nursing process papers retrospectively. The faculty found that the quality of the nursing process papers were similar between the precepted and the traditional groups. Students in both groups struggled with parts of the nursing diagnosis ("related to" statement) and setting measurable expected outcomes. Precepted students demonstrated a better comprehension of the importance of replanning. Another difference between the two groups was timeliness. The precepted students, instructed to turn in their paperwork within a week of completing the shift, tended to fall behind, allowing the paperwork to accumulate.

3.6. Challenges. The research team confronted several challenges during the two-year study. One major challenge was merging the technology of two different institutions via Internet. The information technology (IT) member of the research team worked closely with the two hospitals that participated in the study. The IT personnel from the two

A Comparison of a Traditional Clinical Experience to a Precepted Clinical Experience for Baccalaureate-Seeking
Nursing Students in Their Second Semester

5

hospitals and the university had to breech the "firewall" that existed between institutions. IT teams on both sides were involved and were able to accomplish this task. Once the two systems were connected, the IT member of the research team met with preceptors one-on-one to help them navigate the Blackboard site within the university. The IT personnel discovered that many nurses were not technologically perceptive. The IT member held mini tutorials to help the preceptors learn how to use their institution's intranet, access the university's Blackboard site, and navigate the preceptor course. This challenge was not anticipated by the research team and did require additional time not planned in the original proposal.

Overall, the experiences with the preceptors were positive. Most preceptors had served in the role in the past, orienting new hires on their respective units. One occasion arose where a preceptor placed the student in a dangerous situation (administering medications without being present). The student reported the incident, and working with the institution, the preceptor was replaced with another nurse.

Another challenge was the evaluation process by the preceptors. Although many of the preceptors have mentored new nurses on their units, they had not participated in a formal evaluation process. Some preceptors would circle all the same number on the Likert scale clinical performance evaluation and would not provide any commentary. The members of the research team would meet with preceptors and ask for a verbal evaluation of the student's performance. Questions asked included an assessment of the student's ability to perform a focused review of systems and physical exam, knowledge of medications and their administration, and the potential to use the nursing process to plan appropriate care for the patient, for example. Meeting with preceptors frequently provided more insights into the clinical performance of the student. Reviewing the nursing process papers also provided insights as to how the student was performing in the clinical setting.

4. Discussion

In the last decade, we have seen an increase in the number of applicants to nursing programs, a decline in the number of nurses in the workforce, and a decline in the number of nurses who pursue a career in academia. With the nursing shortage, demands are made on schools to increase enrollment; however, with the shortage of nursing faculty, this demand has been difficult to meet. As a barrier to increasing enrollment has been clinical availability [5], a solution is using nurse preceptors to extend faculty in the clinical setting.

This project examined the use of preceptors, supported by training and technology, to facilitate the clinical experience of students in their second semester medical-surgical course. Precepting students are not a new concept within nursing; however, a preceptor support model for students early in their nursing education has not been fully studied [14]. The purpose of the study was to determine whether students who were precepted performed as well as those

in a traditional clinical group. As there was no significant difference in performance on grades and HESI scores, the premise is upheld. The results suggest that from an academic perspective, providing clinical education when using qualified and trained preceptors did not interfere with the student's ability to master the course content.

The quality of the nursing process papers produced by students was deemed to be equal between the two groups. Students in both groups were provided feedback on their papers and were asked in equal proportion to resubmit work. The quality of the medication information sheets was found to be equivalent. As the main problem encountered was the timeliness of the submission of the paperwork, a solution would be to design a mechanism within the computer-scheduling program that locked out students from posting their schedule until all nursing process paperwork was completed.

Funding

This study was supported by grants from the Health Resource and Service Administration (HRSA 1D64HP01664-01-00) and the Texas Higher Education Coordinating Board (CUS8).

References

[1] "2010-2011 Enrollment and Graduations in Baccalaureate and Graduate Programs in Nursing," American Association of Colleges of Nursing, http://www.aacn.nche.edu/IDS.

[2] M. M. Maag, "Nursing students' attitudes toward technology: a national study," *Nurse Educator*, vol. 31, no. 3, pp. 112–118, 2006.

[3] J. Berry, "A student and rn partnered clinical experience," *Nurse Educator.*, vol. 30, no. 6, pp. 240–241, 2005.

[4] J. Nordgren, S. J. Richardson, and V. B. Laurella, "A collaborative preceptor model for clinical teaching of beginning nursing students," *Nurse Educator*, vol. 23, no. 3, pp. 27–32, 1998.

[5] C. A. Tanner, "Thinking like a nurse: a research-based model of clinical judgment in nursing," *Journal of Nursing Education*, vol. 45, no. 6, pp. 204–211, 2006.

[6] Texas Board of Nurse Examiners, "Rules and regulations," 2004, http://info.sos.state.tx.us/pls/pub.

[7] G. Alspach, "Caring for preceptors: a survey of what they need and want in educational support," *Critical Care Nurse*, vol. 25, no. 8, pp. 10–11, 2005.

[8] O. Yonge and F. Myrick, "Preceptorship and the preparatory process for undergraduate nursing students and their preceptors," *Journal for Nurses in Staff Development*, vol. 20, no. 6, pp. 294–297, 2004.

[9] M. S. Wilkes, J. R. Hoffman, R. Usatine, and S. Baillie, "An innovative program to augment community preceptors' practice and teaching skills," *Academic Medicine*, vol. 81, no. 4, pp. 332–341, 2006.

[10] S. B. Morris-Docker, A. Tod, J. M. Harrison, D. Wolstenholme, and R. Black, "Nurses' use of the internet in clinical ward settings," *Journal of Advanced Nursing*, vol. 48, no. 2, pp. 157–166, 2004.

[11] C. L. Covell, C. Lemay, and D. Gaumond, "Deployment of computer-based training programs via a hospital intranet:

methods used, lessons learned," *Journal for Nurses in Staff Development*, vol. 20, no. 5, pp. 197–210, 2004.

[12] B. W. Thompson, "The transforming effect of handheld computers on nursing practice," *Nursing Administration Quarterly.*, vol. 29, no. 4, pp. 308–314, 2005.

[13] J. M. Johnston, G. M. Leung, K. Y. K. Tin, L. M. Ho, W. Lam, and R. Fielding, "Evaluation of a handheld clinical decision support tool for evidence-based learning and practice in medical undergraduates," *Medical Education*, vol. 38, no. 6, pp. 628–637, 2004.

[14] K. D. Ryan-Nicholls, "Preceptor recruitment and retention," *the Canadian Nurse*, vol. 100, no. 6, pp. 18–22, 2004.

[15] O. A. Freiburger, "A tribute to clinical preceptors. developing a preceptor program for nursing students," *Journal for Nurses in Staff Development*, vol. 17, no. 6, pp. 320–327, 2001.

[16] M. H. Oermann and K. Gaberson, *Evaluation and Testing in Nursing Education*, Springer, New York, NY, USA, 3rd edition, 2006.

[17] L. A. Seldomridge and C. M. Walsh, "Evaluating student performance in undergraduate preceptorships," *Journal of Nursing Education*, vol. 45, no. 5, pp. 169–176, 2006.

Developing Targeted Health Service Interventions Using the PRECEDE-PROCEED Model: Two Australian Case Studies

Jane L. Phillips,[1] John X. Rolley,[2] and Patricia M. Davidson[3]

[1] School of Nursing, The University of Notre Dame Australia, The Cunningham Centre for Palliative Care, St Vincent's & Mater Health Sydney, 170 Darlinghurst Road, Sydney, NSW 2010, Australia
[2] Cardiac Investigation Unit, St Vincent's Hospital, P.O. Box 2900, Fitzroy, VIC 3065, Australia
[3] Cardiovascular Nursing Research, St Vincent's Hospital and Centre for Cardiovascular and Chronic Care, Faculty of Nursing, Midwifery & Health, University of Technology Sydney, Broadway, NSW 2007, Australia

Correspondence should be addressed to Jane L. Phillips, jane.phillips@nd.edu.au

Academic Editor: Sheila Payne

Aims and Objectives. This paper provides an overview of the applicability of the PRECEDE-PROCEED Model to the development of targeted nursing led chronic illness interventions. *Background.* Changing health care practice is a complex and dynamic process that requires consideration of social, political, economic, and organisational factors. An understanding of the characteristics of the target population, health professionals, and organizations plus identification of the determinants for change are also required. Synthesizing this data to guide the development of an effective intervention is a challenging process. The PRECEDE-PROCEED Model has been used in global health care settings to guide the identification, planning, implementation, and evaluation of various health improvement initiatives. *Design.* Using a reflective case study approach, this paper examines the applicability of the PRECEDE-PROCEED Model to the development of targeted chronic care improvement interventions for two distinct Australian populations: a rapidly expanding and aging rural population with unmet palliative care needs and a disadvantaged urban community at higher risk of cardiovascular disease. *Results.* The PRECEDE-PROCEED Model approach demonstrated utility across diverse health settings in a systematic planning process. In environments characterized by increasing health care needs, limited resources, and growing community expectations, adopting planning tools such as PRECEDE-PROCEED Model at a local level can facilitate the development of the most effective interventions. *Relevance to Clinical Practice.* The PRECEDE-PROCEED Model is a strong theoretical model that guides the development of realistic nursing led interventions with the best chance of being successful in existing health care environments.

1. Introduction

Globally, over the past decade there has been increasing recognition of the need for effective management of chronic and complex conditions and less dependence on acute care services [1, 2]. Achieving this magnitude of reform has been difficult because it requires reorientation of health services, a greater focus on primary health care, and an enduring commitment to the delivery of best evidence-based practice. This increased emphasis on evidence-based practice dictates that a systematic and critical analysis of priorities and presumed causes be undertaken to guide health service planning [1, 3]. Yet, health professionals frequently rely solely on intuition or anecdotal information to identify or address a particular health problem at a population level as opposed to empirical research [4].

1.1. Needs Assessment. A Needs Assessment is a complex, multidimensional process which provides information and evidence to inform the objective and valid tailoring of health services or commissioning of new initiatives. The needs assessment process ensures due consideration is given to the quality of the evidence relevant to the risks and benefits of specific interventions [5]. Identifying the priority health problem and analysing the problem is often the catalyst that enables services to reorientate care delivery from being institutionally focused to addressing populations needs [6]. This systematic process facilitates appraisal of a population's health needs, identifies service gaps, the services required and the degree to which the proposed service(s) will be used by those in greatest need [7]. All relevant information, concerning health-related needs, and possible solutions to enable the planning and delivery of cost-effective services or new initiatives are collated [8]. This data enables navigation of a pathway forward, while balancing the clinical, ethical, and economic consideration of "need" [9]. Identifying a number of worthy needs can make determining the health priority the most difficult stage of the needs assessment, particularly as limited resources necessitate prioritisation. Despite various criteria having been put forward to assist prioritising health problems, the absence of an evaluation formula requires decision makers to subjectively determine where to direct health-care resources [10]. The PRECEDE-PROCEED Model endeavors to addresses this limitation.

2. Aim

The purpose of this paper is to demonstrate the applicability of the PRECEDE-PROCEED Model ("Model") to the development of specific chronic care interventions for two distinct Australian populations: a rapidly growing and ageing rural population with unmet palliative care needs (R-PAC Project) and an urban community at higher risk of cardiovascular disease (APRICA 2 Project). The achievement of a comprehensive understanding of the health problem in each population, stakeholder engagement, and the development of tailored interventions signaled the completion of the PRECEDE phases of the process, which is the focus of this paper.

3. Methods

3.1. Applying the PRECEDE-PROCEED Model. This conceptual model minimizes the risk of subjectivity by synthesizing disparate sources of data to ensure that initiatives with the greatest potential of achieving the best health outcomes are implemented [10]. The Model is based on the premise that the determinants of health and health risks are multifactorial and that multifaceted and multisectoral efforts are required to effect behavioural, environmental, and social change [11].

The Model has evolved from a diagnostic tool developed in the 1980s, into a nine-phase model that integrates environmental health factors and evaluation into the process [10]. PRECEDE is an acronym that stands for predisposing, reinforcing, and enabling constructs in education, diagnosis, and evaluation, while PROCEED is the second part of the conceptual model and involves four phases that are focused on implementation and evaluation [10]. These processes work in unison with the PRECEDE phases facilitating the identification of priorities and the setting of objectives, while the PROCEDE phases assist in identifying the criteria for policy implementation and subsequent evaluation [10].

A major strength of this Model is its capacity to facilitate identification of the desired outcomes at the outset of the planning process, which determines the evaluation metrics

[10]. This Model also aids systematic classification of factors by their relative importance and capacity for modification through the use of a ranking system [10]. A ranking system facilitates consideration of the determinants for change at individual, provider, and system levels and allows for the identification, development, and implementation of interventions with the greatest potential of achieving a positive impact. Over the past two decades, the Model has been used internationally by health care planners and researchers to design interventions that acknowledge a wide range of individual and environmental determinants of health [12–15].

3.2. Setting

R-PAC Project. This initiative was undertaken as one component of a larger project, which aimed to strengthen partnerships to improve the coordination and delivery of local palliative care services [16]. This project was undertaken in a regional Australian coastal community, with a population of 67 0000. Over the past 20 years this community has experienced unprecedented population grown due to the internal migration of retirees [17]. It is anticipated that the areas popularity as a preferred retirement destination for baby boomers will continue, with 35% of population growth expected to be in the over 65 age group by 2031 [18]. By this time, estimates suggest that this area will have the highest proportion of over 65-year olds in the state [18].

APRICA 2 Project. This practice improvement intervention was undertaken in the Greater Western Sydney region, which is characterised by a diverse population who experience greater educational disadvantage, lower-levels of employment and employment capacity, and below-average annual income [19]. These determinants all impact adversely on how people perceive their risk for cardiovascular disease (CVD) [20]. The area also has higher proportions of non-English speaking residents [21], with some culturally and linguistically diverse groups being at a potentially greater risk of CVD [22].

The geographical spread of this outer urban community combined with the higher prevalence of socioeconomic disadvantage also adversely impacts on the populations' access to healthcare and appropriate transport [19].

3.3. Governance. The formation of critical reference groups comprising key stakeholders as part of the governance of the R-PAC and APRICA 2 Projects reflects the Models emphasis on assessing the social determinants of the population and engaging community stakeholders. Active stakeholder input ensured that the problems and priorities were defined by the community as opposed to being imposed by external parties.

3.4. Data Sources. Multiple sources of data were considered during the projects, including a comprehensive review of the literature and local policy documents and content emerging from key informant interviews. The Model facilitated the synthesis of the social assessment data which enabled a link between the priority health problems and the communities' needs to be established and focused the planning process.

3.5. Deriving Outcomes. In each project the desired outcomes were identified and defined at the outset of the planning process, which facilitated the development of specific and measurable evaluation metrics at the process (Phase 7), impact (Phase 8), and outcome (Phase 9) evaluation levels. The Model aided systematic classification of factors by their relative importance and capacity for modification for both projects [10, 23]. This ranking system facilitated consideration of the determinants for change at individual, provider, and system levels and allowed for the identification, development, and implementation of tailored interventions with the greatest potential of achieving a positive impact. Evidence suggests that improvement strategies that attend to the highest ranked predisposing, enabling, and reinforcing factors are those most likely to be successful [10, 24, 25]. Adopting this Model to plan health service improvement helps to optimise the use of scarce health resources (time, personnel, services, finances) by developing interventions that are likely to have the most impact, based on importance and changeability [10].

4. Applying PRECEDE-PROCEED Model: Two Case Studies

The Model calls for a deductive approach to assessing populations unmet needs. The complexities associated with the impacts on quality of life, health, behavior, the environment, and factors associated with achieving a desired outcome (predisposing, enabling, and reinforcing factors) for the populations identified as having unmet needs in the two case studies presented in this paper; and how identified health priorities guided subsequent intervention development and evaluation. A summary of the Model's phases as they relate of the R-PAC and APRICIA 2 Projects, are summarized consecutively in the sections below as case studies.

4.1. Phases 1 and 2: Social Assessment and Epidemiological Assessment. Addressing a population unmet needs and improving their quality of life is the Models' aspiration goal. Identifying and evaluating the various social problem(s) which impact on the quality of life of the target populations made undertaking a "social and epidemiological assessment" an important first step towards achieving this goal.

R-PAC Project. To assist with the systematic identification of local palliative care priorities, a focussed needs' assessment was undertaken at the outset of the project [17]. Synthesis of this data established a link between the priority health problems and the communities' needs and identified that improving the delivery of evidence-based palliative care was a key community priority (Figure 1) [17].

APRICA 2 Project. Similarly, the APRICA 2 Projects' needs assessment revealed a need to improve secondary CVD prevention after percutaneous coronary interventions (PCIs)

for a diverse urban population in the outer fringe of Western Sydney. The social determinates of educational disadvantage, underemployment, employment capacity, and below-average annual income have all been identified as impacting adversely on this populations perceived CVD risk [26]. The higher proportions of cultural groups at increased risk of CVD [20], combined with more limited transport and healthcare resources, made focusing on reducing this disadvantaged populations secondary CVD risks a priority for the APRICA 2 Project [21].

4.2. Phase 3: Behavioural and Environmental Assessment. The "behavioural and environmental assessment" facilitated identification of the specific health problems that may contribute to the target populations' quality of life, social goals or problems [10]. This phase assisted in identifying risk factors that deserve priority based on their perceived importance and changeability [10].

R-PAC Project. The evidence that emerged from Phase 1 and 2 suggested that the inward migration of retirees to this regional community was projected to continue and the burden of progressive life limiting diseases would increase in line with population aging, impacting adversely on the capacity of the existing palliative care service to meet growing demand [17]. Many older people requiring palliative care are admitted to the acute or nursing home setting as a result of caregiver burden, living alone and/or their care needs exceed available community services [17]. End-of-life care in nursing homes is provided by nonspecialist providers, for whom care of the dying is not their primary focus making building workforce palliative care capacity a priority [27]. The behavioural issues impacting on the delivery of palliative care to older people exposed a need to increase palliative care access to people with a progressive nonmalignant life limiting illnesses and to enhance palliative care delivery in local nursing homes. Addressing the palliative care needs of older people in aged care was strongly aligned with a national agenda and the release of evidence-based guidelines [27]. Given the availability of funding to strengthen local palliative care partnerships [16], it was considered that positive changes could be achieved during the project period.

APRICA 2 Project. The Phases 1 and 2 data revealed that the area had a higher than state average acute coronary-related admission and readmission rates [22], with people born overseas, who are overweight or obese and smokers being overrepresented [19]. Factors such as smoking, obesity, inactivity, and low uptake and completion rates of secondary prevention programs such as cardiac rehabilitation are all known to contribute to short- and long-term CVD mortality and morbidity [28]. Health professional behaviours inadvertently increasing the population's secondary CVD risks were identified during this process, including poor adherence to evidence-based guidelines and limited followup and promotion of cardiac rehabilitation programs to post, PCI patients. Compounding the populations' secondary CVD risks were environmental factors such as limited access

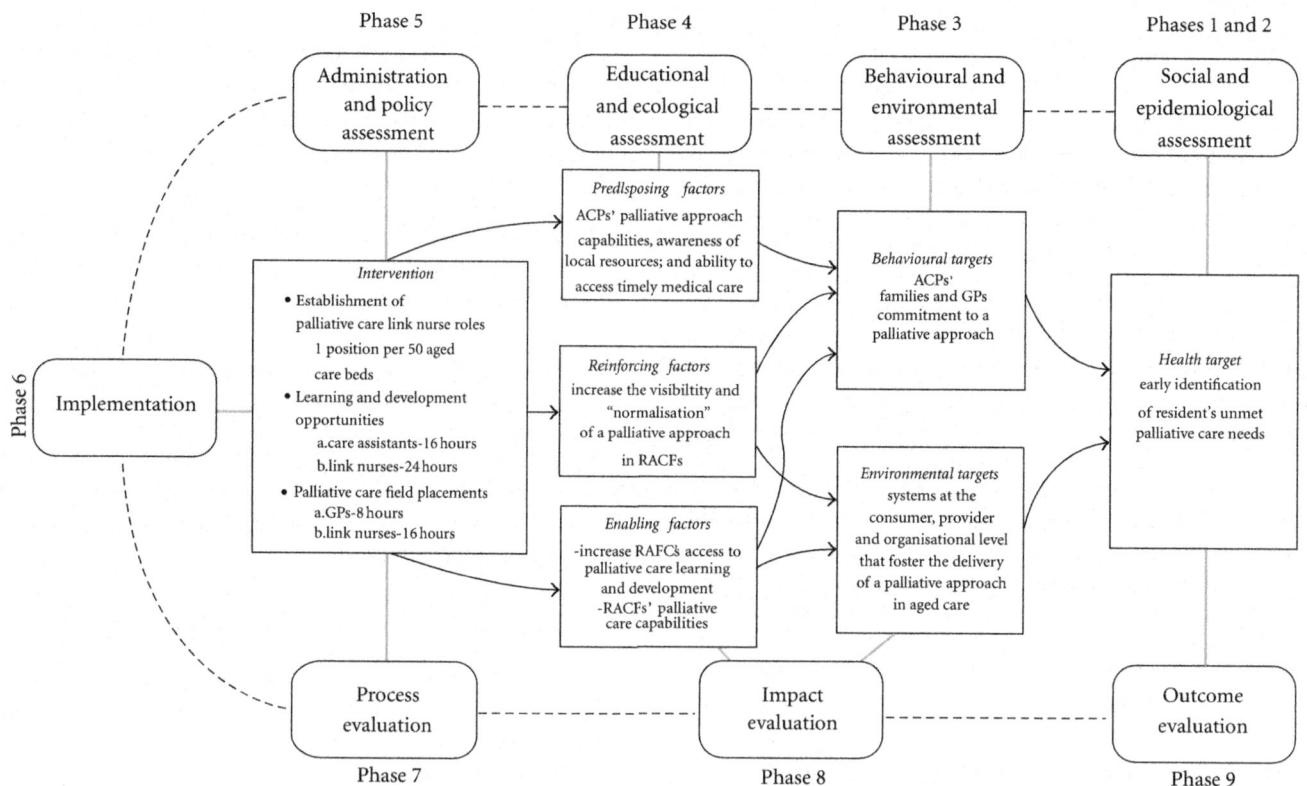

RACF: Residential Aged Care Facility, ACP: Aged Care Provider

FIGURE 1: Overview of the PRECEDE-PROCEED Model as applied to the R-PAC Project.

to appropriate secondary CVD resources, participation in cardiac rehabilitation programs, carer engagement in healthcare decision-making, and secondary prevention activities in the acute care setting.

At the completion of Phase 3, the health priorities for each project were evident, which allowed for the establishment of project objectives, with clearly defined target populations (WHO), desired outcomes (WHAT), and degree to which the target population will benefit (HOW MUCH) within a specific period (WHEN).

4.3. Phase 4: Educational and Ecological Assessment.

An "educational and ecological assessment" facilitates categorising the predisposing, enabling or reinforcing factors contributing to the behaviours previously identified [10]. This phase facilitates systematic identification of health problems and associated risk factors that deserve priority based on their perceived importance and changeability, whilst considering the effective allocation of limited resources [10]. Importantly, this stage focuses on the development of the intervention to address the identified health problem. Having the critical reference groups assess and ranked the predisposing, reinforcing or enabling factors helps drive the change management processes [29, 30].

4.4. Predisposing Factors

R-PAC Project. Predisposing factors ranked highest as acting to either motivate or inhibit the delivery of a palliative approach in local nursing homes, included aged care personnels palliative care awareness, knowledge, competencies, and confidence; access to the specialist palliative care for residents with complex palliative care needs; the number of general practitioners (GPs) prepared to review residents in local nursing homes; residents' and families' awareness of a palliative approach and involvement in care planning [31].

APRICA 2 Project. The highest ranking predisposing factors for the APRIC 2 population were identified as being a pervading sense of being "cured" following PCI [32], inadequate understanding of the need for secondary prevention following PCI, wide diversity in PCI nursing care practices across institutions; inadequate communication between acute and primary care providers, low referral rates to secondary prevention programs, and poor uptake and completion of secondary CVD prevention programs by patients undergoing PCIs.

4.5. Reinforcing Factors

R-PAC Project. In the aged care setting, residents, family members, other health care providers, peers, and educators play a role in reinforcing positive and negative behaviours through rewards, feedback, and punishments [10]. The reinforcing factors considered most important and amenable to change included the need to increase age care personnel's awareness of the specialist palliative care referral process, develop appropriate systems for GPs to be routinely engaged in resident's end-of-life care planning, provide residents and families with information about a palliative approach, and increase the visibility and "normalisation" of a palliative approach in aged care [29].

APRICA 2 Project. The reinforcing factors ranked highest in terms of importance and changeability included the lack of national, state, or local PCI evidence-based nursing care guidelines; no linkage between PCI nursing care delivery in acute care and secondary CVD prevention programs; patients' limited participation in secondary CVD prevention programs.

4.6. Enabling Factors

R-PAC Project. Whereas enabling factors such as: accessibility, availability and skills impacted on the aged care personnel's ability to deliver a palliative approach were the most highly ranked factors. Further analysis revealed that these enabling factors included aged care personnel's capacity to: effectively communicate clinical findings to external health professionals; effectively advocate on behalf of the residents; utilise a common palliative care language, both within aged care and with external health professionals; arrange timely access to palliative care equipment; refer the resident to a specialist palliative care team; acquire greater palliative care competencies and confidence; and access palliative care education opportunities locally [29]. A range of enabling factors were also acting to limit residents' access to palliative care as a result of: a lower ratio of registered nurses as a proportion of the total aged care workforce; aged care personnels limited palliative care knowledge, skills and confidence; under utilisation of the specialist palliative care team; difficulty accessing timely and appropriate GP input, specialist support, medications and equipment; and residents' and families' limited awareness and understanding of a palliative approach [29, 30]. Acknowledging the availability and accessibility of resources along with the competencies required to implement the intervention ensures that the highest ranked factors, in terms of importance and changeability become the focus of the intervention [10].

APRICA 2 Project. Health professionals' willingness to engage in and lead CVD quality improvement activities; the encouragement and support provided by families/carers to enable the patient to reduce their CVD risk; and capacity of the peak cardiovascular organisations to promote a national PCI quality improvement agenda, were identified as being critical enabling factors for change. Integrating relevant data into the Model enabled a comprehensive picture of the cardiovascular health needs of an urban population to be identified and guided identification of the action

required, including: development national PCI evidence-based nursing guidelines integrating secondary prevention [32, 33]; increasing uptake of cardiac rehabilitation post PCIs; informing patients and carers of available social support(s), reinforcing the importance of secondary prevention and details on accessing local CVD secondary prevention information and programs. As risk modification is dependent upon the individual's perception of risk, identifying and ranking these factors was critical to shaping the APRICA Project intervention, in Phase 4 [33].

4.7. Phase 5: Administrative and Policy Assessment

R-PAC Project. The data shaped the development of a multifaceted intervention development focused on increasing aged care personnel's palliative care capacity [34]. The unique learning needs of the various categories of personnel delivering care in the aged care setting dictated the development of tailored learning strategies reflecting their scope of practice [34]. An assessment of the organisational and administrative capabilities allowed for identification of the resources required for the development and implementation of the proposed intervention and consideration of factors that may hinder the proposed change [10]. This process confirmed that the nine participating nursing homes' organisational missions were compatible with the projects goals and the planned intervention objectives [10]. Administrative and policy issues that needed to be factored into the intervention development, including time constraints, change management and the need for a "clinical champion" in each nursing home. Consideration of other dynamics, such as staff shortages, accreditation schedules, commissioning of new beds, and the execution of other initiatives helped determine the extent and speed by which the proposed intervention could be implemented.

APRICA 2 Project. Acute care workforce shortages, frequent patient transfers across institutions, financial pressures, and the need for increased efficiency all had the potential to adversely impact on the implementation of any intervention developed to improve secondary CVD risk after PCI [35]. These complex administrative and policy conditions made the recruitment of local "change champions" to facilitate guideline and intervention implementation and actively engaging Australia and New Zealand's peak cardiovascular nursing organisations in PCI guideline development, important strategies to address these barriers. This reality guided the developed of the subobjectives developed to address these priorities.

4.8. Phase 6: Implementation of the Intervention.
Implementation of the intervention (Phase 6) marks the commencement of the PROCEED component of the Model.

R-PAC Project. The multifaceted intervention implemented sought to work with aged care personnel to increase resident's access to palliative care by creating an enabling and empowering learning environment. The strategies employed included increasing access to specialists' resources and evidence-based information through instituting: a clinical champion "link nurse" role, increasing learning and development opportunities for nurses, care assistants, and GPs, and promoting networking and multidisciplinary care planning processes [34].

APRICA 2 Project. The study has completed the development of a set of evidence-based guidelines for the care of people undergoing PCIs [32]. The implementation of these guidelines is pending. Other clinical interventions arising from this study are being refined for pilot testing in the near future.

4.9. Phases 7, 8, and 9: Evaluation. The completion of the implementation phase signals the transition into the Model's evaluation phase. Process evaluation enables the change process by which the intervention is being implemented to be evaluated. During Phase 8 the "impact evaluation" measures the program effectiveness in terms of the intermediate objectives and changes in the predisposing, enabling, and reinforcing factors. Outcome evaluation is the final evaluation phase of the PRECEDE-PROCEED Model (Phase 9) and measures the overall program goal. Evaluation data from the two projects is reported elsewhere and are beyond the scope of this paper.

4.10. Summary. These case studies demonstrate the applicability of the PRECEDE-PROCEED Model within two discrete population groups. In both settings, unmet needs could have been addressed through implementing existing knowledge; however, applying the Model enabled a focused approach to intervention development that considered a range of relevant factors. As narrowing the evidence-practice gap continues to be a major health reform challenge, it was critical for both projects to take into consideration the obstacles to change for each population in developing effective interventions [36]. As interventions that consider predisposing, enabling, and reinforcing factors have the most success in implementing best practice focusing on these determinants is critical to developing successful interventions, as was demonstrated in these case studies [24, 25]. In the R-PAC Project, focussing the intervention on increasing the competencies of aged care personnel was identified as likely to have the greatest impact on delivery of an evidence-based palliative approach to older people in aged care, while the APRICA 2 Project focussed on improving the outcomes for people undergoing PCI by improving postdischarge care and increasing access to CVD secondary prevention initiatives. This systematic approach to health planning allowed for the setting of priorities and guided the focus of the interventions whilst assisting with delineation of responsibility of those professionals and organisations involved in the process [10]. Applying the Model also ensured that a realistic and applicable evaluation framework was simultaneously developed.

5. Conclusion

As demand for health care resources continues to increase, there is a need to ensure the systematic and critical analysis of priorities and presumed causes is undertaken [3]. The PRECEDE-PROCEED Model takes into account the multiple factors that shape health status and assists health care planners and clinicians to develop programs that intervene on factors that are both important and changeable and encourages participatory research and practice [3, 37]. A key attribute of the Model is its focus on determining the desired outcomes at the outset of the planning process [10]. Applying the Model ensured that all of the relevant environmental and nonbehavioural factors that can act as barriers to health care innovations and practice change were considered, which is an important consideration as they are often overlooked during health intervention planning [10].

A needs assessment is an inexact science with several factors limiting its effectiveness [4, 8, 38]. The PRECEDE-PROCEED Model addresses many of these limitations. This model demands that an inclusive process as opposed to tokenism is utilised, which ensures the active involvement of local communities and consumers in identifying, prioritizing, and responding to these needs [4]. As such, the Model prevents the needs assessment process from being ritualistic and self-justifying, by ensuring that the process is focused on facilitating health care reform [8, 38]. Although, undertaking a needs assessment implies that a change is required, there is little evidence that documenting "need" alone actually leads to effective health system change [9]. In spite of a commitment, many health services have limited capacity to reorientate health priorities and funds into new programs without engaging in a range of far-reaching reforms [6]. In these circumstances, conducting a needs assessment without a commitment to implementing recommended solutions is a lost opportunity to address identified unmet need, resolve issues, and an unnecessary and wasteful strain on scarce resources [6]. The PRECEDE-PROCEED Model challenges health services to change practices and prevents reinforcing a potentially dysfunctional status quo in service or program delivery [4, 8]. This diagnostic method increases the utility of a needs assessment in the real world setting by providing a framework which encourages identification and consideration of the environmental, social, and behavioural factors that may impact on any planned intervention. It enhances the acceptability of interventions by enabling health professionals to develop improvements that act on factors that are not only important but also amenable to the change. These case studies demonstrate the relevance of this multidimensional planning Model in targeting health care improvement strategies in dynamic environments.

Acknowledgments

The authors have no conflict of interests to declare. This research was undertaken, in part, with funding support from the Cancer Institute New South Wales Academic Chairs Program.

References

[1] World Health Organisation, "Building Blocks for Action Innovative Care for Chronic Conditions: Global Report," 2002, http://www.who.int/diabetesactiononline/about/icccglobalreport.pdf.

[2] National Health and Hospitals Reform Commission, "A Healthier Future for all Australians," Final Report of the National Health and Hospitals Reform Commission, Australian Government, Canberra, Australia, 2009.

[3] J. D. Chaney, B. P. Hunt, and J. W. Schultz, "An examination using the PRECEDE model framework to establish a comprehensive program to prevent school violence," *American Journal of Health Studies*, vol. 16, no. 4, pp. 199–204, 2000.

[4] P. Hawe, "Needs assessment must become more change-focused," *Australian and New Zealand Journal of Public Health*, vol. 20, no. 5, pp. 473–478, 1996.

[5] D. L. Sackett, W. M. C. Rosenberg, J. A. M. Gray, R. B. Haynes, and W. S. Richardson, "Evidence based medicine: what it is and what it isn't. It's about integrating individual clinical expertise and the best external evidence," *British Medical Journal*, vol. 312, no. 7023, pp. 71–72, 1996.

[6] A. Agnew, R. Manktelow, B. Taylor, and L. Jones, "Bereavement needs assessment in specialist palliative care: a review of the literature," *Palliative Medicine*, vol. 24, no. 1, pp. 46–59, 2010.

[7] E. Bugge and I. J. Higginson, "Palliative care and the need for education - Do we know what makes a difference? A limited systematic review," *Health Education Journal*, vol. 65, no. 2, pp. 101–125, 2006.

[8] J. Fuller, M. Bentley, and D. Shotton, "Use of community health needs assessment for regional planning in country South Australia," *The Australian Journal of Rural Health*, vol. 9, no. 1, pp. 12–17, 2001.

[9] D. H. Finifter, C. J. Jensen, C. E. Wilson, and B. L. Koenig, "A comprehensive, multitiered, targeted community needs assessment model: methodology, dissemination, and implementation," *Family and Community Health*, vol. 28, no. 4, pp. 293–306, 2005.

[10] L. W. Green and M. W. Kreuter, *Health Program Planning: An Educational and Ecological Approach*, McGraw-Hill Higher Education, New York, NY, USA, 4th edition, 2005.

[11] B. Giles-Corti, "Book review: health promotion planning: an educational and ecological approach," *Health Promotion Journal of Australia*, vol. 10, no. 1, 2000.

[12] A. McAuliffe, "Nursing students' practice in providing oral hygiene for patients," *Nursing Standard*, vol. 21, no. 33, pp. 35–39, 2007.

[13] M. G. Meador and L. A. Linnan, "Using the PRECEDE model to plan men's health programs in a managed care setting," *Health promotion practice*, vol. 7, no. 2, pp. 186–196, 2006.

[14] P. K. H. Mo and W. W. S. Mak, "Application of the PRECEDE model to understanding mental health promoting behaviors in Hong Kong," *Health Education and Behavior*, vol. 35, no. 4, pp. 574–587, 2008.

[15] S. Wang and R. Wang, "Using the PRECEDE model to predict AIDS preventive intentions of junior college students," *Nursing Research*, vol. 8, no. 3, pp. 349–361, 2000 (Chinese).

[16] Australian Divisions of General Practice, "Rural Palliative Care Program," 2004, http://www.agpn.com.au/programs/rural-palliative-care-program.

[17] P. M. Davidson, Y. Salamonson, J. Rolley et al., "Perception of cardiovascular risk following a percutaneous coronary intervention: a cross sectional study," *International Journal of Nursing Studies*, vol. 48, no. 8, pp. 973–978, 2011.

[18] Public Health Information Development Unit, "Population health profile of the Mid North Coast division of general practice," in *Population Profile Series: No 22*, Public Health Information Development Unit, Adelaide, Australia, 2005.

[19] Population Health Division, "Report of the NSW Chief Health Officer," NSW Health, NSW Department of Health, 2008.

[20] F. L. Game and A. F. Jones, "Ethnicity and risk factors for coronary heart disease in diabetes mellitus," *Diabetes, Obesity and Metabolism*, vol. 2, no. 2, pp. 91–97, 2000.

[21] A. Hurni, "Transport and social exclusion in Western Sydney," in *University of Western Sydney and Western Sydney Community Forum*, University of Western Sydney, Sydney, Australia, 2006.

[22] P. M. Davidson, "Do patients following percutaneous coronary intervention perceive a risk of future cardiovascular events?" *Journal of Cardiopulmonary Rehabilitation & Prevention*. In press.

[23] T. G. Hislop, C. Teh, A. Low et al., "Predisposing, reinforcing and enabling factors associated with hepatitis B testing in Chinese Canadians in British Columbia," *Asian Pacific Journal of Cancer Prevention*, vol. 8, no. 1, pp. 39–44, 2007.

[24] D. A. Davis, M. A. Thomson, A. D. Oxman, and R. B. Haynes, "Changing physician performance: a systematic review of the effect of continuing medical education strategies," *Journal of the American Medical Association*, vol. 274, no. 9, pp. 700–705, 1995.

[25] D. H. Solomon, H. Hashimoto, L. Daltroy, and M. H. Liang, "Techniques to improve physicians' use of diagnostic tests: a new conceptual framework," *Journal of the American Medical Association*, vol. 280, no. 23, pp. 2020–2027, 1998.

[26] G. Turrell, L. Stanley, M. de Looper, and B. Oldenburg, *Health Inequalities in Australia: Morbidity, Health Behaviours, Risk Factors and Health Service Use*, Queensland University of Technology & AIHW, Canberra, Australia, 2006.

[27] Australian Department of Health and Ageing and National Health and Medical Research Council, *Guidelines for a Palliative Approach in Residential Aged Care*, E.C. University, Canberra, Australia, 2006.

[28] C. N. Aroney, P. E. Aylward, A. Kelly et al., "Guidelines for the management of acute coronary syndromes," *Medical Journal of Australia*, vol. 184, no. 8, pp. S1–S29, 2006.

[29] J. Phillips, P. M. Davidson, D. Jackson, L. Kristjanson, J. Daly, and J. Curran, "Residential aged care: the last frontier for palliative care," *Journal of Advanced Nursing*, vol. 55, no. 4, pp. 416–424, 2006.

[30] J. L. Phillips, P. M. Davidson, R. Ollerton, D. Jackson, and L. Kristjanson, "Commitment and compassion: survey results from nurses and care assistants working in residential aged care," *International journal of palliative nursing*, vol. 13, no. 6, pp. 282–290, 2007.

[31] J. Phillips, P. M. Davidson, and S. Willcock, "An insight into the delivery of a palliative approach in residential aged care: the general practitioner perspective," *Journal of Applied Gerontology*, vol. 28, no. 3, pp. 395–405, 2009.

[32] J. X. Rolley, Y. Salamonson, C. R. Dennison, and P. M. Davidson, "Nursing care practices following a percutaneous coronary intervention: results of a survey of Australian and New Zealand cardiovascular nurses," *Journal of Cardiovascular Nursing*, vol. 25, no. 1, pp. 75–84, 2010.

[33] R. S. Fernandez, R. Griffiths, C. Juergens, P. Davidson, and Y. Salamonson, "Persistence of coronary risk factor status in participants 12 to 18 months after percutaneous coronary intervention," *Journal of Cardiovascular Nursing*, vol. 21, no. 5, pp. 379–387, 2006.

[34] J. L. Phillips, P. M. Davidson, D. Jackson, and L. J. Kristjanson, "Multi-faceted palliative care intervention: aged care nurses' and care assistants' perceptions and experiences," *Journal of Advanced Nursing*, vol. 62, no. 2, pp. 216–227, 2008.

[35] P. Garling, "Final report of the special commission of inquiry acute care services in NSW public hospitals. Sydney," in *Special Commission of Inquiry: Acute Care Services in NSW Public Hospitals*, N. Health, Sydney, Australia, 2008.

[36] R. Grol and M. Wensing, "What drives change? Barriers to and incentives for achieving evidence-based practice," *Medical Journal of Australia*, vol. 180, no. 6, pp. S57–S60, 2004.

[37] A. C. Gielen and D. Sleet, "Application of behavior-change theories and methods to injury prevention," *Epidemiologic Reviews*, vol. 25, pp. 65–76, 2003.

[38] N. Doyle and D. Kelly, ""So what happens now?" Issues in cancer survival and rehabilitation," *Clinical Effectiveness in Nursing*, vol. 9, no. 3-4, pp. 147–153, 2005.

3

Social Processes That Can Facilitate and Sustain Individual Self-Management for People with Chronic Conditions

Elizabeth Kendall,[1] Michele M. Foster,[2] Carolyn Ehrlich,[1] and Wendy Chaboyer[3]

[1] Centre for National Research on Disability and Rehabilitation Medicine, Griffith Health Institute, Griffith University, Logan Campus, Meadowbrook, QLD 4131, Australia
[2] School of Social Work & Human Services, The University of Queensland, St. Lucia, QLD 4072, Australia
[3] NHMRC Centre of Research Excellence in Nursing Interventions for Hospitalised Patients, Research Centre for Clinical and Community Practice Innovation and Griffith Health Institute, Griffith University, Gold Coast Campus, Southport, QLD 4215, Australia

Correspondence should be addressed to Elizabeth Kendall, e.kendall@griffith.edu.au

Academic Editor: Mi-Kyung Song

Recent shifts in health policy direction in several countries have, on the whole, translated into self-management initiatives in the hope that this approach will address the growing impact of chronic disease. Dominant approaches to self-management tend to reinforce the current medical model of chronic disease and fail to adequately address the social factors that impact on the lives of people with chronic conditions. As part of a larger study focused on outcomes following a chronic disease, this paper explores the processes by which a chronic disease self-management (CDSM) course impacted on participants. Five focus groups were conducted with participants and peer leaders of the course in both urban and rural regions of Queensland, Australia. The findings suggested that outcomes following CDSM courses depended on the complex interplay of four social factors, namely, social engagement, the development of a collective identity, the process of building collaborative coping capacity, and the establishment of exchange relationships. This study highlights the need for an approach to self-management that actively engages consumers in social relationships and addresses the context within which their lives (and diseases) are enacted. This approach extends beyond the psychoeducational skills-based approach to self-management into a more ecological model for disease prevention.

1. Introduction

With a rapid rise in the prevalence of chronic conditions and the ensuing demand placed on health services, the sustainability of most health care systems around the globe has been threatened [1]. During the last decade, the strategy of choice has been to focus on promoting healthy lifestyles and choices [2, 3], the most common method of which has been to promote self-management through the delivery of psychoeducational group programs. This approach has now become an integral component of the Australian and UK healthcare systems. Although there are multiple approaches to the promotion of self-management, the most common approach has been the Lorig [4] model of chronic disease self-management (CDSM). This model is a standardized course delivered over 6 weekly sessions of approximately 2

hours each week. Courses are delivered in community settings and usually facilitated by two trained peer leaders using a highly structured course protocol. Course content introduces participants to a range of topics pertaining to health and well-being (e.g., healthy eating, exercise, relaxation). The process emphasizes group interaction and support and reinforces solution-focused behaviors (e.g., problem solving, goal setting, communication with healthcare team and family) aimed at assisting individuals to actively manage the impact of chronic conditions on all domains of their life (e.g., emotional, physical, and social well-being).

Within this approach, health professionals are primarily responsible for the medical management of the disease or chronic condition, and the individual is responsible for the day-to-day management of his or her condition. The emphasis is on strengthening individuals' skills and confidence

TABLE 1: Focus group participants.

	No. of focus groups	No. of participants	Gender	
			Male	Female
Urban participants	2	16	2	14
Rural participants	2	11	4	7
Peer leaders	1	7	0	7
Total	5	34	6	28

about managing their chronic conditions through supportive group education and improved partnerships between individuals and their health professionals [5]. Self-management remains an individual-level concept framed within a medical model, focused on disease and deficiencies in the person which require education to enable them to comply with health professional advice [6]. In this sense, the CDSM model does not represent a radical shift from traditional approaches to healthcare.

The purpose of this paper was to identify the way in which participants and leaders of the CDSM course described the mechanisms by which it impacted on them and their health.

2. Method

Five focus groups were conducted during the national implementation and evaluation of the CDSM course in Australia. The purpose of this paper was to examine the way in which the course impacted on health from the perspective of participants (e.g., people who had completed the course within the last six months) and peer leaders (e.g., people with chronic conditions who had run a course for others in the last six months). All eligible leaders and participants who had completed a course in one of the two pilot areas were telephoned and asked to participate in a focus group. Initial contact was made by the organization responsible for the delivery of CDSM training in Queensland, Australia. Those who agreed to participate were then contacted by the research team following approval from the University Research Ethics Committee.

Care was taken to ensure reasonable representation of male and female participants from a range of differing course locations and people with a range of chronic conditions. However, as expected given the population of participants and leaders, there was a bias towards female participants and an absence of male peer leaders. All participants were over 50 years of age in accordance with the eligibility requirements established by the organization. The constitution of each focus group is shown in Table 1 and the focus group questions are contained in Table 2.

Focus groups were facilitated by two researchers and were held in the most convenient local building chosen by the leaders of the courses. The focus group discussions were introduced to the participants as having been designed to elicit their perceptions and experiences of the course. Specific prompt questions focused on their awareness and acceptance of self-management as a concept, experiences of

the self-management training (where relevant) and course leadership, interactions among participants and followup with health care providers, perceptions of sustainability of self-management, and overall satisfaction with the program. The focus groups were audio-recorded, transcribed verbatim and analyzed using a collaborative multiwave process.

Two researchers independently coded the transcripts, selecting units of text that contained information about how participants viewed the course and the way in which it had influenced outcomes. Units of text that did not contain any useful information about the course or its influence were discarded (N.B. discarded text usually contained general interactions or comments about benign topics such as the weather, the environment, and personal communications). The units of text selected by these two researchers were compared and discussed to reach agreement about the most important extracts that should be further analysed. Although a few minor pieces of text were discarded as having no meaning for the current study, the two researchers agreed that all other pieces of text should be retained.

Once this first level of data selection was complete, the reduced dataset was analysed by a third researcher to identify the major themes that existed across all selected extracts. The themes that emerged from this second wave of coding were reexamined by another researcher to determine the extent to which the categorization process was transparent and meaningful. Areas of disagreement were minimal but were addressed through discussion. If text added a useful dimension to several themes, it was used in multiple places. Any text that could not easily be categorized was reviewed. If considered by mutual agreement that the text added nothing new to the analysis, it was discarded. Themes reflected both positive and negative articulations of the concept.

To validate the findings, we presented them to a group of peer leaders and trainers as well as national and international experts in the area of CDSM. Feedback indicated that the themes accurately reflected the experience of others in the field. Direct quotes have been replicated verbatim and have been referenced using abbreviations to indicate the source (e.g., U: urban participants, R: rural participants, PL: peer leaders).

3. Results

Participants held strong beliefs about the benefits of the course (e.g., knowledge about chronic disease, self-management skills, problem-solving/coping skills, goal setting and decision-making skills). As expected, they reported that their knowledge increased as a result of the course and that this translated into an increased sense of confidence, greater control over their future, and a positive attitude towards their disease. These findings are presented in more detail elsewhere [7].

Participants in this study reported that some potential attendees had elected not to enroll in the course because they disliked group processes. Similarly, some participants failed to complete the course because they had not enjoyed the group format. This conclusion suggests the possibility of a self-selection bias towards those who valued social

TABLE 2: Focus group prompt questions.

Overall satisfaction with the program	Overall, how satisfied are you with the program?
	What has been the impact (if any) of the program on your life?
Perceptions and experiences of orientation, education, and training	How well were you informed about the program when you first joined?
	What did you know about the program before you commenced?
	What were some of your expectations about the program?
	Overall, how satisfied have you been with the training you received?
	Overall, how satisfied have you been with the postprogram followup?
	What type of support (if any) have you received after program?
	Are there any difficulties you experienced while participating in the program?
	What strategies did you use to overcome these difficulties?
	What kept you coming each week?
Perceived impact of the program	Has the program had an impact on
	the way you manage your condition/s?
	your lifestyle in general?
	How has it changed your lifestyle?
	What are some of the supports/strategies you have used yourself (or are necessary) to make this impact last?
	To what extent did the program leaders answer your questions?
	To what extent do you feel that the program leader gave you adequate information about your condition/s?
	Overall, how would you describe the quality of the program leader

exchanges. Nevertheless, there was little doubt that those who attended the course attributed their gains to the social context of the course. Specifically, self-management appeared to evolve through, and was situated within, a network of social exchanges and support processes that were facilitated by the course. Indeed, the majority of participants who completed the course discussed social processes more often than course content, indicating the importance of these processes to their evaluation of the course. Participants' level of satisfaction with the social processes of their particular group also seemed to be critical to their overall impression of the course. There was evidence that without this contextual feature of the course, the benefits may have been less meaningful to participants. Further, there was evidence that when social processes were negative, the benefits of the course were jeopardized.

The four major social themes that emerged described the importance of the social context to the success of the CDSM course. These themes included

  (i) social engagement;

  (ii) a collective identity;

  (iii) collaborative coping capacity;

  (iv) exchange relationships.

3.1. Social Engagement. An overwhelming theme in the data was the benefit derived purely through social engagement. Participants usually referred to the course as an opportunity for social interaction and described how this interaction addressed the long-term loneliness or social isolation associated with having a chronic condition.

In most cases, the group provided a friendly context within which people learned about each other's experiences but felt no pressure to divulge personal information. This common experience enhanced the likelihood of supportive friendships emerging, even if only temporarily.

> *I found it helpful to mix with people who had similar problems, even though they had different diseases. It was just so supportive (PL).*

> *You make friends with people that go through similar pain as you. Each one of us identified with it (R)...It is the best thing that ever happened to me. Because you make friends and we do not see each other all the time but it is just nice to see their faces again (R).*

Having the time and opportunity to socialize with other group members before and after each session was considered to be a valuable aspect of the course for most participants. Their comments indicated that a great deal of satisfaction accompanied these opportunities for social contact.

> *So when we first arrived which was always good, if you were there a few minutes early you could have a cup of tea...it was really nice to have a drink and a conversation just for five minutes (U).*

In many instances, the chance for social interaction was a major source of motivation not only to join the CDSM program, but also to continue attending sessions and participate in activities designed to impart information and skills.

> *It [course] was the chance of getting out...It does not matter what the group is, it's the*

social interaction [that matters] (U)...As we went along, we got friends and you know we all joined together (U).

The value placed on social engagement was demonstrated in the actions of several participants who made the effort to maintain regular contact with other group members once the course had ended.

We all meet up once a month now and have lunch together and we are going to try and keep it that way (U)...At the follow-up meeting people had actually kept in touch with each other. They seemed to find that very helpful (PL).

Many participants reported that the CDSM course was a significant opportunity to address social isolation. The course not only provided social opportunities, but, enabled them to reevaluate their own self-isolating behaviors and choices.

There's a lot of people who do these courses who are very lonely (U)...I'd done like a similar sort of course. I thought well, it's one way of learning more, and um, and meeting people (U).

We try...and promote the fact that there is social life ahead for you too, we [people with chronic conditions] have a reluctance to even go outside, to catch a bus. I hated to go down to the letterbox because somebody would see me and I would have to talk (PL).

There's that opportunity for social interaction that's important for many people. Because people do tend to feel a bit isolated do not they? Or it's perhaps restricted. It does not matter what group it is. It's the social interaction with it [that matters] (U).

To know that there are other people there and there is a social life...encouragement to do something that we needed more than anything else [to meet people] (R).

In cases where participants' expectations for socialization were not met through the course, the perceived benefits derived by those participants appeared to be reduced, "*I think I was hoping for it to be a little more social for people, like a little more friendly*" (U). Similarly, when participants were dissatisfied with their group, it was often attributed to a lack of social engagement or bonding among participants.

Nobody was sort of friendly or wanted to [get to know each other]...It was a really mixed group of people...I did not feel, like if you had a "cuppa" afterwards there wasn't much talking going on and they did not talk from the way in from the car park. We went out to lunch the last day but...they really had to be forced into it (U).

These findings suggest that the benefits of the course which have previously been attributed to cognitive or educational processes may be equally attributed to the simple process of social engagement that was facilitated by the group setting. There was a dual benefit of social engagement in that it motivated participants to initially engage in self-management but also to continue learning.

3.2. A Collective Identity. Positive changes in confidence and attitude following the course appeared to be associated with the sense of belonging to a cohesive group of people. The cohesion of the groups provided an immediate opportunity to identify shared concerns, to normalize one's difficulties, to gain a sense of accountability to the group, and to be guided by the norms that had been set by the group. This sense of belonging provided a collective identity that encouraged people to view themselves and their situation differently.

A large number of participants commented on the importance of group composition and dynamics to the success of the course and its benefits, "*I think a lot of it has to do with the people who are in the class*" (R). Participants who felt that their group had lacked cohesion reported that this had impacted negatively on their satisfaction and achievements.

The class was excellent, the only thing that I thought about it was that I felt a bit out of it—they [other participants] have all got these beautiful homes, beautiful spas and beautiful pools and exercise bikes. The whole works, and I am coming from a rather grotty home and I would have loved to have lived in their circumstances, I felt life could have been a lot easier. But they were sort of, they all knew each other, it was a bit "clicky" in some ways, I felt it...They were all friends, they all knew each other very well and...In comes a couple of outsiders...(U).

The crucial importance of group membership was summarized by several participants, who pointed out that any group might bring similar benefits if a sense of cohesion could be achieved.

Any group therapy helps you though...it is just a case of getting together and finding other people...You are not on your own (R)...I'm just one of many people with a problem and by coming together as a group you talk and it gives you another outlook on life. You think you're in that one little square, but...there's other people in that little square too (R).

For most participants, the fact that they were "*...answerable to somebody*" was an important source of motivation, because of knowing that "*somebody is sharing an interest in you ... [made you]...more inclined to respond*" (R). For some participants, however, the pressure of being scrutinized by a group compelled them to offer socially desirable responses during feedback sessions rather than admit that they had not achieved their weekly goals. Thus, the influence of the collective on individual behavior was both positive and negative.

The lady I took [to the course], on the way I would say, "How did you go with your weekly plan?" and she would tell me, "I did not do anything" and then we would get there and she would say "Oh yes I [completed my action plan]" (U).

Participants generally agreed that the group norms (e.g., sharing goals and reporting back) meant *"you had that incentive…you had to go back and say when you had done it" (U).* Participants who had not attended to their course requirements (e.g., goal-setting homework) commented that *"…you really felt you were letting the team down to some extent if you did not at least try" (U).* For one person, it was *"like a promise, and you find when you are not there [part of a group] you do not really do it" (R).* Indeed, being a member of a cohesive group instilled motivation for most members to achieve their weekly action plans, *"Over the period of time, I think the group helped one another to try to keep with their activity sheet" (R).*

In summary, our findings suggested that the CDSM group context provided an important opportunity for social comparison, normalization, and a sense of belonging. These benefits appeared to be only achievable through a cohesive group where members shared experiences, motivated each other, and provided opportunities for discussion. When members felt they did not belong, or were unable to meet expectations, the outcomes of the course appeared to be less positive.

3.3. Collaborative Coping Capacity. Participants frequently commented on *"the supportiveness of the group, it was very supportive" (U).* Most participants were in agreement that, *"when around the table with other people…one on one… [it was] much easier to cope with your pain" (U).* Attendance at the group appeared to be associated with increased coping capacity for many participants. The belief that one's coping efforts were being supported and appreciated by others in the group was an important positive outcome for most participants.

However, this effect appeared to have broader implications in that coping became a collective response to a public issue rather than a private response to a hidden problem. With this new approach to coping, many participants gained renewed enthusiasm and energy, facilitating their engagement in self-management. Although it was important to participants to develop more confidence to manage independently, they also identified the need for, and importance of, collective management. For many participants, collective spirit and individual confidence appeared to coexist and complement each other.

Number one [e.g., the most important thing] is better confidence in yourselves [but also] the fact that they're not isolated in their condition and that other people share similar things (R).

The shared experience of being with people who have had similar issues has given them [participants in the course] confidence to tackle stuff that they previously wouldn't have done…they are breaking out of the sick role into more lifestyle issues (U).

Through their shared experience of coping, private pain became a collective experience and was, therefore, perceived as being easier to manage, *"I was not the only one in the community going through pain and disability" (R).* The collective environment provided the necessary opportunity to express fears, concerns, and issues in a way that had not been experienced before. This experience profoundly affected participants' connection to the group and their sense of solidarity as they confronted the shared threat of chronic illness.

I had been to lots of these things [courses] and they left you feeling wrecked…what I found with these meetings is how relaxing they are, how easy it is to gather information. People are given opportunities to be able to speak or express their feelings and where you are given opportunities you are given choices and there is no pressure put on anybody to perform. It is just about people wanting to help somebody else through their daily lives (R).

The group connection was an important starting point for a collective coping response because group members tended to track each other's coping efforts over time and celebrated the successes as a collective.

[It is good] to see how we are growing, in ourselves you know. How we are coping with our lives, yes it [the group] is very important (R).

Conversely, participants described how the presence of negativity in the group impacted on the prevailing collective attitude and had negative consequences for their own psychological well-being and experience, *"A lot of people did their weekly plan [only with] prompting…they never did it [alone]"; "they would make excuses" (U).* The lack of motivation in other group members had negative consequences for several participants. *"[It] made you feel depressed", "oh yes, I did too, I got depressed too" (U).* One participant explained how negativity and lack of motivation in other group members influenced all members of the group:

Some of the people had given up you know just sort of given up and said, "I just cannot do this" …and you just sort of felt, "Am I going to be like that down the line"? (U).

In contrast, one participant explained how exposure to unmotivated individuals fortified her determination to cope and successfully manage her condition in future. The collaborative process motivated this participant to resist the negative influence of another participant, identifying that participant as a deviation from the norm and finding motivation to avoid similar outcomes for herself.

Like I said, once I got out of the group and sort of finished the course, I just sort of kept saying to myself, "There is no way I am going to end up like that, there is no way I am going to end up like that" (U).

This theme described the importance of coping as both an individual and collective process. Participants reported interacting with each other in complementary ways to facilitate better outcomes for all participants. The coping capacity of the entire group influenced individuals and shaped the strategies they applied beyond the group context.

3.4. *Exchange Relationships.* The process of learning from others, swapping ideas within the group, and sharing information about resources was vital to improvements in confidence, sense of control, and positive attitudes. Essential exchange relationships operated throughout the course, and for some participants, continued after course completion. Participants were inspired not only by their capacity to learn from others, but also by their capacity to share with others. The opportunity to provide information as well as gain information from others was a mutually satisfying activity. This two-way learning process was crucial and encouraged participants to conclude that the course was an important adjunct to the current range of available resources

> *Doctors just say go home and look after yourself...whereas if you know there's a group you can go to [the course] and their [other participants'] ideas are so important because one of the persons in that group might have had an illness before and know how to handle situations (PL).*

> *If I can swap something that suits me with somebody else and make it a bit of a benefit out of it then that's the idea of these little groups getting together (U).*

All participants reported sharing resources with each other, indicating the universal nature of this exchange function. Most participants appreciated the exchange of ideas and resources among the group members because it enabled new learning to take place for all parties. It encouraged group members to examine their own role in society and feel that they had contributed to the well-being of others.

> *You might have a certain problem, but if you start talking to one another, "Oh yes I had that and this is how I got around it". In other words, it is a swapping of thoughts (R).*

> *And so, to know that there are other people there and there is a social life for encouragement...that there is a place for us within the community. Not so much...help because I did not realize I needed help, but I'd like to think that my life is [now] a bit more worthwhile (PL).*

The deliberate creation of dyads who could motivate each other and promote the exchange of ideas was useful to many participants. However, there were examples where this "buddy" system did not work well, because not all participants valued such intimate exchanges with another person.

> *Nobody did it [called their buddies] and I felt really silly because I got the attitude when I did*

> *ring that I was a sticky nose that I was interfering. I got that impression from them (U).*

> *I wouldn't participate in that [buddy system] because I am not that kind of person. I'm not a buddy person like that...I mention that because there might be a few other people like me and do not participate in that. I should imagine it works for a lot of people. But I am afraid I am just not that person (U).*

Indeed, the potential for conflict within dyads was evident. One participant relayed a negative encounter that occurred during a session requiring group members to pair up and discuss negative emotions. This experience highlighted the importance of exchange systems that emerged naturally within the broader group process as opposed to forced dyads that could result in damage to one of the parties if the exchange was not mutual.

> *As far as the other people went, we had a major problem with the first or second week, I forget which one. One of the ladies came and she was next to me and I turned around and said to her, "Well would you like to tell me your problems", because that is what we were meant to do [for the activity], and she attacked me. Really attacked me, as if I wouldn't know what a problem was and she had the worst problems and things. I wouldn't have gone back except that they [leaders] said, "Well she [the woman who had been defensive] is not coming back, she is obviously not right for the course". So I thought, "Oh well", I had promised to take [friend] every week so I was forced to go because I had committed myself (U).*

The social rather than interpersonal nature of the group was also highlighted by the fact that participants most commonly reported gaining benefits from processes that engaged the entire group. These activities were viewed as an effective mechanism for social exchange, *"All the work was done on the [white] board and we could all participate"* (U). Participants recognized that practicing new techniques in the group setting, rather than just discussing them, was an important part of the learning process. They noted the values of the immediate performance feedback that could be gained from other participants.

> *They were not just actually telling you about it, they got you down [doing the techniques]. It must make a difference if they take you through it (R).*

> *We all got to see each other [practice the techniques]...I think there was interest and hoping that we would learn something and, be entertained too (U).*

> *You learned something and you were also with a group of people, you know, you weren't just a single person; you were going to learn from others; You exchange experiences, you learn from other*

peoples' way of coping that you hadn't thought of and sometimes you hear much worse problems than your own too and how the other people coped with them (U).

This theme revealed an important social exchange function of the course. Instead of relying only on the information provided through the standardized course content, participants sought a two-way exchange of ideas and social comparison with other participants. This process enabled them to find new strategies, resources, and processes that helped them to manage their conditions. They also gained from the opportunity sharing their successes with others. However, this social exchange process differed from the interpersonal support that might be received through a closer relationship with one person.

4. Discussion

The central argument developed and presented in this paper is that, far from being an individual concept situated in the private lives of people with chronic conditions, self-management is better understood as a social concept embedded within and facilitated by collective processes and supportive systemic contexts. Over the last decade, increasing emphasis has been placed on the social context within which an individual with a chronic condition is located and the important role of social supports, service infrastructure, and social connections [8]. Despite the importance of individual disease treatment, we have previously drawn attention to the limitations of an individual model of self-management [6]. We have also argued that if inadequate attention is given to the social and environmental factors that can facilitate or inhibit health, self-management efforts may be wasted [9].

Our conclusion is further strengthened the key themes that emerged through this analysis of the process by which participants and peer leaders described the impact of the course. Specifically, this study has demonstrated that the social aspect of the group was a crucial factor in the success of the course and that benefits were associated with the interaction of four main social processes. The social context of the course created an environment characterized by collaborative coping, shared learning, and belonging. Most importantly, the course provided a solution to the social isolation that was experienced by many people with chronic conditions. According to participants, these features were linked to the successful outcomes of the course.

This study confirms the raft of evidence that social support is a critical buffer, potentially mitigating the impact of a disabling condition, ameliorating anxiety, and enhancing quality of life [8]. Indeed, there is evidence that high levels of social support are associated with better self-management behaviors [10]. The importance of combining educational and social processes has been found elsewhere [11], suggesting that, although any social gathering might facilitate similar positive outcomes, the course provided the structured interactions that enabled participants to engage in positive ways (e.g., to develop collaborative coping and a collective identity). Choi et al. [12] noted that group members are

exposed to two types of influences: (1) discretionary influences that are available to different group members at different times and in different forms as they interact with other group members (e.g., messages of approval, learning, etc.) and (2) ambient influences that are available to all members and pervade the group setting (e.g., group norms, positive climate, shared ideas, etc.). The current study has articulated these different influences, noting the presence of both ambient (e.g., a collective identity and collaborative coping) and discretionary qualities (e.g., social engagement and exchange relationships).

Despite being delivered in a group setting, the dominant conceptualization of self-management is an individual approach and framed within a medical model. Self-management in this context is defined by three key premises, namely:

(i) the individual is perceived to be dealing with the consequences of disease;

(ii) the individual is perceived to be deficient in skills such as problem solving, decision making and self-confidence;

(iii) the individual is placed in partnerships with a health professional who takes responsibility for medical management [13].

In contrast to this conceptualization, the current study has suggested that self-management is a social concept and that several important social processes might be able to account for the outcomes achieved through CDSM courses. This analysis has defined a "social" model of self-management that may be more sustainable and relevant than the current individual model of self-management. By giving adequate attention to the social aspects of self-management, it is likely that the utility and meaningfulness of the course could be enhanced for a significant proportion of the population.

Self-management as a social concept goes beyond individual interventions and even beyond partnerships with health service providers. It may be better conceptualized as a collaborative concept enacted when individuals come together, although not necessarily in a physical place. The act of coming together creates greater capacity to address the "collective" problems associated with chronic disease. The process of self-management seems to be about sharing approaches to common problems, building resources together, encouraging and motivating each other and transforming private pain into collective responses that would never have emerged in an individualized setting. Thus, health professionals may need to refine their understanding of and support for the social processes that contribute to and sustain self-management outcomes.

The process of social self-management that emerged from this study resembles the notion of cultural health capital [14]. According to Shim [14], cultural health capital accrues as one engages in the repeated enactment of health practices (e.g., consuming information, decision making, self-surveillance, etc.). Thus, cultural health capital has a self-generating quality, accumulating over time through interactions with others. This concept is embedded in social processes and is inherently relational. Rather than placing demands on people to become independent and self-directed managers of their own health through education, the notion of self-management as a form of cultural health capital acknowledges that self-management relies on interdependence and builds over time as people engage with new practices and ideas.

5. Conclusions

The findings of this study revealed that responses to disease and ways of self-managing were clearly situated not only in the private lives of individuals, but also in collective processes. Individuals were encouraged and motivated by the social interactions, engagement, and support they received from coparticipants. These findings suggest a dynamic and multidimensional approach to health and well-being which recognizes the role of context and relational aspects of people's environments. Although not surprising, the current study highlights the fact that the dominant interpretation of self-management adopted by many health professionals may be overly simplistic. The focus on skills, resources, and education about health overlooks the importance of building opportunities to enhance one's cultural health capital through positive social interactions. Our study has suggested that there may be sufficient reason for policy makers and professionals to become concerned with activities and interventions that develop supportive social environments and opportunities in addition to their current focus on lifestyle change at the level of the individual.

However, such a shift will not be easy. Recognition of a social model of self-management will require a fundamental reorientation of professional practice. First and foremost, it will require a shift from the individualistic educational model of self-management towards one based on the application of broad social strategies that can create conditions that foster hope, healing, empowerment, and social connection as well as a positive culture [15]. This shift will require a commitment to new ways of working with clients that reflect the social context within which they function. If health professionals can be encouraged to think about self-management as a form of cultural health capital, accumulated through a vast array of social interactions, they may be able to not only support the social processes that facilitate self-management, but also enact their own role in ways that act as a source of self-management support. The CDSM course appears to be a useful vehicle for facilitating the social processes that emerged from our data. However, it may be possible to promote these social processes more widely within all clinical interactions if a more social view of self-management was propagated. A continued focus on self-management as an individual responsibility that is reliant on the skills and knowledge residing within the individual will encourage health professionals to overlook the social and contextual nature of the concept. It will also enable them to minimize the importance of their own role as a social agent and a facilitator of social processes.

References

[1] D. Yach, C. Hawkes, C. L. Gould, and K. J. Hofman, "The global burden of chronic diseases: overcoming impediments to prevention and control," *Journal of the American Medical Association*, vol. 291, no. 21, pp. 2616–2622, 2004.

[2] N. Gillespie and T. Lenz, "Implementation of a tool to modify behaviour in a chronic disease management program," *Advances in Preventive Medicine*, vol. 2011, Article ID 215842, 5 pages, 2011.

[3] D. Singh, "How can chronic disease management programmes operate across care settings and providers?" WHO Regional Office for Europe and European Observatory on Health Systems and Policies, 2008, http://www.euro.who.int/__data/assets/pdf_file/0009/75474/E93416.pdf.

[4] K. Lorig, "Chronic disease self-management: a model for tertiary prevention," *American Behavioral Scientist*, vol. 39, no. 6, pp. 676–683, 1996.

[5] K. R. Lorig and H. R. Holman, "Self-management education: history, definition, outcomes, and mechanisms," *Annuals of Behavioural Medicine*, vol. 26, no. 1, pp. 1–7, 2003.

[6] E. Kendall and A. Rogers, "Extinguishing the social?: state sponsored self-care policy and the Chronic Disease Self-management Programme," *Disability and Society*, vol. 22, no. 2, pp. 129–143, 2007.

[7] E. Kendall, M. Foster, W. Chaboyer, T. Gee, and T. Catalano, "The sharing health care initiative: a better approach to managing chronic conditions," Tech. Rep., Centre for Work, Leisure and Community Research & Arthritis Queensland. Griffith University, 2004.

[8] H. Muenchberger, E. Kendall, and H. Han, " Human infrastructure in health: a commentary on networks of supports," *Australian Health Review*, vol. 34, no. 3, pp. 1–3, 2010.

[9] E. Kendall, C. Ehrlich, N. Sunderland, H. Muenchberger, and C. Rushton, "Self-managing versus self-management: reinvigorating the socio-political dimensions of self-management," *Chronic Illness*, vol. 7, no. 1, pp. 87–98, 2011.

[10] M. P. Gallant, "The influence of social support on chronic illness self-management: a review and directions for research," *Health Education and Behavior*, vol. 30, no. 2, pp. 170–195, 2003.

[11] T. Catalano, P. Dickson, E. Kendall, P. Kuipers, and T. N. Posner, "The perceived benefits of the chronic disease self-management program among participants with stroke: a qualitative study," *Australian Journal of Primary Health*, vol. 9, no. 2-3, pp. 80–89, 2003.

[12] J. N. Choi, R. H. Price, and A. D. Vinokur, "Self-efficacy changes in groups: effects of diversity, leadership, and group climate," *Journal of Organizational Behavior*, vol. 24, no. 4, pp. 357–372, 2003.

[13] T. Bodenheimer, K. Lorig, H. Holman, and K. Grumbach, "Patient self-management of chronic disease in primary care," *Journal of the American Medical Association*, vol. 288, no. 19, pp. 2469–2475, 2002.

[14] J. K. Shim, "Cultural health capital: a theoretical approach to understanding health care interactions and the dynamics of unequal treatment," *Journal of Health and Social Behavior*, vol. 51, no. 1, pp. 1–15, 2010.

[15] N. Jacobson and D. Greenley, "What is recovery? A conceptual model and explication," *Psychiatric Services*, vol. 52, no. 4, pp. 482–485, 2001.

4

A Data Quality Control Program for Computer-Assisted Personal Interviews

Janet E. Squires,[1,2] Alison M. Hutchinson,[3] Anne-Marie Bostrom,[4,5] Kelly Deis,[6] Peter G. Norton,[7] Greta G. Cummings,[6] and Carole A. Estabrooks[6]

[1] Clinical Epidemiology Program, Ottawa Hospital Research Institute, Ottawa, ON, Canada K1H 8L6
[2] School of Nursing, University of Ottawa, Ottawa, ON, Canada K1H 8M5
[3] Cabrini-Deakin Centre for Nursing Research, School of Nursing and Midwifery, Deakin University and Cabrini Health, Melbourne, VIC 3KM, Australia
[4] Division of Nursing, Department of Neurobiology, Care Sciences and Society, Karolinska Institute, 14183 Huddinge, Sweden
[5] Department of Geriatric Medicine, Danderyd Hospital, 18287 Danderyd, Sweden
[6] Faculty of Nursing, University of Alberta, Edmonton, AB, Canada T6G 1C9
[7] Department of Family Medicine, University of Calgary, Calgary, AB, Canada T2M 0H5

Correspondence should be addressed to Janet E. Squires, jasquires@ohri.ca

Academic Editor: M. H. F. Grypdonck

Researchers strive to optimize data quality in order to ensure that study findings are valid and reliable. In this paper, we describe a data quality control program designed to maximize quality of survey data collected using computer-assisted personal interviews. The quality control program comprised three phases: (1) software development, (2) an interviewer quality control protocol, and (3) a data cleaning and processing protocol. To illustrate the value of the program, we assess its use in the Translating Research in Elder Care Study. We utilize data collected annually for two years from computer-assisted personal interviews with 3004 healthcare aides. Data quality was assessed using both survey and process data. Missing data and data errors were minimal. Mean and median values and standard deviations were within acceptable limits. Process data indicated that in only 3.4% and 4.0% of cases was the interviewer unable to conduct interviews in accordance with the details of the program. Interviewers' perceptions of interview quality also significantly improved between Years 1 and 2. While this data quality control program was demanding in terms of time and resources, we found that the benefits clearly outweighed the effort required to achieve high-quality data.

1. Background

Good data quality is fundamental to survey research; poor data quality can provide misleading results and seriously invalidate study findings. Hence, researchers will often expend considerable effort on quality control procedures. Factors contributing to data quality are numerous, complex, and multidimensional [1]. Sources of error include coverage, nonresponse, sampling, respondent, instrument, and mode of delivery [2]. In the case of face-to-face interview data collection methods, including telephone and computer-assisted personal interviews, the interviewer is also an important part of the process and can be a further source of error.

Two common approaches to survey data quality are the total quality management (TQM) approach and the total survey error (TSE) approach. The TQM approach to data quality focuses on the process of survey production and is based on the assumption that the quality of all elements of the production process contributes to quality of the final dataset [1]. According to this approach, data quality is a function of not only accuracy but also the relevance, comparability, coherence, timeliness, and completeness of the data. Evaluation of quality in the case of TQM addresses process and outcomes.

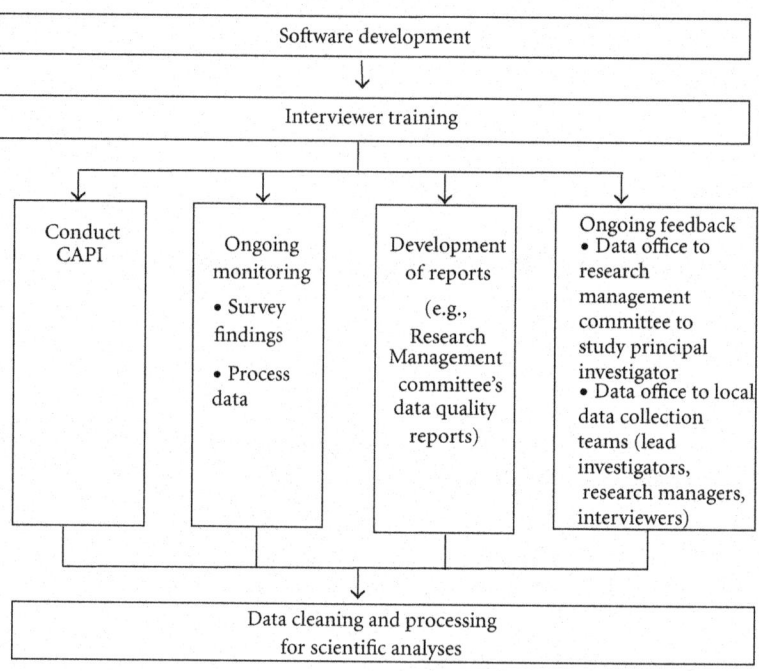

FIGURE 1: Data quality control program.

The TSE approach, on the other hand, describes quality in terms of accuracy and defines data quality "as the relative absence of systematic variable errors" [1, page 66]. Finally, Loosveldt and colleagues emphasize the value of a pragmatic approach to data quality, which focuses on evaluation of the survey process and outcomes as well as on the interviewer tasks, thereby integrating the TQM and TSE approaches [1].

While there is some literature describing quality control and assurance procedures for clinical trials (e.g., Martin and colleagues [3]), this literature is scarce and does not fully apply to survey research. The purpose of this paper is therefore to describe a data quality control program (with elements of TQM and TSE approaches) that was developed to maximize the quality of survey data collected using computer-assisted personal interviews (CAPIs). CAPI involves interviewers reading survey questions aloud to participants and entering responses directly into a survey application using a computer. We illustrate our data quality control program by describing the program and evaluating its usefulness with survey and process data collected in the *Translating Research in Elder Care* (TREC) Study [4, 5]. In TREC, all healthcare aides in 36 nursing homes (in Western Canada) who met the study inclusion criteria were invited to complete the TREC survey (a suite of self-report instruments) annually for two years (June 2008– July 2010). Data collection occurred in quarters with each nursing home having data collected in the same quarter each year. Trained TREC research staff administered the survey to healthcare aides using CAPI. Where it was not possible to use CAPI (e.g., rare situations in which the interviewer could not open the computer software application), a paper survey was completed and data were later entered into the virtual system. Further details on the TREC data collection procedures are reported elsewhere [4].

2. Methods

2.1. The Data Quality Control Program. The data quality control program comprised three phases: (1) software development, (2) an interviewer quality control protocol, and (3) a data cleaning and processing protocol (Figure 1).

2.1.1. Phase 1: Software Development. We contracted the services of a Canadian-based software developer with experience in the development of online surveys and an understanding of the health sector (https://nooro.com/). Our requirements were complex; providing respondent and interviewer access to the survey using a variety of computer systems located within diverse environments across geographically distributed locations and all systems requiring capacity to securely upload individually gathered data to the master dataset located on a remote server. This is typically where Internet accessible surveys would be well suited; however Internet access in our settings was inconsistent and in some communities nonexistent. Without reliable Internet access, our best solution was to purchase several laptop computers (for use by interviewers undertaking data collection concurrently in each setting) and have the survey software installed on each laptop. This allowed for offline survey completion and temporary storage, with subsequent upload of data using a secure file transfer service when internet connectivity was available. Each interviewer was allocated a unique identifier, and each data file had a unique file naming convention.

Important considerations for the software development process included maintenance of confidentiality across the sites and provinces, minimization of error, and expedience in conducting the survey. To help meet these requirements, one feature of the survey software involved predetermined options for certain fields. This feature was linked to the interviewer's unique identifier so that each interviewer would only see options that were relevant to their jurisdiction (e.g., when they selected *facility name*, the common names of the units *only* within that facility would appear). We also recognized that cultural, environmental, and personal experiences could result in differing understandings of terms and phrases used in the survey. To aid understanding, promote standardization, and minimize the influence of interviewer bias, tips and prompts were built into the survey in select places. Interviewers were instructed to use these prompts only if a term or phrase was not clear to the respondent. If a prompt was not available, interviewers were instructed not to say anything additional, to ensure standardization of delivery of the survey.

A risk of CAPI is that the interviewer might inadvertently omit questions, resulting in missing data. To help overcome this, a check and balance system was implemented, whereby at the end of the survey a screen would appear advising the interviewer of the number of questions that remained unanswered and their location within the survey. The interviewer then had the option of returning to the questions concerned to confirm whether they were missed, as opposed to refused by the respondent, and if so, to obtain a response.

Another important consideration in the software development process was the data upload procedure. Development, refinement, and testing of this process took into account the steps required to connect to the server, how soon after data collection the data had to be uploaded, and the type of confirmation that was generated to signal a successful upload. Additionally, system checks were put in place to ensure the same data could be uploaded only once. Testing of the survey and the upload process to ensure each was fully operational and behaving as expected involved internal and external review phases. The internal phase involved a cycle of development, review and testing, and modification, followed by further review and testing. This process took into account the survey content, visual appeal of the survey, and ease of navigation. The former involved checking the question order, completeness of questions, spelling, grammar, and punctuation. The latter involved consideration of overall appearance of the survey, the colors, the format and layout of responses, the number of questions per page, how the questions were separated (different colors and width of lines), the ability to advance or move back in the survey, and the ability to change responses. The external phase involved testing of the software by healthcare aides and evaluation of the overall appearance, functionality, and ease of navigation within the survey.

The final stage of the software development addressed capacity for "real time" monitoring to ensure high-quality data. The software developer provided a private site, accessible only by authorized TREC administration staff, which allowed for generation of live, standardized reports of the number of surveys completed by setting (e.g., province, site). An important feature of the CAPI system is the capacity to generate paradata (data relating to the process of data collection). This data included the number of attempts interviewers had at completing an individual interview, the length of time each interview took, and the time of day the interviews were conducted. Such data enabled tracking of interviewer performance, which is important to achieving high-quality data.

2.1.2. Phase 2: Interviewer Quality Control Protocol. Each of the three provinces participating in the TREC study established a local data team, which was responsible for healthcare aide recruitment and data collection. Each team was led by a site investigator and included a research manager and one or more research assistants and/or professional interviewers.

The data teams participated in intensive interviewer training to ensure standardized technique and the collection of high-quality data. To facilitate this process, an interviewer (procedure) manual and an interviewer quality control protocol were developed and implemented as components of the data quality control program. The interviewer manual contained technical information on the TREC study, the survey, the step-by-step process of conducting a CAPI interview, and an overview of the CAPI software and the processes by which the data were to be handled. The interviewer quality control protocol (Supplementary File 1; see supplementary materials available online at doi:10.1155/2012/303816) was central to the quality control program and contained three core components: (1) characteristics of a successful interviewer, (2) training, and (3) tracking and monitoring processes.

(1) Characteristics of a Successful Interviewer. Four broad categories of characteristics of a successful interviewer were identified based on a review of existing literature and our experience with conducting face-to-face structured interviews. The four categories were (1) physical attributes, (2) personal characteristics, (3) technical skills, and (4) compliance with interview procedures. Physical attributes included open posture, consistent eye contact (with interviewee), and comfort with conducting the interview. Personal characteristics included a personable demeanor, engaging with the interviewee, appropriate speed of talking and clear and audible speech, appropriate (professional) dress and hygiene, and ability to problem-solve (e.g., technological problems) during interviews. Technical skills included ability to log on to the computer, ability to open and launch the virtual server CAPI software, ability to navigate through the survey, acceptable typing speed, ability to conduct the interview while entering responses with minimal delays, and ability to connect to the virtual server to allow data synchronization and upload following the interview.

(2) Interviewer Training. The interviewer training consisted of two core elements: (1) a field school or orientation session, depending on date of hire of the interviewer, and (2)

practice interviews. Explicit steps were taken to standardize interviewer techniques in order to maximize consistency between interviewers. Initial training included attendance at a two-day "CAPI Field School." All existing and newly hired staff (research managers and research assistants) who could potentially be assigned to conduct CAPI interviews for the study were required to attend the field school. The study principal investigator, provincial investigators, administrative staff, and research trainees also attended the field school, which took place one month prior to initiation of data collection. The intent of the field school was threefold to ensure interviewers (1) had a shared understanding of the study, (2) understood how to use the CAPI software, and most importantly (3) received the same (standardized) training with respect to *how* to conduct CAPI. Interviewers hired after the field school were required to attend an orientation session in their province, hosted by the provincial research manager, which incorporated the important elements of the field school.

The field school was developed to be informative, interactive, fun, and a team building process. Sessions focused on (1) getting to know the research team, (2) providing information on the TREC study and survey (including an item-by-item review of the survey to ensure all potential interviewers understood the items in the same way) and the CAPI and software process, and (3) practice interviews. Prior to practicing their interviewing skills, field school participants observed "good and easy" and "bad and difficult" interviews as role-played by TREC administrative staff and research trainees. A "bad and difficult" interview was role-played first. Participants were then asked to provide feedback in terms of what could have been done differently. The same role players then conducted a "good" interview to highlight the way in which data could be collected more efficiently and effectively. Following role-playing, participants were assigned to small groups where they were asked to rotate through the roles of interviewer, interviewee, and observer. A senior investigator circulated throughout the groups observing, giving feedback, and answering questions. To conclude the initial (field school) training, all team members were invited to share their experiences with the group.

Following attendance at the field school or orientation session and prior to conducting formal data collection, each interviewer was required to complete a minimum of five practice interviews in which they demonstrated an acceptable level of competence and the characteristics of a good interviewer. Three interviews were done with people other than other interviewers (e.g., investigators) and two were with other interviewers. A minimum of two of these interviews was required to be observed by the provincial research manager who provided feedback on the interviewer's performance using standard forms: an *interviewer checklist* (which outlines the characteristics of a good interviewer) and an *interviewer monitor form* (which lists interviewer techniques, delivery, and data entry skills) (both in Supplementary File 1). In some cases, the research manager also attended the first few "real" interviews to ensure compliance with the interviewer quality control protocol.

(3) Monitoring and Feedback. Information on the quality of the survey data collected in the CAPI interviews and the process of conducting the interviews was monitored throughout the data collection period. Monitored information included survey findings (e.g., missing data, skewness) and process-related data (e.g., travel time, time on site, number of interviews completed/in progress/refused) collected using standardized forms, which were submitted to and verified by the central office for the TREC study. In the event of discrepancies or errors with the process data, the data manager for the study would contact the research manager for the indicated province for resolution. Once verified, the information was entered (and double checked for accuracy) into a statistical database where it was analyzed and used to generate quality reports. Security and confidentiality policies were enforced for all reports (e.g., forms had to be sent by bonded courier; courier packages had to be received by an identified person in central office and were documented and stored in a locked cabinet). Also as a part of the quality control program, following each interview (once the respondent (healthcare aide) left the room), interviewers were asked to complete a series of questions (the *interviewer checklist*, Supplementary File 1) on the interview process. This also allowed for a better understanding of the circumstances in which each survey was completed. These data were analyzed regularly (quarterly) to further assess quality of the interviews and compliance with the quality control interviewer protocol. This information was fed back to the interviewers when necessary.

Regular feedback on the quality of the data to the TREC Research Management Committee and the local (provincial) data collection teams was a critical component of the interviewer quality control protocol. The Research Management Committee was composed of the study's principal investigator, senior investigators, and decision makers. The committee met quarterly. A CAPI data quality report was prepared for and reviewed at each Research Management Committee Meeting throughout data collection. This report included, for example, for each interviewer the number of interviews completed, missing data by survey item, item skewness and kurtosis, and instances where survey responses were significantly different for one interviewer compared to other interviewers within a facility and/or province. Table 1 and Figures 2 and 3 comprise a sample table and graphs from a data quality report.

Ongoing feedback was also provided to the local data collection teams. Interviewers were given feedback starting the first day after data collection and regularly thereafter. Details of the feedback provided at each time interval (i.e., weekly, quarterly, yearly) are summarized in the quality control interviewer protocol (Supplementary File 1). In addition to this feedback, data-related issues such as missing data and survey item responses that differed significantly from other interviewers were also fed back to the provincial lead investigator in each province who discussed the issue with their research manager and interviewers.

2.1.3. Phase 3: Data Cleaning and Processing Protocol. The third and final phase of our quality control program was

TABLE 1: Number of interviews for data collector by province and nursing home, partial wave 2 (July 16th, 2009–November 23th, 2009).

Data collector	Province 1 Facility									Province 2 Facility					Province 3 Facility				Total
	S3	A2	T5	E5	B9	H3	G7	D2	Total	R7	W9	F3	K4	Total	Z8	T9	Q8	Total	
1	11		27					36	74										74
15					8	4	24		36										36
16					28	16	41		85										85
29	2								2										2
30	12	10	20	2				26	70										70
35		9	37	8					54										54
26										9	4	13		26					26
34										25	16	22	13	76					76
13															6		7	13	13
18															28	6	17	51	51
27															21	9	6	36	36
Total	25	19	84	10	36	20	65	62	321	34	20	35	13	102	55	15	30	100	523

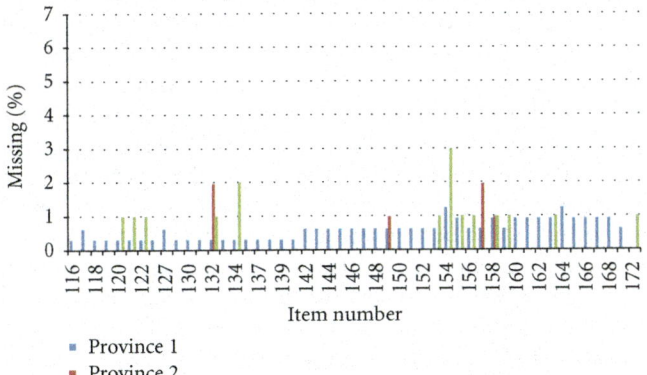

FIGURE 2: Missing values by item for all provinces (July 16th, 2009–Nov 23rd, 2009).

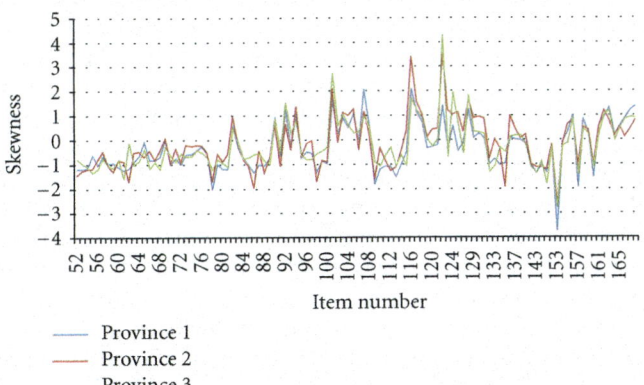

FIGURE 3: Skewness by item for all provinces (July 16th, 2009–November 23rd, 2009). Comment presented in the report: The skewness graph indicates if the answers to any item are skewed or not. Negative is left skewed (tend to have small values) and positive is right skewed (tend to have large values). In the skewness it shows that there is no significant difference among all three provinces.

a data cleaning and processing protocol (Supplementary File 2). The protocol consisted of six steps and was implemented quarterly by a data analyst for the study: (1) systematic data entry, (2) data cleaning, (3) prederivation processing, (4) derivation of scale scores, (5) descriptive assessment of derived scores, and (6) assessment of missing data. Throughout this process, a four-part report was produced for the study lead investigators: steps 1-2 (report A), step 3 (report B), steps 4-5 (report C), and step 6 (report D). Each report was reviewed and approved by the study principal investigator before the data analyst proceeded to the next phase of cleaning and processing.

3. Results

3.1. Survey Data

3.1.1. Missing Data. Data were collected from 3004 healthcare aides (1494 and 1510 in Years 1 and 2, resp.). Missing data was minimal with 99% of healthcare aides having 5% or less missing data (Table 2). Individually, all cases with >10% missing data (i.e., missing on at least 19 of the 192 survey items) were explored to inform a decision regarding retention. A total of 12 cases (0.4% of the sample) had >10% missing data; 8 of these cases were deleted because data were missing for several core domains that were essential to the testing of the study's main hypotheses. One additional case was also deleted from the data because the participant did not meet the eligibility criteria. This resulted in a final sample size of 2,995 (99.7% of all healthcare aides interviewed).

3.1.2. Systematic Data Errors. Systematic data errors (i.e., errors that tend to shift all measurements in a systematic way [2, 6]) were corrected within the data as they were discovered. Such errors were minimal ($n = 6$) and most ($n = 5$ of 6) related to miscoding of missing and/or not applicable responses. Outside these coding errors, only one

TABLE 2: Missing data over the two years of the TREC Project 1.

Missing rate	Year 1		Year 2		Total (Year 1 + Year 2)		
	Frequency	Percent	Frequency	Percent	Frequency	Percent	Cumulative percent
No missing	0	0	1135	75.2	1135	37.8	37.9
0%~1%	0	0	222	14.7	222	7.4	45.3
1%~2%	0	0	95	6.3	95	3.2	48.5
2%~3%	1010	67.6	33	2.2	1043	34.7	83.3
3%~4%	381	25.5	8	0.5	389	13.0	96.3
4%~5%	70	4.7	8	0.5	78	2.6	98.9
5%~10%	26	1.7	3	0.2	29	1.0	99.9
>10%	6	0.4	6	0.4	12	0.4	100.0
Total	1493	100.0	1510	100.0	3003	100.0	

systematic error was detected. The responses for one set of six items were all 1's across all data. After consultation with our software developer, it was discovered that the original codes for the item set were imported incorrectly into the software; a new code was written by the software developer to correct the error.

3.1.3. Random Data Errors. We also assessed for random data entry errors where paper surveys were used. Random error, also known as variable or chance error, is caused by chance factors that confound measurement [2]. A total of 70 paper surveys were completed (43 in Year 1 and 27 in Year 2). Annual "random" data entry error rates were low: 13% and 1.6% for Years 1 and 2, respectively. The annual random error rate was calculated using the following formula: number of errors/[(192 items)(X surveys)]. Since we checked all entries on all paper surveys, we also corrected all random errors.

3.1.4. Distributions. As a part of our ongoing monitoring of the survey data, we also examined each item (and scale scores) quarterly for mean and median values, standard deviation, skewness, and kurtosis. All mean and median values and standard deviations were within acceptable limits. Skewness and kurtosis was minimal with the majority of items displaying an approximate normal distribution.

3.2. Process (Interviewer) Data. Process-related data collected from the interviewers included, for example, whether or not a paper-based survey was used. These data indicated that the proportion of paper-based surveys used was small and fell over time (from 2.9% in Year 1 to 1.8% in Year 2; chi-square, $P = 0.040$): an indication that the procedure for enabling software updates overnight (to prevent computer start-up delays during the daytime) was functioning well and the interviewers were confident in using the software. Data were also collected on whether or not the interviewers were able to set up the interview according to protocol. Overall, in only 3.4% (Year 1) and 4% (Year 2) of cases was the interviewer unable to set up in accordance with the protocol. On most occasions, the interview was conducted in a private location as per protocol (72% in Year 1 and 78% in Year 2).

Frequently the location was also visible to other staff (65% in Year 1 and 75% in Year 2) and close to resident care (68% in Year 1 and 86% in Year 2). Interruptions during data collection, which could potentially threaten the quality of the data, were also monitored. The majority of the interviews were conducted without interruption (76% in Year 1 and 84% in Year 2). Another possible threat to data quality was pauses (where the interview had to be stopped and restarted). The majority of interviews proceeded that required a pause (91% in Year 1 and 95% in Year 2). Interviewers were also asked to rate the overall quality of the interview from 1 (terrible) to 5 (wonderful). Their perceptions of overall quality improved between Year 1 (mean 3.84) 2 (mean 4.11); this improvement was statistically significant (chi square, $P < 0.001$) which could reflect improved competence and confidence from training and feedback provided in the data quality control program and as they gained experience in conducting the interviews.

We also examined survey data in relation to the individual who conducted the interview. This was part of the quarterly quality reports. In particular, we assessed the data (by interviewer) for missing data and skewness to determine if we had any "interviewer problems." Overall, few issues were noted. Some instances that were detected are as follows. In one instance, we discovered skewed healthcare aide responses for a particular item set for the majority of the interviews conducted by one interviewer in one quarter. The information was feed backed to the local team and the provincial research manager then observed the interviewer conducting their next set of interviews. This revealed that the interviewer was delivering (reading) the questions too quickly, resulting in the healthcare aides not having sufficient time to answer the questions with accuracy. The interviewer was given feedback accordingly and the skewness of his or her data was monitored in future reports. No further problems were observed, illustrating the importance of our quality assessment and providing ongoing feedback to the interviewers. In another instance, high levels of missing data for specific variables, across interviewers and provinces, were detected. Investigation revealed that this issue was related to a security update performed by the software provider, which had affected specific data fields during the survey upload process. This problem was rectified and the correct data were restored. In another example, a quality report highlighted the existence of relatively high rates of missing data on the interviewer checklist across several interviewers. The checklist data were very important for assessment of the overall quality of the interviews. In response to identification of this discrepancy, the research managers stressed to the interviewers the importance of completing the checklist. Subsequent reports found almost no missing data for the interview checklists.

4. Discussion

Our efforts to adopt the CAPI method, to provide interviewer training, and to implement a rigorous quality control program were motivated primarily by a desire to promote efficiency in the collection and processing of the survey data, maximizing the quality of the data, facilitating data processing, and saving time. The upfront cost (in terms developing the software and training the interviewers) and ongoing investment (in terms of staff and investigator person hours required to develop the quality reports and clean/process the data) was not insignificant. For instance, approximately 500 hours of paid staff time (combined data analyst, data manager, and data research assistant) were required to compile the quarterly quality reports and clean and process one year of CAPI data. However, despite this investment of time and resources, our results demonstrate that the CAPI method combined with our data quality control program was successful overall, which for us made this investment worthwhile. Missing data was minimal with only 8 cases (out of a possible 3004) requiring deletion due to excessive (>10%) missing data; we believe this result can be attributed to a combination of the survey method, the software design, interviewer skills, and regular monitoring. Our ongoing monitoring process (e.g., quality reports and data cleaning and processing reports) further enhanced our ability to produce high-quality data for the study. The generation of the quality reports was unique to the TREC study. These reports were highly beneficial in highlighting aspects of data quality that required further investigation such as high levels of missing data for specific variables and/or across interviewers. In several cases, had a quarterly quality report not been generated, it is unlikely that certain issues would have been detected and thus corrected.

As recommended by Loosveldt and colleagues [1], we adopted a pragmatic approach to the promotion of data quality, integrating the TQM and TSE approaches to focus on evaluation of the survey process, outcomes, adnd interviewer tasks. Interviewer skills cannot be assumed to be of high-quality, and variability in interviewer proficiency presents a significant risk to data quality. While training can address interviewer skills, variability between interviewers cannot be overcome by training alone [7–11]. Thus, use of a standardized approach to data quality control that addressed process as well as outcome measures provided us with ongoing monitoring of the quality of our survey data and

enabled us to intervene when deviations or discrepancies were identified. Additionally, the use of CAPI enabled further standardization and control of the interview process by allowing for automated skip patterns and embedded prompts. Additionally, prompts at the completion of the survey to alert the interviewer to any unanswered questions helped to promote completeness of the data. In combination, we found that these strategies maximized the quality of the survey data we collected.

5. Challenges Encountered

Despite the benefit of acquiring high-quality data, our quality control program was not without its challenges. Internet access, interviewer training, maintaining security of the data, and the monitoring and tracking of the data presented a range of challenges for the investigatory team to overcome. These challenges were not insurmountable, but they did require a substantial lead-time to address them adequately prior to the commencement of data collection. For example, the decision to adopt the CAPI approach to data collection presented challenges with respect to Internet access. Because reliable Internet connections could not be guaranteed, the software had to be developed to enable delayed transmission of collected data. Data security was of a high priority for data stored on laptop computers until such time as the interviewer could access the Internet to upload their data. As a result, strict procedures and protocols were required to promote consistency in handling of the computer equipment and transfer of the data in order to reduce the risk of a security breach or loss of data. Further, computers purchased within each of the provinces had different operating systems and there were varying security arrangements across the sites. This resulted in the software developer being responsible for specific installations and instructions for each software user to ensure all computers functioned correctly.

While interviewer training was labor intensive, it was a vital element of the quality control process. This training involved not only development of interpersonal and interviewing skills but also skills in use of the equipment, navigation of the survey, and transmission of the data following the interview. An unplanned delay for two of the three participating provinces between the field school and the commencement of the interview data collection phase enabled interviewers to practice, but was a threat to skill retention. Field school was only offered at the startup of the interview data collection phase, and ongoing training of interviewers who were dispersed over three provinces had to be undertaken at the provincial level. This requirement had the potential for some variation in training, even though a standard training manual was provided. Additionally, as new interviewers were employed, training had to be provided on an ad hoc basis, as required. A further challenge was that interviewers only had access to the software developer during normal business hours. Therefore, if difficulties were encountered in the field, outside business hours, interviewers often could not achieve a resolution in a timely manner. This, however, was rare.

6. Conclusion

The quality of survey data is of methodological importance and can be addressed using a comprehensive, standardized quality control and improvement process. Our findings indicate that the data quality control program developed in the TREC study can have a positive influence on data quality. While there are many challenges associated with achieving high survey data quality, the benefits outweigh the effort required to achieve high-quality data.

Conflict of Interests

The authors declare that they have no conflict interests.

Authors' Contribution

C. A. Estabrooks, P. G. Norton, and G. G. Cummings participated in conceptualizing the TREC program and in securing the grant that provided its funding. J. E. Squires, C. A. Estabrooks, P. G. Norton, and G. G. Cummings participated in conceptualizing Project 1 and J. E. Squires, C. A. Estabrooks, P. G. Norton, and G. G. Cummings in Project 1 data collection. All authors (J. E. Squires, A. M. Hutchinson, A. M. Bostrom, K. Deis, P. G. Norton, G. G. Cummings, and C. A. Estabrooks) contributed to developing and implementing the quality control program described in this paper. J. E. Squires and A. M. Hutchinson drafted the paper. All authors provided critical comments on the manuscript and approved the final version.

Acknowledgments

The authors also acknowledge the *Translating Research in Elder Care* (TREC) Study, which was funded by the Canadian Institutes of Health Research (CIHR) (MOP #53107). The TREC Team (at the time of this study) include Carole A. Estabrooks (PI), Investigators: Greta G. Cummings, Lesley Degner, Sue Dopson, Heather Laschinger, Kathy McGilton, Verena Menec, Debra Morgan, Peter Norton, Joanne Profetto-McGrath, Jo Rycroft-Malone, Malcolm Smith, Norma Stewart, and Gary Teare; Decision-Makers: Caroline Clarke, Gretta Lynn Ell, Belle Gowriluk, Sue Neville, Corinne Schalm, Donna Stelmachovich, Gina Trinidad, Juanita Tremeer, and Luana Whitbread; Collaborators: David Hogan Chuck Humphrey, Michael Leiter, Charles Mather; Special Advisors: Judy Birdsell, Phyllis Hempel (deceased), Jack Williams, and Dorothy Pringle (Chair, Scientific Advisory Committee). C. A. Estabrooks is supported by a CIHR Canada Research Chair in Knowledge Translation. G. G. Cummings holds CIHR New Investigator and Alberta Heritage Foundation for Medical Research (AHFMR) Population Health Investigator awards. C. A. Estabrooks is the principal investigator and G. G. Cummings and P. G. Norton are co-investigators in the TREC program. At the time of this study, K. Deis was the Administrative Director of the TREC Program; J. E. Squires was a doctoral student in the TREC program funded by a CIHR fellowship in KT, AHFMR studentship, and Killam Predoctoral Scholarship; A. M. Hutchinson and A. M. Bostrom were postdoctoral fellows in the TREC program funded by the CIHR, and AHFMR Fellowships.

References

[1] G. A. Loosveldt, A. Carton, and J. Billiet, "Assessment of survey data quality: a pragmatic approach focused on interviewer tasks," *International Journal of Market Research*, vol. 46, no. 1, pp. 65–82, 2004.

[2] C. F. Waltz, O. L. Strickland, and E. R. Lenz, *Measurement in Nursing and Health Research*, Springer, New York, NY, USA, 2005.

[3] R. J. Martin, D. K. Kephart, A. M. Dyer, J. Fahy, and M. Kraft, "Quality control within the Asthma Clinical Research Network," *Controlled Clinical Trials*, vol. 22, no. 6, supplement 1, pp. 207S–221S, 2001.

[4] C. A. Estabrooks, J. E. Squires, G. G. Cummings, G. F. Teare, and P. G. Norton, "Study protocol for the translating research in elder care (TREC): building context—an organizational monitoring program in long-term care project (project one)," *Implementation Science*, vol. 4, no. 1, article 52, 2009.

[5] C. A. Estabrooks, A. M. Hutchinson, J. E. Squires et al., "Translating research in elder care: an introduction to a study protocol series," *Implementation Science*, vol. 4, no. 1, article 51, 2009.

[6] J. Nunnally and I. Bernstein, *Psychometric Theory*, McGraw-Hill, New York, NY, USA, 1994.

[7] M. A. Demitrack, D. Faries, J. M. Herrera, D. J. DeBrota, and W. Z. Potter, "The problem of measurement error in multisite clinical trials," *Psychopharmacology Bulletin*, vol. 34, no. 1, pp. 19–24, 1998.

[8] K. A. Kobak, A. D. Feiger, and J. D. Lipsitz, "Interview quality and signal detection in clinical trials," *American Journal of Psychiatry*, vol. 162, no. 3, p. 628, 2005.

[9] K. A. Kobak, J. D. Lipsitz, J. B. W. Williams, N. Engelhardt, and K. M. Bellew, "A new approach to rater training and certification in a multicenter clinical trial," *Journal of Clinical Psychopharmacology*, vol. 25, no. 5, pp. 407–412, 2005.

[10] N. Engelhardt, A. D. Feiger, K. O. Cogger et al., "Rating the raters: assessing the quality of Hamilton rating scale for depression clinical interviews in two industry-sponsored clinical drug trials," *Journal of Clinical Psychopharmacology*, vol. 26, no. 1, pp. 71–74, 2006.

[11] K. A. Kobak, N. Engelhardt, and J. D. Lipsitz, "Enriched rater training using Internet based technologies: a comparison to traditional rater training in a multi-site depression trial," *Journal of Psychiatric Research*, vol. 40, no. 3, pp. 192–199, 2006.

5

Implementation of Stroke Dysphagia Screening in the Emergency Department

Stephanie K. Daniels,[1] **Jane A. Anderson,**[2] **and Nancy J. Petersen**[3]

[1] Research Service Line, Department of Communication Sciences and Disorders, Michael E. DeBakey VA Medical Center and University of Houston, 2002 Holcombe Boulevard, Houston, TX 77030, USA
[2] Health Services Research and Development Center of Excellence, Department of Neurology, Michael E. DeBakey VA Medical Center and Baylor College of Medicine, 2002 Holcombe Boulevard, Houston, TX 77030, USA
[3] Health Services Research and Development Center of Excellence, Department of Medicine, Michael E. DeBakey VA Medical Center and Baylor College of Medicine, 2002 Holcombe Boulevard, Houston, TX 77030, USA

Correspondence should be addressed to Stephanie K. Daniels; skdaniels@uh.edu

Academic Editor: Deborah Vincent

Early detection of dysphagia is critical in stroke as it improves health care outcomes. Administering a swallowing screening tool (SST) in the emergency department (ED) appears most logical as it is the first point of patient contact. However, feasibility of an ED nurse-administered SST, particularly one involving trial water swallow administration, is unknown. The aims of this pilot study were to (1) implement an SST with a water swallow component in the ED and track nurses' adherence, (2) identify barriers and facilitators to administering the SST through interviews, and (3) develop and implement a process improvement plan to address barriers. Two hundred seventy-eight individuals with stroke symptoms were screened from October 2009 to June 2010. The percentage of patients screened increased from 22.6 in October 2009 to a high of 80.8 in March 2010, followed by a decrease to 61.9% in June (Cochran-Armitage test $z = -5.1042$, $P < 0.0001$). The odds of being screened were 4.0 times higher after implementation compared to two months before implementation. Results suggest that it is feasible for ED nurses to administer an SST with a water swallow component. Findings should facilitate improved quality of care for patients with suspected stroke and improve multidisciplinary collaboration in swallowing screening.

1. Introduction

A well-established best practice in the care of patients with stroke is the early detection of dysphagia as it allows for immediate intervention thereby reducing morbidity, length of stay, and healthcare costs [1–3]. The essential first step to ensure early detection of dysphagia, and to prevent dysphagia-related morbidity, is to screen all stroke patients for signs of swallowing impairment prior to oral intake [1]. When a swallowing screening protocol is implemented, there is a decrease in morbidity over each year that the protocol is in place [4]. Moreover, when hospitals implement a formal swallowing screening protocol for patients with stroke, there is improvement in clinicians' adherence with

screening swallowing prior to oral intake [2], and the first dose of aspirin is administered earlier [5].

These findings have led the American Heart Association/American Stroke Association (AHA/ASA) to include screening of swallowing prior to the administration of food, liquid, or medication in individuals presenting with stroke symptoms as part of their guidelines on the early management of adults with acute stroke [6]. Within the Veterans Health Administration (VHA) the importance of dysphagia screening in patient with stroke is reflected in the issuance of multiple directives. The Office of the Inspector General (OIG) issued VHA Directive 2006-032 mandating that the initial nurse assessment must include screening of swallowing, and in 2011 the VHA Directive for Treatment of Acute

Ischemic Stroke (AIS) required that all VHA facilities include dysphagia screening in their stroke care protocols and track performance as a measure of quality stroke care [7].

Completion of dysphagia screening prior to administration of oral intake was a Joint Commission (JC) required performance measure for Primary Stroke Center Certification until 2010 when it was removed due to a lack of systematically defined standards for what constitutes a valid screening tool for swallowing [8]. The discontinuation by the JC, however, does not indicate that screening swallowing in patients with stroke is no longer a best practice. Rather, it suggests that further research is warranted to obtain consensus on validated swallowing screening tools (SSTs).

Dysphagia screening protocols for patients with stroke, nevertheless, should include SSTs that incorporate evidence-based swallowing screening items (SSIs). Evidence-based SSIs have been validated for identifying aspiration in patients with stroke based on instrumental evaluation as the reference standard. A process for identifying evidence-based SSIs is described elsewhere [9] and is considered by the authors to be a legitimate interim approach until consensus is reached on specific SSTs or until a VHA-specific stroke SST is identified. Implementation strategies should also include effective training on administration and interpretation of the SST to ensure reliable results and sustainable swallowing screening skills among nurses and other clinicians administering the dysphagia screening protocol. Finally, it is equally important that SSTs are feasible for implementation in various practice settings because even the most valid and reliable SST will not be used if it is not feasible to administer in practice.

In response to the AHA/ASA guidelines and for compliance with stroke quality performance measures outlined in VHA directives, many VHA facilities have implemented locally developed SSTs for nurses to administer as part of stroke dysphagia screening protocols. There is debate on the need to incorporate trial water swallows with nonswallowing screening items as opposed to using purely nonswallowing screening items in locally developed SSTs. While most SSTs within VHA do not currently include trial swallows [10, 11], water swallows are standard in many SSTs used outside the VHA [12–14]. Furthermore, research provides strong evidence that suggests a water swallow component is critical when screening for dysphagia in individuals with suspected stroke [1, 9]; thus, a water swallow component appears to be an important item to include as part of an evidence-based SST.

Some contend, however, that administration of trial water swallows may compromise patient safety when administered by clinicians without specific expertise in dysphagia screening, such as nurses. There is also the perception that including a trial water swallow component will require extra time to administer thus creating a time constraint that will affect the feasibility of administering the SST. This may be especially true in the emergency department (ED) where there is pressure to complete rapid evaluation and treatment of individuals presenting with suspected stroke. These factors, as well as other unknown barriers, may impede the feasibility of implementing an SST that includes a trial water swallow component.

1.1. Purpose of the Study. Since screening of swallowing is a best practice that is essential for safe, high-quality care in individuals presenting with suspected stroke and the VHA has established the OIG and AIS directives, it is paramount that evidence-based mechanisms for screening for dysphagia in veterans with stroke are developed and implemented across VHA. Moreover, a swallowing screening protocol for veterans presenting with symptoms of stroke must be efficient and feasible for use by clinicians in any care delivery setting. The overall objective of this performance improvement study was to identify strategies for effective implementation of swallowing screening in patients with stroke symptoms that presented to the ED at a large VHA facility.

2. Methods

2.1. Design. A process improvement approach using a before/after design and qualitative methods was applied to determine the feasibility of implementing an evidence-based SST that included a water swallow component in the ED. The following questions were addressed: (1) Among nurses administering a stroke dysphagia screening protocol in a VHA facility ED, what are the barriers and facilitators to administering an SST with a water swallow component? (2) Does nurses' adherence with screening swallowing prior to oral intake in patients with stroke increase over time after applying process improvement strategies to implement an evidence-based SST with a water swallow component in the ED?

2.2. Setting and Sample. The study took place at the Michael E. DeBakey Veterans Affairs Medical Center (MEDVAMC) located in Houston, TX. The MEDVAMC is certified by the JC as a Primary Stroke Center and has the largest number of stroke admissions within the VHA. The ED is staffed with 20 registered nurses (RNs) and 3 emergency medicine physicians. A convenience sample of ED nurses ($N = 8$) was recruited to participate in semistructured interviews to obtain feedback on barriers and facilitators to implementing an SST with water swallow in the ED. Participants were recruited via personal invitation and email solicitation, and they all provided written consent prior to participation. The study was approved by the Institutional Review Board at Baylor College of Medicine and by the Research and Development Committee at the MEDVAMC.

2.3. Planning and Assessing the Implementation. In meeting study objectives, Plan, Do, Study, Act (PDSA) cycles were applied to identify process improvement strategies for implementation of an evidence-based SST with water swallow in the ED. The PDSA cycle is a well-established process improvement methodology that can be used to implement quality improvement changes in the "real-world" practice setting [15]. Prior to establishing an evidence-based nurse-administered stroke SST, swallowing screening for stroke patients was conducted in a nonstandardized fashion primarily by ED physicians and neurology residents, and infrequently by nurses.

TABLE 1: Michael E. DeBakey Veterans Affairs Medical Center stroke swallowing screening tool.

Non-swallowing items
Somnolent-difficult to maintain arousal/alertness with vigorous stimulation
Wet, gurgly voice quality-hear audible secretions in the throat with speech or respiration
Dysarthria-slurred speech
Drooling or pooling of saliva in oral cavity-difficulty managing saliva in the mouth
Coughing, choking on saliva
Patient/family reports patient with current difficulty swallowing
Swallowing items
5 mL water ×2
10 mL water ×2
20 mL water ×2

The first step, "Plan" was accomplished by a multidisciplinary team of speech pathologists and nurses with expertise in stroke and dysphagia. From June–September 2009, the team developed an evidence-based stroke SST that included a water swallow component. Items incorporated in the stroke SST were based on literature review [16–19] and expert consensus agreement (Table 1). A stroke dysphagia screening protocol was then developed to guide administration of the SST and clinical interventions based on screening results. The protocol required that nonswallowing "observational" items be administered first. If any nonswallowing item was evident, the screening was discontinued. The patient continued nil per os (NPO), that is, nothing by mouth including medication, and speech pathology was consulted. If none of the observational items were present, trial water swallows were initiated starting with a 5 mL volume. Each volume was administered twice. If cough, throat clear (audible attempt to clear material out of the throat), or wet voice was evident after any water trial, the screening was stopped and no further water was administered. The patient continued NPO status, and speech pathology was consulted. If cough, throat clear, or wet voice was not evident, the patient was considered to have no risk of dysphagia and oral intake was initiated.

The second step, "Do" involved implementing the swallowing screening protocol in the ED at the MEDVAMC. Implementation strategies began with initial education sessions from December 2009 to mid-January 2010 for all ED nurses in which information was presented on (1) the current guideline-derived best practices for swallowing screening in patients with stroke [6, 7], (2) how to administer the stroke SST with water swallow [16], and (3) specific protocol actions required based on whether the patient passed or failed the SST [6, 7]. After training sessions were completed, the ED nurses implemented the SST with a water swallow component as part of the stroke dysphagia screening protocol starting in December 2009.

The third step, "Study" involved tracking of nurses' adherence to the swallowing-screening protocol as it was implemented over time and also conducting semistructured interviews with ED nurses to identify barriers and facilitators encountered during implementation of the swallowing-screening protocol. Semistructured interviews were conducted in March 2009 and were designed to elicit feedback from the nurses responsible for administering the SST with water swallow. The interviews lasted 20 minutes and were audio recorded for transcription. Participants were asked to describe their experience in administering the SST including barriers and facilitators to completing the screening including the water swallow section, what they liked and disliked about the SST, and what facilitated and impeded documentation in the electronic health record (EHR) and to provide ideas on how to make the process of administering the SST better for ED nurses. Audiotapes from the interview sessions were transcribed and coded using content analysis. Words and word phrases were categorized as being indicative of either a barrier or a facilitator to administering the SST [20]. From March to April, minimal contact with the ED nurses was made as data were analyzed; however, SST implementation continued.

The final step, "Act" was initiated in April 2009 and included implementing multiple strategies and lessons learned based on feedback from ED nursing staff. This involved the application of rapid PDSA cycles [15] to target identified barriers and was an iterative process completed over a 3-month period. One important product was the development of a Stroke Dysphagia Screening Bundle (SDSB) that included (1) an evidence-based SST with water swallow, (2) EHR order sets that automated NPO status and consultation to speech pathology for patients with a positive SST and diet orders for patients with a negative SST, and (3) electronic templates that automated documentation of the entire dysphagia screening process in the EHR.

To address implementation barriers, the same process of PDSA cycles was applied, and implementation methods and education modules were developed and tailored to address the needs of the nurses administering the SDSB. Implementation tools and education modules were made accessible via a web interface for easy access and for booster training as needed.

2.4. Data Analysis of Pre-/Postimplementation Measures. Adherence with implementing an evidence-based SST with water swallow in the ED was assessed before and after implementation of the SDSB. This was accomplished by reviewing the EHRs of patients admitted to MEDVAMC with stroke symptoms and tracking if these patients received screening of swallowing prior to oral intake. EHRs were reviewed from October and November 2009 (the two months prior to implementing the SDSB) with continuation to June 2010 to identify the percent of patients screened each month in the ED post-SDSB implementation. The Cochrane-Armitage test was used to test if there was a trend in the percent of patients screened over the 9 months. Logistic regression was used to calculate the odds of being screened in the 7 months following implementation compared to the 2 months before implementation.

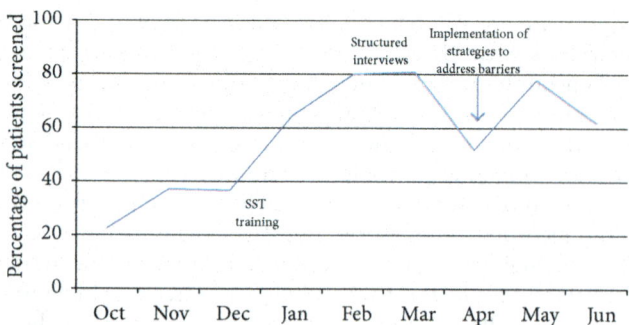

FIGURE 1: Percentage of patients screened in the emergency department from October 2009 to June 2010.

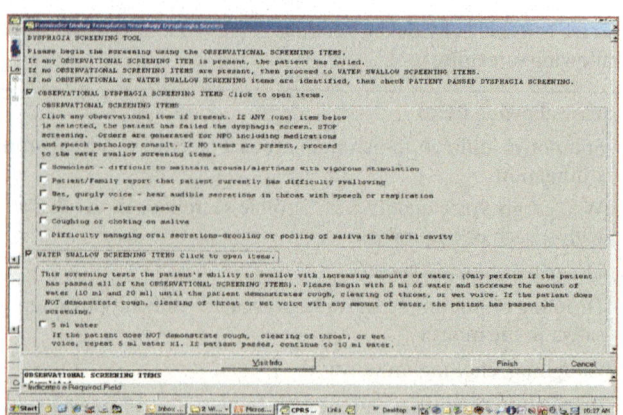

FIGURE 2: Template of swallowing screening in the electronic health record system.

3. Results

A total of 278 individuals with stroke symptoms were screened in the ED from October 2009 to June 2010. The percentage of patients screened increased from 22.6% in October 2009 to a high of 80.8% in March 2010, followed by a decrease to 61.9% in June 2010. Following implementation of the SST, the percentage of patients screened decreased to its lowest point of 51.9% in April 2010 but rebounded to 77.8% in the following month after implementing strategies to address identified barriers. There was a significant increase in the percentage of patients screened in the ED over time (Cochran-Armitage test $z = -5.1042$, $P < 0.0001$) (Figure 1). The odds of being screened was 4.0 times higher after implementation (95% CI, 2.2 to 7.3), compared to the 2 months before implementation.

Barriers identified from nurses' interview sessions were (1) difficulty finding time to document screening results in the EHR, (2) difficulty recalling all screening items during administration of the SST, (3) inconsistent administration of the SST, and (4) inaccurate interpretation of screening items, (e.g., confusing the item somnolence with the assessment of a patient's level of orientation or administering a patient 5 mL of water using a syringe instead of having the patient drink water from a cup).

Key facilitator themes that were subsequently applied in developing implementation strategies were (1) more education on dysphagia and evidence-based screening of swallowing, (2) efficient processes to support SST administration and interpretation, and (3) multidisciplinary team cooperation and support from ED administrators. The time it took to administer the SST was not formally recorded. However, during interview sessions, nurses reported, on average, the SST took approximately 5 minutes. Interestingly, no nurse reported that administration of the water swallow component was a barrier to completing the SST.

To facilitate the incorporation of the SDSB into daily practice, implementation methods and education materials were tailored to address identified barriers. Pocket cards were provided as a reminder aid (e.g., listed all SST items and steps for administration), and electronic tools (order sets and templates) were developed in the EHR to automate the steps of the SDSB and to facilitate documentation of SST results

(Figure 2). An online video training module was produced to illustrate appropriate administration and interpretation of the SST, and booster education sessions were tailored to the specific needs of the nurse and targeted areas of identified deficit.

4. Discussion

This current performance improvement study was designed to determine the feasibility of implementing a nurse-administered stroke SST with a water swallow component and to identify strategies for effective implementation of a dysphagia-screening protocol for patients with stroke symptoms who present to the ED. We are unaware of any previous research that has assessed the feasibility of a nurse-administered SST, particularly an SST for use in the ED. The three major findings of this implementation study were as follows (1) an SST with a water swallow component was feasible for nurses to complete in patients presenting to the ED with symptoms of stroke; (2) an SDSB was created and swallowing screening significantly improved over time after implementation; (3) tailored implementation and education methods with booster sessions improved the sustainability of nurses' adherence with implementing the SDSB. Thus, the bundling of evidence-based SST items, swallowing screening processes, and clinical interventions with tailored implementation and education methods significantly improved stroke dysphagia screening at our facility.

Screening swallowing prior to oral intake in individuals presenting to the hospital with stroke symptoms is an important best practice described in AHA/ASA guidelines [6]. Since many patients with stroke symptoms first present to the ED, screening swallowing in the ED is most appropriate. This is based on the rationale that screening swallowing early, at the first point of patient contact, has the greatest potential to prevent administration of oral intake or oral medications prior to completing dysphagia screening. It is not uncommon for stroke patients in the ED to require immediate interventions to control blood pressure, discomfort, and other medical concerns that are often treated with oral medications.

The ED, however, is extremely busy, with nurses responsible for multiple care processes in the stroke work-up, and completing an SST that includes a water swallow component will add to nurses' responsibilities. Yet, all nurses in this study welcomed the opportunity to objectively determine the feasibility of implementing an SST with water swallow and to identify strategies for effective stroke dysphagia screening in the ED.

4.1. Focused Implementation Strategies. We engaged nursing staff in identifying facilitators and barriers for administration of an SST with water swallow in the ED and sought their input in developing strategies to address identified implementation barriers. Two implementation strategies emerged: (1) "bundling" dysphagia screening processes and (2) "tailoring" implementation and education methods. The multiple sequential actions involved in administering the SST and the required clinical interventions were bundled into an all inclusive SDSB.

Bundles are defined as a set of evidence-based interventions for a specific patient population and setting that when implemented together result in significantly better outcomes than when implemented individually [21]. The Institute for Healthcare Improvement and other groups recommend the use of "care bundles" to improve patient care and clinical outcomes [22]. Bundles have been most effective in improving the quality of care for mechanically ventilated patients by improving healthcare providers' compliance with relevant evidence-based practices. Bundles have also been shown to improve effective assessment of pain, appropriate use of blood transfusions, appropriate sedation, appropriate peptic ulcer prevention, and appropriate deep vein thrombosis prophylaxis [21].

The application of the bundle concept to improve dysphagia screening in patients with stroke is well suited because the primary purpose of a bundle is to pull together the essential evidence-based interventions (SST and associated clinical actions) that target a specific patient population (patients with stroke) undergoing a particular procedure (dysphagia screening) to ensure the best possible patient care and outcomes (prevent dysphagia-associated morbidity/mortality). The essential evidence-based interventions needed to develop an SDSB are as follows: (1) maintain the patient on a NPO status (including medications) until administration and interpretation of an evidence-based SST [6], (2) administer an evidence-based SST and interpret findings, (3) initiate oral diet without dysphagia modifications and initiate oral medications if SST results are negative, (4) continue NPO status and consult speech pathology to complete a swallowing assessment if screening results are positive, and (5) document completion of each SDSB component in the EHR.

Tailoring involves adapting or modifying interventions, implementation strategies, and educational resources to fit a specific population or context. Tailoring appears to be a critical factor related to effective implementation and is associated with improvements in process and patient outcomes [23, 24]. Effective tailoring requires engagement of stakeholders in developing implementation strategies to address identified

barriers. For example, when the nurses in this study reported it was difficult to remember each screening item and the specific steps for the water swallow component included in the SST, they suggested developing a pocket card that listed each screening item with instruction on how to administer the water swallow component. Tailoring supports the unique needs of health care providers delivering the intervention but also makes possible adjustments in the intervention based on specific needs [23, 24]. Consistent administration of the SST and documentation of the administration process and findings in the EHR were an identified barrier. Nurses recommended developing an electronic template in the EHR that provided the step-by-step process used to administer the SST and would simultaneously document each step of the SST that was completed as the nurse interacted with the template. Later in the implementation process when the SDSB was developed, automated data sets were also incorporated into the EHR.

In terms of education, tailored strategies included providing ongoing training to nursing staff when deficits were identified. Performance monitoring and feedback that included the percentage of SSTs completed each month was reported to nursing staff in the ED and was used as an incentive and as an indicator of learning need. The investigators produced a video-training module of the SST procedure and made it accessible to all nursing staff on a facility intranet site. This provided easy access for booster training sessions when performance monitoring showed decreases in swallowing screening rates or when learning needs were identified by nursing staff.

4.2. Sustainability. The MEDVAMC receives the largest number of admissions for suspected stroke compared to other VHA facilities. In Fiscal Year 2009, approximately 20 patients with stroke symptoms were admitted monthly. Even with this high volume, an individual nurse may have the opportunity to complete an SST only once a month, so maintaining consistent and reliable administration and interpretation of the SST is challenging and may affect sustainability as evidenced by our fluctuating numbers in screenings during the study period. Consistently high screening numbers were observed following initiation of the screening protocol when education was fresh and the initiative was a new endeavor and again when nurses were engaged in developing strategies to address identified implementation barriers.

This finding is in line with much of the literature on the adoption of innovation which claims that adoption of a best practice or innovation is not a one-time occurrence, but rather a complex process that develops over time [25]. Adoption can be described in three stages: preadoption, early use, and established use [26]. The first stage, preadoption, occurs early on with the first introduction to a new innovation. Adoption of the innovation builds as the intended adopters have sufficient knowledge about what the innovation is, how it is used, and how it benefits them. The next stage, early use, includes periods of fluctuation as adoption builds to more consistent use. This occurs when adopters are provided continued access to information about the innovation and receive sufficient training to support innovation tasks. During the final phase, established use becomes more evident and is related to adopters receiving adequate feedback on performance and sufficient opportunity to adapt and refine the innovation to improve its fit based on setting and context.

The fluctuation seen in the adoption of the SST by ED nurses in this study is most indicative of the stages of preadoption and early use. During the first few months of this 9-month pilot study, nurses were first introduced to the SST and received ongoing information about the SST, training on how to use it, and opportunities to adapt and develop implementation strategies. During the final 3 months of the project, targeted strategies developed by the ED nurses were initiated.

Another trend that may be attributed to the fluctuation in swallowing screening rates is that increases in swallowing screening were observed after periods of engagement with ED nurses (i.e., training and interview sessions) and decreases were observed in swallowing screening during times of minimal engagement with the ED staff. This finding strongly suggests that periodic engagement of the ED staff and availability of educators to answer questions and to provide ongoing booster sessions are important for sustained adoption. Moreover the involvement of the ED staff throughout the implementation process appeared critical to success and sustainability. Although fluctuation in screening adoption was evident, it is important to note that screening adherence never dropped to preimplementation levels further supporting the implementation of an ED nurse-administered SST with a water swallow component.

Since completion of this pilot study, we have continued to track performance with dysphagia screening and provide performance feedback to ED staff. The SDSB has been adopted at the MEDVAMC to implement evidence-based dysphagia screening and now includes ongoing booster education when deficiencies in dysphagia screening are identified. To date, the SDSB has been effective for consistent implementation of evidence-based dysphagia screening for patients admitted with suspected stroke with sustained screening rates between 93% and 100%. These data support adoption of the SDSB at the stage of established use. Subsequent steps are to test the effectiveness of developing site-specific SDSBs and tailored implementation methods and education in multiple VHA facilities.

4.3. Limitations. The time period evaluated was approximately 9 months. Continued longitudinal research is warranted to determine if results are maintained. Furthermore, implementation of this procedure should be completed at large and small medical centers to determine if the implementation process and results are similar. The time to administer any SST is an important focus of future research to ensure feasibility.

Every ED may not be able to complete a stroke SST given high-volume patient load, rapid transfer to patient wards, and/or limited staff. In cases where screening cannot be completed in the ED, it is unclear if this implementation process would work on a hospital ward and requires further research.

While the SST developed for the MEDVAMC is evidence based, it has not been validated. Work is in progress to develop and validate a VHA stroke SST in a separate study. Since several VHA directives have charged VHA facilities with implementing and monitoring dysphagia screening protocols for patients with stroke, evidence-based SSTs and effective implementation strategies are needed now. Thus, implementation studies should be completed in parallel with validation studies and once an SST is validated, effective implementation processes will be in place.

5. Conclusions

It is well established that patient outcomes are improved when dysphagia screening is completed prior to oral intake in individuals with stroke symptoms. This body of work supports the feasibility of nurses screening swallowing using an SST with water swallow in patients with stroke symptoms that present to a busy ED. Engaging nursing staff in the process of identifying barriers and targeted solutions resulted in the development of an SDSB and tailored implementation and education methods that significantly improve dysphagia screening adherence over time. Continued interaction and booster education sessions on administering and interpreting the SST are required for sustained improvement and consistent practice.

Acknowledgments

The project reported here was supported by the Department of Veterans Affairs, Veterans Health Administration, Health Services Research and Development Service Quality Enhancement Research Initiative (RRP-09-182), the Houston VA HSR&D Center of Excellence (HFP90-020), and by the Rehabilitation Research & Development Service of the VA Office of Research and Development (1I01RX000121). Dr. Daniels received funding from RRP-09-182 and 1I01RX000121, and Dr. N. J. Petersen was funded by RRP-09-182 and by HFP90-020. For Dr. J. A. Anderson, no conflict of interests was declared. The views expressed in this paper are those of the authors and do not necessarily represent the views of the Department of Veterans Affairs.

References

[1] R. Martino, G. Pron, and N. Diamant, "Screening for oropharyngeal dysphagia in stroke: insufficient evidence for guidelines," *Dysphagia*, vol. 15, no. 1, pp. 19–30, 2000.

[2] J. A. Hinchey, T. Shephard, K. Furie, D. Smith, D. Wang, and S. Tonn, "Formal dysphagia screening protocols prevent pneumonia," *Stroke*, vol. 36, no. 9, pp. 1972–1976, 2005.

[3] I. R. Odderson and B. S. McKenna, "A model for management of patients with stroke during the acute phase: outcome and economic implications," *Stroke*, vol. 24, no. 12, pp. 1823–1827, 1993.

[4] I. R. Odderson, J. C. Keaton, and B. S. McKenna, "Swallow management in patients on an acute stroke pathway: quality is cost effective," *Archives of Physical Medicine and Rehabilitation*, vol. 76, no. 12, pp. 1130–1133, 1995.

[5] M. L. Power, S. P. Cross, S. Roberts, and P. J. Tyrrell, "Evaluation of a service development to implement the top three process indicators for quality stroke care," *Journal of Evaluation in Clinical Practice*, vol. 13, no. 1, pp. 90–94, 2007.

[6] H. P. Adams Jr., G. del Zoppo, M. J. Alberts et al., "Guidelines for the early management of adults with ischemic stroke: a guideline from the American heart association/American stroke association stroke council, clinical cardiology council, cardiovascular radiology and intervention council, and the atherosclerotic peripheral vascular disease and quality of care outcomes in research interdisciplinary working groups:," *Stroke*, vol. 38, no. 5, pp. 1655–1711, 2007.

[7] B. Bates, J. Y. Choi, P. W. Duncan et al., "Veterans Affairs/ Department of Defense clinical practice guideline for the management of adult stroke rehabilitation care: executive summary," *Stroke*, vol. 36, no. 9, pp. 2049–2056, 2005.

[8] K. Lakshminarayan, A. W. Tsai, X. Tong et al., "Utility of dysphagia screening results in predicting poststroke pneumonia," *Stroke*, vol. 41, no. 12, pp. 2849–2854, 2010.

[9] S. K. Daniels, J. A. Anderson, and P. C. Willson, "Valid items for screening dysphagia risk in patients with stroke: a systematic review," *Stroke*, vol. 43, no. 3, pp. 892–897, 2012.

[10] Department of Veterans Affairs, Quality Enhancement Research Initiative (QUERI), "Nursing admission dysphagia screening tool," 2009, http://www.queri.research.va.gov/tools/ stroke-quality/dysphagia.cfm.

[11] J. A. Hind, J. Robbins, and B. Priefer, "Development of a multidisciplinary evidence-based dysphagia screening for all acute care admissions," *Perspectives on Swallowing and Swallowing Disorders (Dysphagia)*, vol. 18, no. 4, pp. 134–139, 2009.

[12] J. Edmiaston, L. T. Connor, L. Loehr, and A. Nassief, "Validation of a dysphagia screening tool in acute stroke patients," *American Journal of Critical Care*, vol. 19, no. 4, pp. 357–364, 2010.

[13] R. Martino, F. Silver, R. Teasell et al., "The toronto bedside swallowing screening test (TOR-BSST) development and validation of a dysphagia screening tool for patients with stroke," *Stroke*, vol. 40, no. 2, pp. 555–561, 2009.

[14] D. M. Suiter and S. B. Leder, "Clinical utility of the 3-ounce water swallow test," *Dysphagia*, vol. 23, no. 3, pp. 244–250, 2008.

[15] G. L. Langley, K. M. Nolan, T. W. Nolan, C. L. Norman, and L. P. Provost, *The Improvement Guide: A Practical Approach To Enhancing Organizational Performance*, Jossey-Bass Publications, San Francisco, Calif, USA, 2nd edition, 2009.

[16] S. K. Daniels, K. Brailey, D. H. Priestly, L. R. Herrington, L. A. Weisberg, and A. L. Foundas, "Aspiration in patients with acute stroke," *Archives of Physical Medicine and Rehabilitation*, vol. 79, no. 1, pp. 14–19, 1998.

[17] J. Horner, E. W. Massey, J. E. Riski, D. L. Lathrop, and K. N. Chase, "Aspiration following stroke: clinical correlates and outcome," *Neurology*, vol. 38, no. 9, pp. 1359–1362, 1988.

[18] P. Linden, K. V. Kuhlemeier, and C. Patterson, "The probability of correctly predicting subglottic penetration from clinical observations," *Dysphagia*, vol. 8, no. 3, pp. 170–179, 1993.

[19] G. H. McCullough, J. C. Rosenbek, R. T. Wertz, S. McCoy, G. Mann, and K. McCullough, "Utility of clinical swallowing examination measures for detecting aspiration post-stroke," *Journal of Speech, Language, and Hearing Research*, vol. 48, no. 6, pp. 1280–1293, 2005.

[20] R. P. Weber, *Basic Concept Analysis*, Sage, Newbury Park, Calif, USA, 2nd edition, 1990.

[21] Institute of Heathcare Improvement, "Evidence-based care bundles," http://www.ihi.org/knowledge/Pages/Changes/default. aspx.

[22] S. W. Aboelela, P. W. Stone, and E. L. Larson, "Effectiveness of bundled behavioural interventions to control healthcare-associated infections: a systematic review of the literature," *Journal of Hospital Infection*, vol. 66, no. 2, pp. 101–108, 2007.

[23] F. Cheater, R. Baker, C. Gillies et al., "Tailored interventions to overcome identified barriers to change: effects on professional practice and health care outcomes," *Cochrane Database of Systematic Reviews (Online)*, no. 3, Article ID CD005470, 2005.

[24] S. R. Kirsh, R. H. Lawrence, and D. C. Aron, "Tailoring an intervention to the context and system redesign related to the intervention: a case study of implementing shared medical appointments for diabetes," *Implementation Science*, vol. 3, no. 1, article 34, 2008.

[25] E. M. Rogers, *Diffusion of Innovation*, Free Press, New York, NY, USA, 1995.

[26] G. E. Hall and S. M. Hord, *Change in Schools*, State University of New York Press, Albany, NY, USA, 1987.

6

Horizontal Violence and the Quality and Safety of Patient Care: A Conceptual Model

Christina Purpora[1] and Mary A. Blegen[2]

[1] School of Nursing and Health Professions, University of San Francisco, 2130 Fulton Street, San Francisco, CA 94117, USA
[2] Department of Community Health Systems, School of Nursing, University of California, San Francisco, 2 Koret Way, P.O. Box 0608, San Francisco, CA 94143, USA

Correspondence should be addressed to Christina Purpora, cmpurpora@usfca.edu

Academic Editor: Shellie Simons

For many years, nurses in international clinical and academic settings have voiced concern about horizontal violence among nurses and its consequences. However, no known framework exists to guide research on the topic to explain these consequences. This paper presents a conceptual model that was developed from four theories to illustrate how the quality and safety of patient care could be affected by horizontal violence. Research is needed to validate the new model and to gather empirical evidence of the consequences of horizontal violence on which to base recommendations for future research, education, and practice.

1. Introduction

For several decades, clinical and academic nurses have written about horizontal violence among nurses in clinical settings and its consequences. Horizontal violence is behavior that is directed by one peer toward another that harms, disrespects, and devalues the worth of the recipient while denying them their basic human rights [1]. Examples include nonverbal behavior, such as ignoring a peer, verbal behavior, such as making sarcastic comments to them or talking behind their back, and/or physical acts like shoving someone or slamming things [1]. Other similar terms used to label negative behavior among nurses at work include nurse-on-nurse aggression [2, 3], bullying [4–8], verbal abuse [9–11], lateral violence [12–14], incivility [15], and lateral or horizontal hostility [16, 17]. The term horizontal violence was used in this paper because, unlike the other terms, horizontal violence is drawn from oppression theory, one of the four theories used to develop the model described herein. Research articles [2, 3, 5–7, 18, 19] and opinion pieces [20–22] from Australia, New Zealand, the United Kingdom, and the United States suggest that nurses share an ongoing and growing concern about horizontal violence and its

consequences for nurses, nursing, healthcare organizations, and particularly for patients.

Many researchers have described horizontal violence among nurses working in hospitals [2, 3, 5, 6, 10, 11, 14, 18, 23, 24]. Nurses suffer consequences as a result of their experiences such as sadness, anxiety, mistrust, diminished self-esteem and self-confidence [7, 10, 18], job dissatisfaction [10], and negative effects on peer relationships [10]. Some describe their experiences as painful [24] and far more distressing than when similar behaviors are directed toward them by physicians or patients [2, 3]. Some nurses intend to leave their current job to find work elsewhere [5, 6, 8, 11] while others consider leaving nursing altogether [5, 18]. Some nurses believe that horizontal violence threatens the safety of patients [18] and diminishes the quality of their care [10].

When behavior similar to horizontal violence occurs among healthcare providers from different disciplines, the term disruptive behavior is often used to name the behavior. Rosenstein and O'Daniel [25, 26] reported that doctors and nurses in hospitals perceive that disruptive behavior, such as use of rude tone of voice or threatening body language, decreases their communication. Communication decreases when individuals feel too intimidated to communicate with members of the healthcare team who are known instigators of these negative behaviors [26, 27]. The Joint Commission [28] reports that 60% of actual or potential harm to patients can be linked to insufficient communication in healthcare organizations. Yet, no direct empirical links among horizontal violence or disruptive behavior, communication, and patient care have been made. The dearth of research about the impact of horizontal violence on nurses' relationships and communication with each other and the concern about consequences for patients in the presence of horizontal violence call for studies of horizontal violence among nurses in hospitals, its effect on their relationships and communication, and the consequences for patient care.

To date, some researchers who study horizontal violence among nurses used Freire's [29] theory of oppression as a framework. Those who used it did so implicitly by using the term horizontal violence, one of its concepts [18, 30], while others did so explicitly [6, 14, 23, 24]. Conceptual models are important because of their utility for explaining situations and for guiding research [31], yet, none of the studies proposed a model to explain horizontal violence and its consequences for patient care.

This paper presents a conceptual model that illustrates how the quality and safety of patient care could be affected by horizontal violence. The paper begins with a description of the model in which Freire's oppression theory [29], Maslow's theory of human motivation [32], DeVito's essential human communication model [33], and Reason's Swiss cheese model of system accidents [34] are linked. Then, implications for research are provided.

2. Conceptual Model for Horizontal Violence and the Quality and Safety of Patient Care

A conceptual model is an illustration of proposed causal relationships among a group of variables hypothesized to be associated with a problem [35]. The proposed horizontal violence and the quality and safety of patient care model displayed elsewhere [36] are shown in Figure 1. Directionality of the model flows from left to right.

2.1. Oppression. In his theory of oppression, Freire postulated that the Brazilian people he observed were living in a "situation of oppression" ([29, page 55]). They were dominated by others who had violently obstructed them from living their lives freely as human beings ensconced in their unique beliefs and values. Freire [29] contends that a situation of oppression can be changed because it results from an imbalanced social structure, not fate.

Building on the work of Freire and others, Roberts [37] posited that nurses have worked in a situation of oppression since the early 1900s when they began caring for patients in hospitals controlled by male physicians and administrators. Ashley [38] and Reverby [39] describe nurses in the mid 1800s to early 1900s doing the work traditionally thought of as the work of women in hierarchical hospitals. Their practice

was controlled either by groups with more power that are held in higher esteem or by the systems in which they work. Power is defined as "... the ability to influence the decision and actions of others" ([40, page 38]). Today, nurses continue to bear a great deal of responsibility caring for patients whose lives are in their hands; yet they have little power compared to physicians and administrators [41].

2.2. Internalized Dominant Values and Horizontal Violence. Freire [29] theorized that oppressed people internalize their situation by adopting the dominant group's beliefs and values while minimizing their own. Oppressed people manifest what they internalize by acting like those who oppress them while remaining submissive to them. As the oppressed align with the oppressor, they develop hatred for their own group. This hatred is manifested when the oppressed themselves become oppressors of their group. The oppressed become fearful of fighting for freedom at the risk of more violence from those who oppress them who are threatened by the oppressed's struggle to break free from oppression [29]. Freire further postulates that the oppressed suffer from duality; they yearn for freedom and yet fear it. Duality splits the group, preventing them from engaging in a struggle for freedom.

Roberts [37] suggested that nurses have internalized the dominant physician values while minimizing those of nursing. She supports her argument by pointing to the prominence and value placed on the medical model over nursing. She further postulates that oppressed nurses manifest what they have internalized by exhibiting poor self-esteem, feelings of inferiority, aversion for nurses who are most often, but not always, women, dissatisfaction with the primarily female profession, disunity, and lack of professional identity.

Working with Roberts and others, DeMarco et al. [42] used the concepts "oppressed self" and "oppressed group" to explain how nurses' exhibit internalized dominant values while minimizing their own ([42, page 299]). Oppressed self demonstrates a person's beliefs about their individual worth. When people minimize their own worth, they may stay quiet rather than contribute their opinion in situations. Oppressed group represents beliefs about women, most nurses in hierarchical hospitals are women, and how they may be inclined to act together. When beliefs are negative, their collective contribution as women or nurses is minimized.

Freire used the term "horizontal violence" ([29, page 62]) to name a behavior he observed among oppressed Brazilians and a behavior first described by Fanon's [43] observation of oppressed Algerians. The concept was originally defined as acts of violence such as killing, burning each other's houses, and pulling knives on one another. Freire postulated that the oppressed feel aggressive but remain submissive toward those who oppress them and these violent acts occur as one way that oppressed people relieve mounting situational tension among them. Blanton and colleagues [1] used Freire's [29] work as well as others to develop the definition of horizontal violence used in the model proposed in this paper, the only one known to be derived from Freire's theory. Though the acts described by Blanton et al. between coworkers are

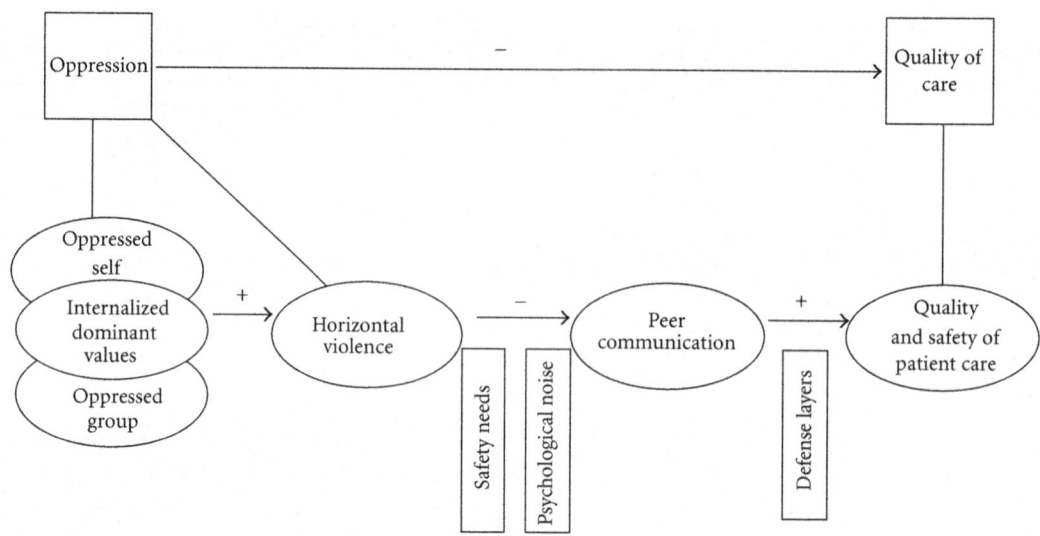

FIGURE 1: A conceptual model for horizontal violence and the quality and safety of patient care.

not the same acts of horizontal violence defined by Freire, the concept is useful, nonetheless, for explaining behavior among nurses who are also thought to be oppressed.

In the model, horizontal violence represents the harmful behavior oppressed nurses are at risk for engaging in to relieve mounting frustration from working in hierarchical hospitals where they have great responsibility but little power. While there are many factors that influence nurses' work-related behavior, oppression is central and understudied. Other factors could include age, education, and experience. An assumption that nurses may engage in horizontal violence because they are oppressed has persisted in the nursing literature for at least three decades [6, 9, 24, 37]. The purpose of using the concepts of oppression, oppressed group, oppressed self, and horizontal violence in the proposed model is not to fault nurses [42, 44] but instead to explain, theoretically, why, as a group, nurses may be considered oppressed and, thus, at risk for engaging in horizontal violence. The proposition in the proposed model is that internalized dominant values are positively related to experiences of horizontal violence, that is, as internalized dominant values when exhibited as oppressed group or oppressed self increase, so does horizontal violence.

2.3. Horizontal Violence and Peer Communication. In his theory of human motivation, Maslow [32] explained how adult human behavior is motivated by several basic needs. Safety needs are centered on a human being's need to be free from physical and emotional harm. When a person's safety needs are met, they feel safe enough to relate to others. Conversely, a person who perceives the world as unsafe may believe their physical and emotional well-being are at risk for harm and may react to this threat by not relating to others. The concept is useful for explaining how nurses who have suffered psychological harm from horizontal violence may perceive threats to their emotional safety in work environments. Their hesitation or resistance to interacting with others may be in response to perceived threats to

their emotional wellbeing including fear of more horizontal violence and more psychological harm.

Experiencing threats to one's well-being and fear of future horizontal violence interferes with communication. DeVito [33] illustrates communication between people and the factors that promote or impede it in his essentials of human communication model. He defines communication as the interpersonal exchange of verbal and nonverbal messages between people [33]. He explains that, at one extreme, a sender's message will not reach an intended recipient at all because of psychological noise, a factor that impedes communication. Psychological noise includes thoughts about or beliefs and attitudes formed in advance of the communication and/or strong negative feelings about how that communication may occur.

In the proposed model displayed in Figure 1, safety needs and psychological noise provide the link between horizontal violence and peer communication; nurses who have experienced horizontal violence may avoid interacting with their peers because of perceived threats to psychological wellbeing and preconceived notions about how the communication exchange will play out. Using safety needs and psychological noise to link them, the proposition is that horizontal violence is negatively related to peer communication; that is, as horizontal violence increases, peer communication decreases.

2.4. Quality of Care. Quality of care is the extent to which care delivered to patients increases the chance of meeting their needs [45]. Good quality of care is culturally sensitive and clearly communicated care that is delivered competently while involving the patient in decisions about their care. Further, the first dimension of high-quality care is that it is safe and does not result in injury to patients [45].

2.5. Peer Communication and Quality and Safety of Patient Care. Reason's [34] Swiss cheese model of system accidents illustrates how people and things get harmed in technologically sophisticated organizations including healthcare.

He developed the model to promote evaluation of bad outcomes by considering what failed in a system's defense layers rather than simply blaming people for the errors. In his conceptualization, these layers protect people and things from harm. They consist of people, such as nurses and pilots, technology such as alarms, and policies and procedures that each play a vital part and, collectively, are usually protective. Conversely, when these layers are compromised, an opportunity for an error to cause harm exists. The defense layer of interest is the one comprised of people that, in healthcare, consists of those caring directly for patients including their communication with each other. Without open communication among caregivers or the people in the defense layer, the potential for detecting and preventing harm is reduced.

In the proposed model displayed in Figure 1, peer communication is hypothesized as one of many important contributors to protecting patients from harm. Communication among nurses is conceptualized as sharing information related to the care of patients including asking each other questions, providing feedback to each other, giving each other advice or seeking clarification, or validation of care. Decreased peer communication is hypothesized to threaten the integrity of the defense layer.

The concept of the quality and safety of patient care is used to name the process of delivering care that meets the needs of an individual where patient harm is evaded and averted [45, 46]. In the model, using defense layers to link them, peer communication is positively related to the quality and safety of patient care, that is, as peer communication decreases, so does the quality and safety of patient care.

3. Implications for Research

The horizontal violence and the quality and safety of patient care model offers a framework to guide research where there is a paucity of empirical evidence on a topic of growing concern among nurses internationally. The model and its propositions generate research hypotheses for testing. Hypothesis one: the model suggests that as internalized dominant values exhibited as oppressed group or self increase, so does horizontal violence. Hypothesis two: the model suggests as horizontal violence increases, peers communication decreases. Hypothesis three, the model suggests that as peer communication decreases, so does the quality and safety of patient care. Mounting evidence of empirical links, or lack thereof, validates and provides opportunity for improvement of the model [36, 47]. Evidence of empirical links creates a new call for research to inform strategies for addressing horizontal violence and its consequences for patients.

4. Conclusion

This paper presented the horizontal violence and the quality and safety of care model. Four theories linked for the first time illustrate how horizontal violence arises and its effect on the quality and safety of patient care. Internationally, nurses share concern about horizontal violence and its consequences. Studies suggest that nurses suffer consequences as a result of their experiences with horizontal violence; yet little, if anything, is known about consequences for patients and no known framework exists to explain or guide research on the topic. The new model begins to fill this gap. However, research is needed to validate the new model. Empirical evidence gathered from studies guided by the model will establish the foundation of practice and education recommendations.

Acknowledgment

The first author would like to thank the Gordon and Betty Moore Foundation for the Betty Irene Moore Doctoral Fellowship.

References

[1] B. A. Blanton, C. Lybecker, and N. M. Spring, "A horizontal violence position statement," July 1998, http://proactivenurse.com/index.php?option=com_content&Itemid=22&id=83.

[2] G. A. Farrell, "Aggression in clinical settings: nurses' views," *Journal of Advanced Nursing*, vol. 25, no. 3, pp. 501–508, 1997.

[3] G. A. Farrell, "Aggression in clinical settings: nurses' views—a follow-up study," *Journal of Advanced Nursing*, vol. 29, no. 3, pp. 532–541, 1999.

[4] R. G. Hughes and C. M. Clancy, "Complexity, bullying, and stress: analyzing and mitigating a challenging work environment for nurses," *Journal of Nursing Care Quality*, vol. 24, no. 3, pp. 180–183, 2009.

[5] S. L. Johnson and R. E. Rea, "Workplace bullying: concerns for nurse leaders," *Journal of Nursing Administration*, vol. 39, no. 2, pp. 84–90, 2009.

[6] S. Simons, "Workplace bullying experienced by massachusetts registered nurses and the relationship to intention to leave the organization," *Advances in Nursing Science*, vol. 31, no. 2, pp. E48–E59, 2008.

[7] J. Randle, "Bullying in the nursing profession," *Journal of Advanced Nursing*, vol. 43, no. 4, pp. 395–401, 2003.

[8] J. A. Vessey, R. F. DeMarco, D. A. Gaffney, and W. C. Budin, "Bullying of staff registered nurses in the workplace: a preliminary study for developing personal and organizational strategies for the transformation of hostile to healthy workplace environments," *Journal of Professional Nursing*, vol. 25, no. 5, pp. 299–306, 2009.

[9] H. Cox, "Verbal abuse nationwide, part I: oppressed group behavior," *Nursing Management*, vol. 22, no. 2, pp. 32–35, 1991.

[10] M. M. Rowe and H. Sherlock, "Stress and verbal abuse in nursing: do burned out nurses eat their young?" *Journal of Nursing Management*, vol. 13, no. 3, pp. 242–248, 2005.

[11] L. Sofield and S. W. Salmond, "Workplace violence. A focus on verbal abuse and intent to leave the organization," *Orthopaedic Nursing*, vol. 22, no. 4, pp. 274–283, 2003.

[12] M. Griffin, "Teaching cognitive rehearsal as a shield for lateral violence: an intervention for newly licensed nurses," *Journal of Continuing Education in Nursing*, vol. 35, no. 6, pp. 257–263, 2004.

[13] N. Sheridan-Leos, "Understanding lateral violence in nursing," *Clinical Journal of Oncology Nursing*, vol. 12, no. 3, pp. 399–403, 2008.

[14] K. M. Stanley, M. M. Martin, Y. Michel, J. M. Welton, and L. S. Nemeth, "Examining lateral violence in the nursing workforce," *Issues in Mental Health Nursing*, vol. 28, no. 11, pp. 1247–1265, 2007.

[15] D. M. Felblinger, "Incivility and bullying in the workplace and nurses' shame responses," *Journal of Obstetric, Gynecologic, and Neonatal Nursing*, vol. 37, no. 2, pp. 234–242, 2008.

[16] S. P. Thomas, "Horizontal hostility nurses against themselves: how to resolve this threat to retention," *The American Journal of Nursing*, vol. 103, no. 10, pp. 87–91, 2003.

[17] G. Alspach, "Critical care nurses as coworkers: are our interactions nice or nasty?" *Critical Care Nurse*, vol. 27, no. 3, pp. 10–14, 2007.

[18] B. G. McKenna, N. A. Smith, S. J. Poole, and J. H. Coverdale, "Horizontal violence: experiences of registered nurses in their first year of practice," *Journal of Advanced Nursing*, vol. 42, no. 1, pp. 90–96, 2003.

[19] L. Quine, "Workplace bullying in nurses," *Journal of Health Psychology*, vol. 6, no. 1, pp. 73–84, 2001.

[20] G. Georgiou, "Anti-bullying tactics make a difference," *RCM Midwives*, vol. 10, no. 6, p. 268, 2007.

[21] M. Moye, "Nursing hostility: what is causing horizontal violence between nurses and what steps can individuals take to bring it to an end? Advance for nurses," 2010, http://nursing.advanceweb.com/Editorial/Content/PrintFriendly.aspx?CC=214570.

[22] S. Stewart, "Confronting bullying," *Nursing New Zealand*, vol. 16, no. 3, p. 23, 2010.

[23] H. Dunn, "Horizontal violence among nurses in the operating room," *AORN journal*, vol. 78, no. 6, pp. 977–988, 2003.

[24] L. N. Skillings, "Perceptions and feelings of nurses about horizontal violence as an expression of oppressed group behavior," in *Critique, Resistance, and Action*, J. L. Thompson, D. D. Allen, and L. Rodrigues-Fisher, Eds., pp. 167–185, National League for Nursing Press, New York, NY, USA, 1992.

[25] A. H. Rosenstein and M. O'Daniel, "Disruptive behavior and clinical outcomes: perceptions of nurses and physicians," *The American Journal of Nursing*, vol. 105, no. 1, pp. 54–65, 2005.

[26] A. H. Rosenstein and M. O'Daniel, "A survey of the impact of disruptive behaviors and communication defects on patient safety," *Joint Commission Journal on Quality and Patient Safety*, vol. 34, no. 8, pp. 464–471, 2008.

[27] Institute for Safe Medication Practices, *Results from ISMP survey on workplace intimidation*, March 2004, https://www.ismp.org/survey/surveyresults/survey0311.asp.

[28] The Joint Commission, "Sentinel event data: root causes by event type 2004-third quarter2011," 2011, http://www.jointcommission.org/assets/1/18/Root_Causes_Event_Type_2004-3Q2011.pdf.

[29] P. Freire, *Pedagogy of the Oppressed*, The Continuum International Publishing Group, New York, NY, USA, 30th edition, 2003.

[30] J. Longo, "Horizontal violence among nursing students," *Archives of Psychiatric Nursing*, vol. 21, no. 3, pp. 177–178, 2007.

[31] A. I. Meleis, *Theoretical Nursing Development & Progress*, Lippincott Williams & Wilkins, Philadelphia, Pa, USA, 4th edition, 2007.

[32] A. H. Maslow, "A theory of human motivation," *Psychological Review*, vol. 50, no. 4, pp. 370–396, 1943.

[33] J. A. DeVito, *Essentials of Human Communication*, Pearson Allyn and Bacon, Boston, Mass, USA, 6th edition, 2008.

[34] J. Reason, "Human error: models and management," *British Medical Journal*, vol. 320, no. 7237, pp. 768–770, 2000.

[35] J. A. Earp and S. T. Ennett, "Conceptual models for health education research and practice," *Health Education Research*, vol. 6, no. 2, pp. 163–171, 1991.

[36] C. Purpora, M. A. Blegen, and N. A. Stotts, "Horizontal violence between hospital staff nurses related to oppressed self or oppressed group," *Journal of Professional Nursing*. In press.

[37] S. J. Roberts, "Oppressed group behavior: implications for nursing," *Advances in Nursing Science*, vol. 5, no. 4, pp. 21–30, 1983.

[38] J. Ashley, *Hospitals, Paternalism, and the Role of the Nurse*, Teachers College Press, New York, NY, USA, 1976.

[39] S. M. Reverby, *Ordered to Care: The Dilemma of American Nursing*, Cambridge University Press, New York, NY, USA, 1987.

[40] A. Cicchetti, "Networks: between markets and hierarchies," *Strategic Management Journal*, vol. 7, no. 1, pp. 37–51, 1986.

[41] A. N. Garman, D. C. Leach, and N. Spector, "Worldviews in collision: conflict and collaboration across professional lines," *Journal of Organizational Behavior*, vol. 27, no. 7, pp. 829–849, 2006.

[42] R. DeMarco, S. J. Roberts, A. Norris, and M. K. McCurry, "The development of the nurse workplace scale: self-advocating behaviors and beliefs in the professional workplace," *Journal of Professional Nursing*, vol. 24, no. 5, pp. 296–301, 2008.

[43] F. Fanon, *The Wretched of the Earth*, Grove Press, New York, NY, USA, 1963.

[44] P. Keen, "Caring for ourselves," in *Caring and Nursing: Exploration in Feminist Perspectives*, R. M. Neil and R. Watts, Eds., pp. 173–188, National League for Nursing, New York, NY, USA, 1991.

[45] The Institute of Medicine, *Crossing the Quality Chasm: A New Health System for the 21st Century*, National Academy Press, Washigton, DC, USA, 2001.

[46] Agency for Healthcare Research and Quality, *Hospital Survey on Patient Safety*, 2004, http://www.ahrq.gov/qual/patientsafetyculture/hospscanform.pdf.

[47] C. Purpora, *Horizontal Violence among Hospital Staff Nurses and the Quality and Safety of Patient Care*, Doctoral dissertation, University of California, San Francisco, Calif, USA, 2010.

7

Multidisciplinary Treatments, Patient Characteristics, Context of Care, and Adverse Incidents in Older, Hospitalized Adults

Leah L. Shever[1] and Marita G. Titler[2]

[1] *Nursing Research, Quality, and Innovation, University of Michigan Health System,*
300 North Ingalls, Room NI 5A07, Ann Arbor, MI 48109-5446, USA
[2] *University of Michigan School of Nursing and University of Michigan Health System,*
400 North Ingalls, Suite 4170, Ann Arbor, MI 48109-5482, USA

Correspondence should be addressed to Leah L. Shever, sheverl@med.umich.edu

Academic Editor: John Daly

The purpose of this study was to examine factors that contribute to adverse incidents by creating a model that included patient characteristics, clinical conditions, nursing unit context of care variables, medical treatments, pharmaceutical treatments, and nursing treatments. Data were abstracted from electronic, administrative, and clinical data repositories. The sample included older adults hospitalized during a four-year period at one, academic medical facility in the Midwestern United States who were at risk for falling. Relational databases were built and a multistep, statistical model building analytic process was used. Total registered nurse (RN) hours per patient day (HPPD) and HPPDs dropping below the nursing unit average were significant explanatory variables for experiencing an adverse incident. The number of medical and pharmaceutical treatments that a patient received during hospitalization as well as many specific nursing treatments (e.g., restraint use, neurological monitoring) were also contributors to experiencing an adverse incident.

1. Background

The Institute of Medicine (IOM) report *To Err is Human* [1] revealed the number and significance of adverse events and errors that occur during hospitalization. The report was a call to action to transform healthcare systems to ensure patient safety and higher quality care. In one step toward healthcare transformation, the Centers for Medicare and Medicaid (CMS) no longer reimburses institutions for the care, or treatment, associated with certain hospital-acquired conditions [2].

Understanding what factors contribute to adverse incidents during hospitalization is essential to developing effective counter measures. In order to improve factors that are modifiable within a hospital structure or with healthcare delivery, it is important to first have an understanding of what is broken. There are a number of potential contributing factors that need to be considered such as the patient's condition, the care the patient receives, and the environment in which they receive care [3, 4].

Battles and Lilford [3] provide a conceptual model for patient safety that includes antecedent conditions, which would include the patient's comorbid conditions, the primary reason the patient was admitted to the hospital, and characteristics the patient possessed before entering the hospital. Their model also includes the structure, or environment, in which the patient receives care such as the hospital, or nursing unit. Also acting within the structure are the processes of care (the interventions or treatments) delivered by the multidisciplinary team caring for the patient in the hospital. None of these components exist in isolation, which is why it is important to examine all of these factors and how they interact [3].

2. Purpose

The purpose of this study was to examine factors that contribute to adverse incidents that occur during hospitalization by creating a model that included patient characteristics, clinical conditions, nursing unit context of care variables,

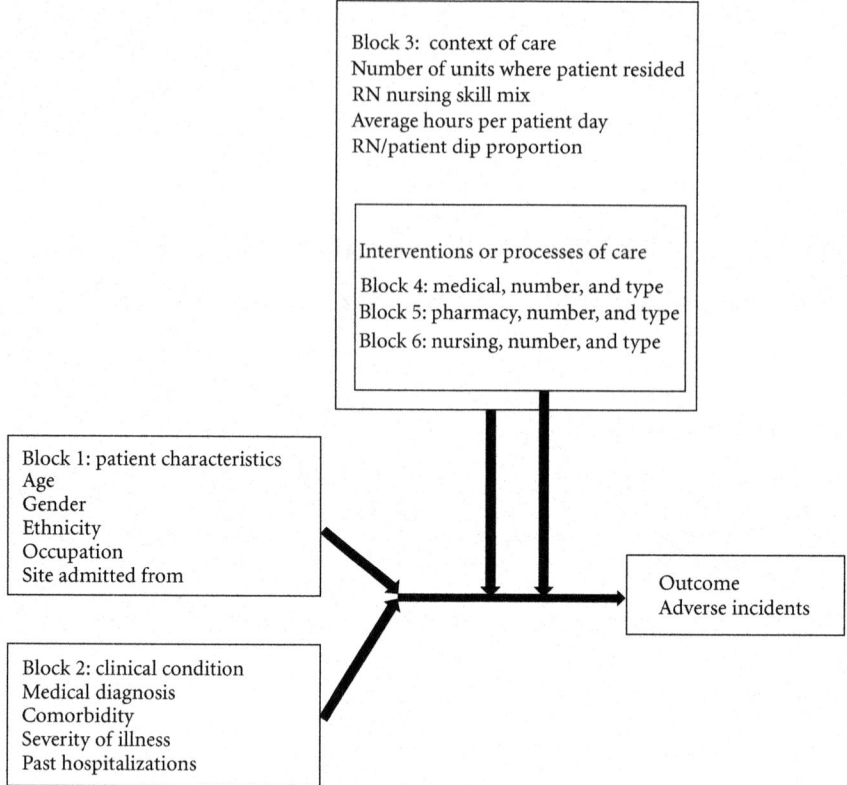

FIGURE 1: Model for predicting adverse incidents in the hospital.

medical treatments, pharmaceutical treatments, and nursing treatments. The research question addressed in this study is: what patient characteristics, clinical conditions, context of nursing care variables (e.g., nursing hours per patient day, RN skill mix, number of units resided on during hospitalization), and treatments (medical, pharmaceutical, and nursing treatments) explain the occurrence of adverse incidents for hospitalized, older adults at risk for falling? A model that has been used successfully to guide multidisciplinary effectiveness research in the hospital setting can be seen in Figure 1 [5, 6].

3. Methods

Data for this exploratory study came from a large, health service effectiveness grant [7] and was approved by the institution's Human Subjects review board. Data from a four-year period (July 1, 1998 to June 31, 2002) were extracted for the primary study from one large Midwestern academic medical center. Data sources came from nine electronic data repositories, including the nursing information system that used the Nursing Interventions Classification (NIC) [8] to electronically document nursing care delivered. Detail of the nine electronic repositories and methods to assure validity and reliability are discussed elsewhere [5]. Extracted data were stored in a structured query language (SQL) server and relational databases were built using a unique subject number.

3.1. Sample. The inclusion criteria were hospitalizations to one Midwestern tertiary care hospital over a four-year period, patients 60 years of age or older upon admission, and at risk of falling. Patients were determined to be at risk of falling based on a fall risk assessment [6] that was completed upon admission or when the patient received the nursing intervention of Fall Prevention as recorded in the electronic documentation system. Patients at risk for falling were selected with the rationale that they would be at risk for experiencing one adverse incident (i.e., falling), and therefore interventions would be initiated to prevent the adverse incident. In addition, the hospitalizations were selected as the unit of analysis rather than individual patients and a variable was included to control for patients who had more than one hospitalization.

3.2. Study Variables. Conceptual and operational definitions for the independent variables included in the explanatory model are displayed in Table 1 and organized by the conceptual model seen in Figure 1 (patient characteristics, clinical conditions, context of care, and treatments). When appropriate, the source used to guide coding of variables is provided; for example, pharmaceutical treatments, or medications, were coded using the American Hospital Formulary Service (AHFS) codes [9].

The dependent variable for this analysis was the first occurrence of an adverse incident during an episode of hospitalization. Adverse incidents were defined as any undesired

Multidisciplinary Treatments, Patient Characteristics, Context of Care, and Adverse Incidents in Older, Hospitalized Adults

45

TABLE 1: Independent variable definitions.

Variable name	Variable definition and coding source	Variable type and operational definition
Patient characteristics		
Gender	The behavioral, cultural, and psychological traits typically associated with one's sex.	Categorical: M = male, F = female, D = deferred (not determined yet).
Age	Age when patient was admitted to hospital.	Continuous; measured in years.
Occupation	Activity pursued as a livelihood.	Categorical: 1 = retired, 2 = working/employed, 3 = homemaker, 4 = not retired/not employed.
Ethnicity	Race: a group of people united by certain characteristics.	Categorical: 1 = Caucasian, 2 = all others (includes the categories of African American, Hispanic, Native American/Alaskan Native; Asian/Pacific Islander, and other).
Site admitted from	The site from which the patient was admitted to the hospital.	Categorical: 1 = hospital, 2 = care facility, 3 = home/other routine admission.
Clinical conditions		
Primary medical diagnosis	The primary medical diagnoses came from the International Classification of Diseases, 9th Revision (Clinical Modification) (ICD-9-CM) codes [10] found in MRA diagnostic codes and have been classified into Clinical Classification Software (CCS) categories [11].	Dichotomous: 0 = no, the diagnosis (i.e., as represented by a particular CCS category) is not the primary diagnosis, 1= yes, the diagnosis (i.e., as represented by a particular CCS category) is the primary diagnosis.
Severity of illness	A rating assigned to each hospital visit retrospectively to measure organ system loss of function or physiological decompensation. Coded using the All Patient Refined Diagnosis Related Groups (APR-DRGs) [12].	Integral: 1 = mild, 2 = moderate, 3 = major, 4 = severe.
Comorbid conditions	Clinical conditions that exist before admission are not related to the principal reason for hospitalization and are likely to be significant factors influencing mortality and resource use [13].	Each of 30 comorbid medical conditions is treated as a dichotomous variable: 0 = no, the condition was not present at time of admission, 1 = yes, the condition was present at the time of admission.
Past hospitalizations during the study period	The number of previous hospitalizations that the patient experienced during the study period.	Integral: 0 = no previous hospitalizations, 1 = 1 previous hospitalization, 2 = 2 previous hospitalizations, 3 = 3 previous hospitalizations, and 4 = 4 or greater previous hospitalizations.
Context of care variables		
Average CGPR-RN	For an entire visit, the average number of all hourly CGPR RN values [14] for the visit. The hourly CGPR RN values serve as the building blocks for this variable and are calculated by dividing the total RN hours for a one-hour period by the total patient hours for that same 1-hour time period.	For each 1 hour of the visit, calculate: total no. of RN hours for a 1-hour time period total no. of patient hours for that same hour and then calculate: sum of hourly CGPR RN values for the entire hospitalization total hours of hospitalization. The average of the hourly RN values was obtained by dividing the total number of RNs for all hours by the total number of hours for the hospital visit. The average of the total caregiver hours was obtained by dividing the total number of caregivers for all hours by the total number of hours for the hospital visit.
Nursing skill mix	Proportion of RNs to all nursing direct caregivers for a specified time period.	

TABLE 1: Continued.

Variable name	Variable definition and coding Source	Variable type and operational definition
CGPR RN dip variable	The extent to which the minimum amount of RN care falls below the average of all the hourly CGPR values for the entire visit. This represents the variability in the amount of RN care that is available, specifically the extent to which the amount of RN care available drops below the average amount of RN care available for the hospital visit.	Average CGPR-RN minus the average of the three lowest hourly CGPR RN values for the visit. The larger this value is, the more the minimum CGPR RN fell below the average for the visit.
Number of units resided on	The sum of the number of units on which treatment was provided to an individual patient during the course of the hospital visit.	Integral: 1 = 1 unit, 2 = 2 units, 3 = 3 units, 4 = 4 units, 5 = ≥ 5 units
Treatments		
Number of medical treatments	Medical procedures performed during a hospital visit to diagnose and treat a given patient based upon a physician's judgment and knowledge to promote or maintain health, cure diseases, or palliate incurable diseases. Coded using ICD-9-CM codes [10] from the medical record abstraction (MRA) and regrouped into multilevel CCS categories [11].	Continuous: a count on the number of medical treatments that were performed during the course of a hospital visit, this is not the number of unique medical treatments.
Types of medical treatments	Any procedure that, based upon a physician's judgment and knowledge, is necessary to promote or maintain health, cure diseases, or palliate disease processes that are incurable. Coded using ICD-9-CM codes [10] from the MRA and regrouped into multilevel CCS categories [11].	Dichotomous: 0 = no the treatment (i.e., as represented by a particular CCS category) was not received during hospitalization, 1 = yes, the treatment (i.e., as represented by a particular CCS category) was received at least once during hospitalization.
Number of unique medications	The count per visit of unique generic drug names for drugs administered at least once during a visit. Medication types were coded using the American Hospital Formulary Service's (AHFS) three-level system [9].	Continuous: a count of the number of unique medications delivered during a hospital visit.
Pharmacy treatments	Medications used in the care of patients during a hospital visit. Medication types were coded using the AHFS three-level system [9].	Dichotomous: 0 = no medication from the AHFS class was administered during the hospital visit, 1 = yes, at least one medication from the AHFS class was administered at least once during the hospital visit.
Number of unique nursing treatments	The number of unique nursing treatments delivered during the hospital visit. Captured using NIC [8, 15].	Continuous: a count of the unique nursing treatments delivered during the hospital visit.
Nursing treatments	Any treatment nursing personnel performed to enhance patient outcomes. Captured using NIC [8, 15].	Categorical: (multilevel) [16]. (a) NIC used in >95% of visits; divided into quartiles 1 = 1–25% (lowest use rates, includes 0 use), 2 = 26–50% quartile, 3 = 51–75% quartile, 4 = 76–100% quartile (highest use rates). (b) NIC used in ≤95% and >5% of visits; divided into thirds: 0 = NIC not used, 1 = 1–33% lowest third, 2 = 34–67% middle third, 3 = 68–100% top third. (c) NIC used in <5% of the visits 0 = did not receive the NIC, 1 = did receive the NIC.

Multidisciplinary Treatments, Patient Characteristics, Context of Care, and Adverse Incidents in Older, Hospitalized Adults

47

circumstance that lead to, or could have led to, personal harm. Adverse incidents were collected by the internal incident reporting system at the institution. Adverse incidents included falls, medication errors, procedure-related events (e.g., wrong patient, wrong procedure or test), equipment-related events (e.g., equipment malfunction, unplanned removal, improper set-up), and new conditions (e.g., skin breakdown).

4. Analytic Procedures

Due to the large number of study variables, a four-step model building process using logistic regression was used to answer the research question.

4.1. Step One. Each independent variable included in the analysis was tested independently using a bivariate analysis and a Score Statistic to determine the association with occurrence of an adverse incident. In this bivariate analysis, no other variables were statistically controlled for. Variables with P values ≤ 0.15 were retained for step two. A P value ≤ 0.15 was used as the criterion to guard against eliminating variables too soon in this exploratory analysis.

4.2. Step Two. The variables retained in step one (P values ≤ 0.15) were then analyzed within their respective conceptual variable blocks (i.e., patient characteristics, clinical conditions, context of care, medical treatments, pharmaceutical treatments, and nursing treatments) using logistic regression. A backward elimination process was used, indicating that the variable with the largest P value was eliminated and the analysis was rerun on the remaining variables within the block. This procedure was repeated until all variables within the block had a P value ≤ 0.15. A P value of ≤ 0.15 during step two was chosen to guard against eliminating variables too soon because they might yet prove to have a statistically significant effect when combined with variables from other conceptual blocks.

4.3. Step Three. A model integrating all of the conceptual variable blocks was built in a progressive fashion using the variables that were retained in step two. The significant variables were added to the model by their respective blocks. Starting with the significant variables in block one (patient characteristics) and block 2 (clinical conditions), a model was built using the backward elimination process described in step two until the only variables remaining in the model were those with a P value ≤ 0.15. The significant variables from block three (context of care) were then added to what remained of blocks one (patient characteristics) and two (clinical conditions) in the model. Once again, a backward elimination process was performed until the only variables remaining in the model were those with values ≤ 0.15. This process of adding blocks and using the backward elimination continued until the last block (nursing treatments) was added. At this point, when the significant variables from the final block were added and backward elimination was performed, the criterion for significance was decreased to a P value ≤ 0.05. This resulted in a final model containing only those variables with a P value ≤ 0.05. In step three, variables with a P value ≤ 0.05 in the logistic regression indicated that variables were significantly related to the dependent variable (occurrence of an adverse incident) after controlling for the other variables in the model.

4.4. Step Four. Covariates used for risk adjustment included age, severity of illness, and number of hospitalizations during the study period (see Table 2). Step four added these covariates used for risk adjustment (severity of illness, age, and more than one hospitalization during the study period) to the model to those that were significant in step three. Categorical variables with more than two categories were analyzed by comparing each level to a reference category. For example, severity of illness (four levels from minor to severe) was analyzed by comparing each of the three upper level categories to the lowest level of severity of illness (i.e., minor).

5. Results

There were 10,157 hospitalizations included in this analysis, comprised of 7,851 unique patients. The mean age was 73.7 years; most were retired (74.4%), Caucasian (93.5%), female (52.6%), and admitted from home (64.4%). This patient group, defined primarily by receiving the nursing treatment Fall Prevention, was medically diverse. The most common primary medical diagnoses were diseases of the circulatory system (28.5%), neoplasms (13.8%), and injury, including fractures, or poisoning (11.5%).

There were 1,568 hospitalizations that experienced at least one adverse incident in this sample. The most commonly experienced adverse incident for this patient group included medication errors (37%), falls (27%), and equipment-related events (14%).

Results of the model building process are illustrated in Table 2 by variable blocks. The bivariate correlations completed in step one are not included in Table 2 due to space constraints but are available from the authors upon request. The second column in Table 2 illustrates variables retained from step one that were analyzed within blocks with P values ≤ 0.15 (step two of model building) and thus retained for step three. The third column includes P values from the third part of the modeling building process, prior to adding covariates used for risk adjustment to the final model (step four). The final model is illustrated in Table 3.

Five patient characteristics entered step one of the model building process but none were significant beyond step two. *Age*, although not significant in any of the three model building steps, was entered in the final model for risk adjustment [17]. *Age* was not significant in the final model (see Table 3).

Nine primary medical diagnoses were retained from step two, four were retained from step three, and three were retained ($P \leq 0.05$) in the final model (see Tables 2 and 3). As the results in Table 3 indicate, *other nervous system disorders, other primary cancer* and *senility and organic mental disorders* were all significant ($P \leq 0.05$) in the final model. *Other nervous system disorders* was the only

TABLE 2: Results from the model building process for determining explanatory variables of experiencing an adverse incident.

Variable	Significant P values ($P \leq 0.15$) for within block correlations	Significant P values ($P \leq 0.05$) for the final model
Patient characteristics		
Ethnicity	0.0029	
Site admitted from	<0.0001	
Clinical conditions		
Primary medical diagnoses (% of sample)		
Cancer, other primary (1.7)	<0.0001	0.0010
Maintenance chemotherapy, radiotherapy (1.1)	0.1408	
Fluid and electrolyte disorder (1.6)	0.0172	
Senility & organic mental disorders (3.0)	<0.0001	0.0140
Affective (2.1)	0.0007	
Other nervous system disorders (1.1)	0.0686	0.0176
Respiratory (3.1)	0.0687	
Chronic obstructive pulmonary (1.8)	0.0332	
Symptoms, signs, and ill-defined conditions (1.8)	0.1034	
Severity of illness	<0.0001	
Congestive heart failure (11.8)	0.0155	
Other neurological disorders (3.6)	0.1218	
Diabetes (17.7)	0.0347	
Peptic ulcer disease without bleeding (4.4)	0.0985	
Rheumatoid arthritis/collagen vas (4.0)	0.0918	
Psychoses (5.7)	0.0211	
Depression (6.6)	0.0237	
Severity of illness		
Severity of illness	<0.0001	
Elixhauser comorbid conditions (% of sample)		
Congestive heart failure (11.8)	0.0155	
Other neurological disorders (3.6)	0.1218	
Diabetes (17.7)	0.0347	
Peptic ulcer disease without bleeding (4.4)	0.0985	
Rheumatoid arthritis/collagen vas (4.0)	0.0918	
Psychoses (5.7)	0.0211	
Depression (6.6)	0.0237	
Past hospitalizations		
Past hospitalizations	0.0199	
Context of care variables		
Number of units resided on	<0.0001	
CGPR dip proportion	<0.0001	0.0092
Skill mix	0.0003	
Average caregiver patient ratio	<0.0001	<0.0001
Treatments		
Medical treatments		
Total number of procedures	<0.0001	0.0059
Types of medical treatments (% of sample)		
Incision and excision of CNS (2.0)	0.0059	
Incision of pleura, thoracentesis, chest drainage (3.8)	0.0637	
Coronary artery bypass graft (CABG) (3.1)	<0.0001	

Multidisciplinary Treatments, Patient Characteristics, Context of Care, and Adverse Incidents in Older, Hospitalized Adults

49

TABLE 2: Continued.

Variable	Significant P values ($P \leq 0.15$) for within block correlations	Significant P values ($P \leq 0.05$) for the final model
Diagnostic cardiac catheterization, coronary arteriography (7.9)	0.0007	
Other therapeutic procedures, hemic and lymphatic system (2.8)	0.1205	
Upper gastrointestinal endoscopy, biopsy (6.6)	0.0062	
Gastrostomy, temporary and permanent (1.5)	0.1035	
Oophorectomy, unilateral & bilateral (1.3)	0.0062	
Partial excision bone (1.5)	0.0769	
Treatment of fracture or dislocation (2.3)	0.0513	
Arthroplasty (3.0)	0.0014	
Amputation of lower extremity (1.1)	0.1257	
Spinal fusion (1.0)	0.0089	
Debridement of wound, infection or burn (1.5)	0.0395	
Arterio or venogram (not heart or head) (2.2)	0.0091	
Diagnostic ultrasound (33.5)	0.0048	
Radioisotope scan (6.6)	0.0667	
Physical therapy (4.7)	<0.0001	0.0015
Psychological and psychiatric evaluation and therapy (1.8)	<0.0001	
Enteral and parenteral nutrition (9.5)	0.0063	
Pharmaceutical treatments		
Number of unique medications	<0.0001	<0.0001
Types of pharmaceutical treatments (% of sample)		
Sympathomimetic (adrenergic) agents (17.3)	0.0241	
Anticholinergic agents (13.5)	0.0054	
Skeletal muscle relaxants (5.4)	0.0140	
Cardiac drugs (64.8)	0.0445	
Hypotensive agents (37.7)	0.0882	
Psychotherapeutic agents (35.0)	<0.0001	
Succinimides (27.8)	<0.0001	0.0015
Miscellaneous central nervous system agents (3.9)	0.0923	
Opiate antagonists (1.4)	0.0669	
Anorexigenic agents and respiratory & cerebral stimulants (1.4)	0.0146	
Caloric agents (51.8)	0.0244	0.0128
Irrigating solutions (7.3)	0.0414	
Ammonia detoxicants (2.7)	0.0785	0.0274
EENT anti-infectives (42.2)	0.0002	0.0148
EENT carbonic anhydrase inhibitors (2.2)	0.0404	
Miscellaneous GI drugs (59.8)	0.1098	
Parathyroid (1.4)	0.0228	
Anti-infectives (21.5)	0.0346	
Anti-inflammatory agents (6.8)	0.0438	
Multivitamin preparations (18.7)	0.0425	
Vitamin B complex (7.4)	0.1130	
Unclassified therapeutic agents (34.0)	0.0619	
Tetracyclines (1.3)	0.1135	
Opiate agonists (64.0)	0.0034	
Barbiturates (2.8)	0.0014	
Benzodiazepines (56.2)	0.0024	

TABLE 2: Continued.

Variable	Significant P values ($P \leq 0.15$) for within block correlations	Significant P values ($P \leq 0.05$) for the final model
Misc. anxiolytics, sedatives, & hypnotics (17.8)	0.0022	
Nursing treatments		
Nursing treatment types (% of sample)		
Fluid management (99.5)	0.0098	
Bathing (93.5)	0.0600	
Pressure ulcer care (91.5)	<0.0001	0.0005
Bowel management (88.2)	0.1049	
Teaching (81.5)	0.0003	
Discharge planning (76.0)	0.0042	
Routine care: adult (56.2)	0.0626	
Health screening (48.8)	<0.0001	<0.0001
Sleep enhancement (47.7)	0.0572	
Oxygen therapy (42.4)	0.0008	
Post-op care (27.8)	<0.0001	
Wound care (21.4)	0.0137	
Neurologic monitoring (20.2)	0.0002	0.0003
Analgesic administration (17.2)	0.0723	
Fluid/electrolyte monitoring (15.1)	0.0365	
Medication management (12.2)	0.0678	
Nutrition management (11.3)	0.0022	
Embolus precautions (9.4)	0.0687	
Infection protection (8.9)	0.0182	
Enteral tube feeding (9.4)	0.0042	
Blood products administration (8.6)	0.0004	0.0192
Restraint (8.5)	<0.0001	<0.0001
Postprocedure care (5.6)	0.0219	
Specimen management (5.3)	0.0079	0.0098
Active listening (4.8)	0.0161	0.0003
Surgical preparation (4.1)	0.1281	0.0441
Total parenteral nutrition (TPN) administration: adult (3.4)	0.0033	
Aspiration precautions (3.2)	0.0233	
Anger control assistance (2.8)	0.0177	
Mood management (2.5)	0.0091	0.0004
Self-care assistance (2.2)	0.1323	
Procedure preparation (2.1)	0.1079	
Dementia management (1.6)	0.0816	
Electroconvulsive therapy (1.6)	0.0290	
Cast care: maintenance (1.1)	0.0035	0.0037
Splinting (1.1)	0.0086	
Music therapy (1.1)	0.0036	0.0019
Medical immobilization (0.9)	0.0356	

primary medical diagnosis of the three inversely associated with experiencing an adverse incident (O.R. = 0.43), indicating that hospitalizations with this medical diagnosis were less likely to suffer an adverse incident compared to hospitalizations that did not have this condition. Other *primary cancer* and *senility and organic mental disorders*

were both positively associated with experiencing an adverse incident with odds ratios of 1.94 and 1.57, respectively.

Severity of illness, although not significant in step three, was entered into the final model for risk adjustment [17]. *Severe* and *major* severity of illness categories were significantly ($P \leq 0.05$) and positively associated with

Multidisciplinary Treatments, Patient Characteristics, Context of Care, and Adverse Incidents in Older, Hospitalized Adults

51

TABLE 3: Final model for the explanatory variables of experiencing an adverse incident.

Variable names	Estimate	Standard error	P value	Odds ratio	95% C.I.	
Patient characteristics						
Age at admission	−0.0001	0.00375	0.9735	1.000	0.993	1.007
Clinical conditions						
Primary medical diagnoses						
Other nervous system disorders	−0.8502	0.3623	0.0189	0.427	0.210	0.869
Cancer, other primary	0.6602	0.1957	0.0007	1.935	1.319	2.840
Senility and organic mental disorders	0.4532	0.1704	0.0078	1.573	1.127	2.197
Severity of illness						
Severe/extreme	0.3116	0.1530	0.0417	1.366	1.012	1.843
Major	0.2795	0.1379	0.0427	1.322	1.009	1.733
Moderate (*mild is reference category*)	0.1513	0.1355	0.2644	1.163	0.892	1.517
Past hospitalizations						
Four or more previous hospitalizations	−0.1976	0.2580	0.4437	0.821	0.495	1.361
Three previous hospitalizations	−0.0810	0.2460	0.7419	0.922	0.569	1.494
Two previous hospitalizations	−0.1733	0.1625	0.2864	0.841	0.611	1.156
One previous hospitalization (*no previous hospitalizations is reference*)	0.0133	0.0888	00.8809	1.013	0.852	1.206
Context of Care						
Average CGPR RN for Hospitalization (mean RN HPPD = 9.47) [Best Staffing]	−0.2817	0.1002	0.0049	0.755	0.620	0.918
Average CGPR RN for hospitalization (mean RN HPPD = 6.64)	−0.4737	0.1007	<0.0001	0.623	0.511	0.758
Average CGPR RN for hospitalization (mean RN HPPD = 5.56)	−0.0861	0.0917	0.3480	0.918	0.767	1.098
Average CGPR RN for hospitalization (mean RN HPPD = 4.07) [worse staffing]						
CGPR RN dip proportion	0.6771	0.2647	0.0105	1.150 (per 0.2 increments)	1.172	3.307
Treatments						
Medical treatments						
Number of medical treatments	0.0279	0.0140	0.0460	1.028	1.000	1.057
Physical therapy	0.4192	0.1307	0.0013	1.521	1.177	1.965
Pharmacy treatments						
Number of unique medications	0.0431	0.00438	<0.0001	1.044	1.035	1.053

TABLE 3: Continued.

Variable names	Estimate	Standard error	P value	Odds ratio	95% C.I.	
Succinimides	0.2175	0.0707	0.0021	1.243	1.082	1.428
Caloric agents	0.2002	0.0792	0.0115	1.222	1.046	1.427
Ammonia detoxicants	−0.4192	0.1811	0.0206	0.658	0.461	0.938
EENT anti-infectives	0.1705	0.0730	0.0195	1.186	1.028	1.368
Nursing treatments						
Pressure ulcer care						
High use (68–100%) 0.92 use rate	0.00989	0.1555	0.9493	1.010	0.745	1.370
Medium use (34–67%) 0.41 use rate	0.3385	0.1390	0.0149	1.403	1.068	1.842
Low use (1–33%) 0.25 use rate	0.3472	0.1361	0.0107	1.415	1.084	1.848
Health screening						
High use (68–100%) 0.72 use rate	−0.2464	0.1366	0.0713	0.782	0.598	1.022
Medium use (34–67%) 0.21 use rate	−0.0938	0.0969	0.3332	0.910	0.753	1.101
Low use (1–33%) 0.08 use rate	0.2803	0.0776	0.0003	1.323	1.137	1.541
Neurologic monitoring						
High use (68–100%) 7.56 use rate	−0.1478	0.1462	0.3119	0.863	0.648	1.149
Medium use (34–67%) 4.46 use rate	0.0110	0.1308	0.9328	1.011	0.782	1.306
Low use (1–33%) 1.96 use rate	0.4180	0.1062	<0.0001	1.519	1.234	1.870
Blood products administration						
High use (68–100%) 3.70 use rate	−0.1061	0.1847	0.5657	0.899	0.626	1.292
Medium use (34–67%) 0.89 use rate	0.4029	0.1465	0.0060	1.496	1.123	1.994
Low use (1–33%) 0.17 use rate	0.1758	0.1498	0.2405	1.192	0.889	1.599
Restraint						
High use (68–100%) 16.47 use rate	0.7698	0.1554	<0.0001	2.159	1.592	2.928
Medium use (34–67%) 4.79 use rate	0.6229	0.1471	<0.0001	1.864	1.397	2.487
Low use (1–33%) 1.19 use rate	0.4595	0.1423	0.0012	1.583	1.198	2.092
Specimen management						
High use (68–100%) 1.68 use rate	−0.1680	0.2255	0.4564	0.845	0.543	1.315
Medium use (34–67%) 0.34 use rate	0.3912	0.1879	0.0374	1.479	1.023	2.137
Low use (1–33%) 0.10 use rate	0.4334	0.1767	0.0142	1.543	1.091	2.181
Active listening 1.79 use rate	0.4895	0.1385	0.0004	1.631	1.244	2.140
Mood management 3.09 use rate	0.6080	0.1748	0.0005	1.837	1.304	2.587
Cast care maintenance 5.31 use rate	0.6905	0.2335	0.0031	1.995	1.262	3.153
Music therapy 0.21 use rate	0.7102	0.2287	0.0019	2.034	1.300	3.185

experiencing an adverse incident compared to the lowest severity of illness category (i.e., mild) (see Table 3).

Seven comorbid conditions were retained from step two for inclusion in step three but none were significant and thus were not retained for inclusion in the final model. Past hospitalizations during the study period were significant in step two but not in step three (see Table 2). However, this variable was entered into the final model to adjust for patients that had experienced more than one hospitalization during the study period. In the final model (Table 3) past hospitalizations were not significant.

Four context of care variables, the *number of units the patient resided on during hospitalization*, the *dip proportion (falling below the unit's average staffing)*, *skill mix*, and the *average Caregiver Patient Ratio (CGPR)* [14], were significant in step two (see Table 2) but only two variables, the *dip proportion* and *average CGPR*, were significant in step three and retained for the final model (see Table 2). Both were significant in the final model (step four) as illustrated in Table 3. The *average CGPR* (RN hours per patient day (HPPDs)) was categorized as quartiles to enable comparison and interpretation for this nonlinear variable. The two highest *average CGPR* quartiles (9.5 RN HPPDs and 6.6 RN HPPDs) were significantly ($P \leq 0.05$) and inversely associated with experiencing an adverse incident, indicating that when compared to the lowest quartile of staffing (4.1 RN HPPDs), the odds of experiencing an adverse incident decreased in the highest two quartiles of nursing hours per patient day. The odds of experiencing an adverse incident for hospitalizations with the highest *average CGPR* quartile (9.5 RN HPPDs) were 0.76 of the odds for hospitalizations that experienced the lowest *average CGPR* quartile (4.1 RN HPPDs). The odds of experiencing an adverse incident for hospitalizations with the second highest *average CGPR* (6.6 RN HPPDs) were 0.62 of the odds for hospitalizations in the lowest *CGPR average* quartile.

The CGPR dip proportion was significantly ($P = 0.011$) and positively associated with experiencing an adverse incident. The results shown in Table 3 are in terms of 0.2 increments of change and indicate that for each 20% fall in staffing below the average, the odds of experiencing an adverse incident increase by 15% (O.R. = 1.15).

The number of medical treatments received during hospitalization and 20 types of medical treatment were significant in step two (see Table 2) and were therefore included in step three. In step three of the analysis, the number of medical treatments received during hospitalization and one medical treatment type, *physical therapy*, were significant ($P \leq 0.05$) and retained for the final model. Both were positively associated with experiencing an adverse incident (see Tables 2 and 3). The results indicate that for each additional medical treatment received during hospitalization, the odds of experiencing an adverse incident increased by approximately 3% (O.R. = 1.03). Hospitalizations that received the medical treatment *physical therapy* were 52% (O.R. = 1.52) more likely to experience an adverse incident than hospitalizations that did not receive this medical treatment.

The number of unique medications received during hospitalization and 27 specific pharmaceutical treatments (i.e., medications types) were significant in step two of the analysis ($P \leq 0.15$) and thus retained for step three. The number of unique medication types and four types of medications were significant in step three (see Table 2) and all were significant in the final model (see Table 3). The number of unique medications was positively associated ($P < 0.001$) with experiencing an adverse incident (O.R. = 1.04). Receipt of *succinimides, caloric agents,* and *EENT anti-infectives* during hospitalization increased the odds of an adverse incident. *Ammonia detoxicants* were inversely associated ($P = 0.021$) with experiencing an adverse incident (O.R. = 0.46).

In step two of the analysis, the number of unique nursing treatments received during hospitalization was not significant but 38 types of nursing treatments were significant ($P \leq 0.15$) and entered into step three (see Table 2). Eleven were significant at step three and ten were significant in the final model (see Tables 2 and 3). *Surgical preparation* was not significant in the final model. The nursing treatment *pressure ulcer care*, received by 91.5% of the sample, was divided into thirds based on the average number of times per day it was delivered (see Table 1). The results for the three categories of use are interpreted in comparison to hospitalizations that did not receive the nursing treatment. The middle and low use categories of *pressure ulcer care* were significantly ($P \leq 0.05$) and positively associated with experiencing an adverse incident, indicating that hospitalizations that received *pressure ulcer care* a little less than once every other day (use rate = 0.41) or once every four days (use rate = 0.25) were more likely to experience an adverse incident than hospitalizations that did not receive *pressure ulcer care*. A similar pattern emerged with the nursing treatment of *specimen management*. The medium (use rate = 0.34) and low (use rate = 0.10) categories were significantly ($P \leq 0.05$) and positively associated with experiencing an adverse incident (see Table 3).

Both *health screening* and *neurologic monitoring* had low use categories that were significantly ($P \leq 0.05$) and positively correlated with experiencing an adverse incident. The results indicate that hospitalizations that received the low use of these two nursing treatments were more likely to experience an adverse incident than hospitalizations that did not receive the associated nursing treatment (see Table 3).

The medium use category of *blood products administration* (use rate = 0.89) was significantly ($P \leq 0.05$) and positively (O.R. = 1.49) associated with experiencing an adverse incident. Hospitalizations that received *Blood Products Administration* a little less than once a day were almost 50% more likely to experience an adverse incident than hospitalizations that did not receive *blood products administration*.

All three categories of use for the nursing treatment *Restraint* were significantly ($P < 0.01$) and positively associated with experiencing an adverse incident (see Table 3). The high use category had an average delivery of 16.47 times a day and hospitalizations that received high use of *restraint* had more than double the odds (O.R. = 2.16) of experiencing an adverse incident compared to hospitalizations that did not receive this nursing treatment. Hospitalizations that received *restraint* approximately four and a half times a day (medium use category) had almost double the odds (O.R. = 1.86) of experiencing an adverse incident compared to hospitalizations that did not receive *restraint*. The lowest category of use was delivered an average a little more than once a day and increased the likelihood of experiencing an adverse incident by 58% (O.R. = 1.58) compared to no use.

The remaining significant nursing treatments were delivered to less than 5% of the sample and were therefore operationalized as dichotomous variables so that hospitalizations that received the nursing treatment at least once are compared to hospitalizations that did not receive the treatment (see Table 1 for definition). *Active listening* received at least once by 4.8% of the sample was significantly (*P* < 0.001) and positively (O.R. = 1.63) associated with experiencing an adverse incident.

Mood management was received by only 2.5% of the sample but was delivered an average of 3.1 times per day when it was delivered. Hospitalizations that received *mood management* almost doubled their odds (O.R. = 1.84) of experiencing an adverse incident compared to hospitalizations that did not receive *mood management*.

Cast care maintenance was another nursing treatment that was delivered frequently (more than five times a day on average) when hospitalizations required it. Receiving this nursing treatment doubled the odds (O.R. = 2.00) of experiencing an adverse incident compared to hospitalizations that did not receive this nursing treatment.

Slightly more than one percent of the sample received the nursing treatment *music therapy*. The average use rate for hospitalizations that received this treatment was slightly more than once every ten days (use rate = 0.21). The odds of experiencing an adverse incident were double (O.R. = 2.03) for hospitalizations that received this nursing treatment compared to hospitalizations that did not receive *music therapy* (see Table 3).

6. Discussion

None of the patient characteristics were significant, indicating that patient characteristics were not explanatory variables of adverse incidents, given the other variables that entered the model. Also nonsignificant were two clinical conditions: number of past hospitalizations during the study period and comorbid medical conditions. This indicates that after controlling for other variables in the model, patient characteristics of this sample of older adults were not significant for experiencing an adverse incident during hospitalization.

Three primary medical diagnoses were significant explanatory variables associated with experiencing an adverse incident. *Other nervous system disorders* were inversely associated with experiencing an adverse incident. This inverse relationship may be explained by considering the type of nursing unit these patients are typically admitted to. A primary medical diagnosis of *nervous system disorder*, which is composed of peripheral and central nervous system disorders along with more generic symptoms of a nervous system disorder [11], would likely warrant admission to a

neurology unit in this academic medical setting where the nursing personnel are skilled in the care of these patients and may recognize the need for increased surveillance. This heightened surveillance for these specialized patients may decrease adverse incidents.

Other primary cancer was positively associated with experiencing an adverse incident. Patients hospitalized with the primary medical diagnosis of *other primary cancer* are on high-risk medications, some that call for double-checks, and that may increase the number of medication errors that are discovered. The third primary medical diagnosis, *senility and organic mental disorders*, appears similar in nature to *other nervous system disorders* but is positively associated with experiencing an adverse incident, unlike *other nervous system disorders*. This may be because patients who have *senility and organic mental disorders* are less capable of using safety equipment in their environment like call lights and hand rails and are more likely to be dispersed among a variety of general medical or surgical units. The environment and specialized nursing expertise may not be readily available to meet the unique care demands of individuals with this primary medical condition. In the final model, the top two severities of illness categories (i.e., severe and major) were significantly and positively associated with experiencing an adverse incident. This is not surprising, as patients who are sicker often have complex care issues which may place them at greater risk to experience an adverse incident.

Related to the structure of care (context of care), the two highest categories of the *average CGPR* (RN HPPDs) were significantly and inversely associated with experiencing an adverse incident compared to the lowest quartile, indicating that when there are more nursing hours per patient day, there is a decreased likelihood of preventing an adverse incident. This is consistent with findings from previous research [18–24].

The *CGPR RN dip proportion* was positively associated with adverse incidents. The more the RN staffing fell below the nursing unit average, the more likely an adverse incident was to occur during that hospitalization. This finding indicates that not only is the number of nurses, or HPPDs, an important predictor of adverse incidents but so is staffing below the average on a nursing unit. This may indicate that units develop effective processes dependent upon their average staffing and when the staffing is altered, the processes are impacted. Staffing below the unit average places the patient at greater risk for having an adverse incident

Processes of care included medical, pharmaceutical, and nursing treatments. Both the number of medical treatments and the number of unique medications received during hospitalization were positively associated with experiencing an adverse incident. As the number of procedures and medications increased so did the odds of having an adverse incident (e.g., medication error, wrong site surgery, trauma, etc.).

There was one medical treatment, *physical therapy*, and two medication types, *succinimides* and *ammonia detoxicants*, that were significantly associated with experiencing an adverse incident, which may be related to falls. The positive association between *physical therapy* and adverse

Multidisciplinary Treatments, Patient Characteristics, Context of Care, and Adverse Incidents in Older, Hospitalized Adults

55

incidents may be a reflection of patients with decreased functional status who are at greater risk for falling. Similarly, *succinimides* are anticonvulsives and are in the same AHFS class as *barbiturates* and *benzodiazepines* [9], which are positively associated with falls [25]. *Ammonia detoxicants* was the only pharmaceutical treatment in the final model inversely associated with experiencing an adverse incident (see Table 3). Patients who require *ammonia detoxicants* often have conditions associated with liver dysfunction, which makes it more difficult for them to excrete ammonia that builds up in their body. Patients that have high ammonia levels are often confused, disoriented, difficult to direct, and are at great risk for falling for these reasons.

The nursing treatments associated with adverse incidents were diverse. There was one nursing treatment, *pressure ulcer care*, that is used to treat an adverse incident (i.e., pressure ulcer). There were also a number of nursing treatments positively associated with adverse incidents where providing the treatment showed that the patient likely had greater exposure to an adverse incident than patients who did not receive the treatment. One example is the nursing treatment *specimen management* where a patient is more likely to have a mislabeled lab as an adverse incident than a patient who did not receive this treatment. The same could be true for *blood product administration* and *cast care maintenance*.

Similarly, all three categories of *Restraint* were significantly and positively associated with experiencing an adverse incident. Only 8.5% of the hospitalizations in this sample received *restraint* at least once but the use rates were relatively high, especially the high use category with an average delivery of 16.47 times per day. These findings also show that use of restraints does not prevent adverse incidents (e.g., falls) and in fact may contribute to them as has been demonstrated in other research [26, 27].

Active listening, *mood management*, and *music therapy* may be used as complementary therapies for patients who are distressed, confused, or combative when other treatments have not worked. Hospitalizations that require these nursing treatments may be at greater risk for falling because the patient is unable to follow commands, is impulsive or unable to communicate effectively.

7. Limitations

This study was conducted at one academic medical center and therefore further multisite research is needed. Although the effectiveness research model used in this study includes many important, patient and multidisciplinary components, there were important aspects of care that impact patient safety such as the individual characteristics of the clinicians involved in care (e.g., experience, education) and how they interact with one another (e.g., teamwork, communication) that were not included in this study [28].

8. Conclusion

This study examined a number of patient conditions, structural variables, and process of care variables to better understand what factors contribute to adverse incidents during hospitalization. This is one of the first studies to show that delivered nursing treatments help explain adverse incidents in hospitalized, older adults. This study also used a multidisciplinary model that considered medical and pharmaceutical components of treatment, which are critical when providing care of the older adult in acute care. With this more robust multidisciplinary model, RN staffing was still an important explanatory variable for adverse incidents, which is congruent with findings from other research [29, 30].

Acknowledgment

This research was supported by a Grant from NIH (PI: Titler. NINR 1 R01 NR05331).

References

[1] Institute of Medicine, *To Err Is Human: Building a Safer Health System*, National Academy of Sciences, Washington, DC, USA, 2000.

[2] U.S. Department of Health and Human Services Centers for Medicare and Medicaid Services, Hospital Acquired Conditions. http://www.cms.gov/HospitalAcqCond/06_Hospital-Acquired_Conditions.asp.

[3] J. B. Battles and R. J. Lilford, "Organizing patient safety research to identify risks and hazards," *Quality and Safety in Health Care*, vol. 12, supplement 2, pp. ii2–ii7, 2003.

[4] M. Duckers, M. Faber, J. Cruijsberg, R. Grol, L. Schoonhoven, and M. Wensing, "Safety and risk management interventions in hospitals: a systematic review of the literature," *Medical Care Research and Review*, vol. 66, supplement 6, pp. 90S–119S, 2009.

[5] M. Titler, J. Dochterman, X. J. Xie et al., "Nursing interventions and other factors associated with discharge disposition in older patients after hip fractures," *Nursing Research*, vol. 55, no. 4, pp. 231–242, 2006.

[6] M. Titler, J. Dochterman, D. M. Picone et al., "Cost of hospital care for elderly at risk of falling," *Nursing Economics*, vol. 23, no. 6, pp. 290–306, 2005.

[7] M. Titler, "Nursing interventions and outcomes effectiveness in 3 older populations," Tech. Rep. NR05331-02, National Institute of Nursing Research (NINR), Rockville, Md, USA, 2000.

[8] J. M. Dochterman and G. M. Bulechek, *Nursing Interventions Classification (NIC)*, Mosby, St. Louis, Mo, USA, 4th edition, 2004.

[9] G. K. McEvoy, *American Hospital Forumlary Service (AHFS) Drug Information 2000*, American Society of Health System Pharmacists, Bethesda, Md, USA, 2000.

[10] Public Health Service and Health Care Financing Administration, *ICD-9-CM: International Classification of Diseases, 9th Revision, Clinical Modification*, Public Health Service, Washington, DC, USA, 1994.

[11] Agency for Healthcare Research and Quality (AHRQ), *Healthcare Cost and Utilization Project (HCUP)*, Clinical Classifications Software (CCS) for ICD-9-CM, Rockville, Md, USA, 2002.

[12] 3M Health Information Systems, *All Patient Refined Diagnosis Related Groups (APR-DRGs)*, 3M Health Information Systems, Wallingford, Conn, USA, 1993.

[13] A. Elixhauser, C. Steiner, D. R. Harris, and R. M. Coffey, "Comorbidity measures for use with administrative data," *Medical Care*, vol. 36, no. 1, pp. 8–27, 1998.

[14] G. Budreau, R. Balakrishnan, M. Titler, and M. J. Hafner, "Caregiver-patient ratio: capturing census and staffing variability," *Nursing Economics*, vol. 17, no. 6, pp. 317–324, 1999.

[15] M. Titler, J. Dochterman, and D. Reed, *Guideline for Conducting Effectiveness Research in Nursing and Other Health Services*, The University of Iowa, College of Nursing, Center for Nursing Classification & Clinical Effectiveness, Iowa City, Iowa, USA, 2004.

[16] D. Reed, M. G. Titler, J. M. Dochterman, L. L. Shever, M. Kanak, and D. M. Picone, "Measuring the dose of nursing intervention," *International Journal of Nursing Terminologies and Classifications*, vol. 18, no. 4, pp. 121–130, 2007.

[17] L. Iezzoni, *Risk Adjustment for Measuring Health Care Outcomes*, Health Administration Press, Chicago, Ill, USA, 3rd edition, 2003.

[18] S. H. Cho, S. Ketefian, V. H. Barkauskas, and D. G. Smith, "The effects of nurse staffing on adverse events, morbidity, mortality, and medical costs," *Nursing Research*, vol. 52, no. 2, pp. 71–79, 2003.

[19] N. Dunton, B. Gajewski, R. L. Taunton, and J. Moore, "Nurse staffing and patient falls on acute care hospital units," *Nursing Outlook*, vol. 52, no. 1, pp. 53–59, 2004.

[20] L. M. Hall, D. Doran, and G. H. Pink, "Nurse staffing models, nursing hours, and patient safety outcomes," *Journal of Nursing Administration*, vol. 34, no. 1, pp. 41–45, 2004.

[21] P. Potter, N. Barr, M. McSweeney, and J. Sledge, "Identifying nurse staffing and patient outcome relationships: a guide for change in care delivery," *Nursing Economics*, vol. 21, no. 4, pp. 158–166, 2003.

[22] M. D. Sovie and A. F. Jawad, "Hospital restructuring and its impact on outcomes: nursing staff regulations are premature," *Journal of Nursing Administration*, vol. 31, no. 12, pp. 588–600, 2001.

[23] L. Unruh, "Licensed nurse staffing and adverse events in hospitals," *Medical Care*, vol. 41, no. 1, pp. 142–152, 2003.

[24] G. R. Whitman, Y. Kim, L. J. Davidson, G. A. Wolf, and S. L. Wang, "The impact of staffing on patient outcomes across specialty units," *Journal of Nursing Administration*, vol. 32, no. 12, pp. 633–639, 2002.

[25] J. C. Woolcott, K. J. Richardson, M. O. Wiens et al., "Meta-analysis of the impact of 9 medication classes on falls in elderly persons," *Archives of Internal Medicine*, vol. 169, no. 21, pp. 1952–1960, 2009.

[26] J. V. Agostini, D. I. Baker, and S. T. Bogardus Jr, "Prevention of falls in hospitalized and institutionalized older people," in *Making Health Care Safer: A Critical Analysis of Patient Safety Practices. Evidence Report/Technology Assessment no. 43*, K. G. Shojania, B. W. Duncan, and K. M. McDonald, Eds., Agency for Healthcare Research and Quality (AHRQ), Rockville, Md, USA, 2001.

[27] D. Evans, J. Wood, and L. Lambert, "A review of physical restraint minimization in the acute and residential care settings," *Journal of Advanced Nursing*, vol. 40, no. 6, pp. 616–625, 2002.

[28] T. Hoff, L. Jameson, E. Hannan, and E. Flink, "A review of the literature examining linkages between organizational factors, medical errors, and patient safety," *Medical Care Research and Review*, vol. 61, no. 1, pp. 3–37, 2004.

[29] R. L. Kane, T. Shamliyan, C. Mueller, S. Duval, and T. J. Wilt, "Nurse staffing and quality of patient care," *Evidence Report/Technology Assessment*, no. 151, pp. 1–115, 2007.

[30] D. M. Picone, M. G. Titler, J. Dochterman et al., "Predictors of medication errors among elderly hospitalized patients," *American Journal of Medical Quality*, vol. 23, no. 2, pp. 115–127, 2008.

8

Health Literacy Influences Heart Failure Knowledge Attainment but Not Self-Efficacy for Self-Care or Adherence to Self-Care over Time

Aleda M. H. Chen,[1] **Karen S. Yehle,**[2,3,4] **Nancy M. Albert,**[5] **Kenneth F. Ferraro,**[3,6] **Holly L. Mason,**[7] **Matthew M. Murawski,**[7] **and Kimberly S. Plake**[3,4,8]

[1] *Assistant Professor of Pharmacy Practice, School of Pharmacy, Cedarville University, 251 N. Main Street, Cedarville, OH 45314, USA*

[2] *School of Nursing, Purdue University, 502 N. University Street, JNSN 238, West Lafayette, IN 47907, USA*

[3] *Center on Aging and the Life Course, Purdue University, West Lafayette, IN 47907, USA*

[4] *Regenstrief Center for Healthcare Engineering, Purdue University, West Lafayette, IN 47907, USA*

[5] *Office of Research & Innovation, Nursing Institute and CNS, Kaufman Center for Heart Failure, Heart and Vascular Institute, Cleveland Clinic, 9500 Euclid Avenue, J3-4, Cleveland, OH 44195, USA*

[6] *Distinguished Professor of Sociology, Purdue University, Bill and Sally Hanley Hall, 1202 W. State Street, West Lafayette, IN 47907, USA*

[7] *Pharmacy Administration, College of Pharmacy, Purdue University, Heine Pharmacy Building, 575 Stadium Mall Drive, West Lafayette, IN 47907, USA*

[8] *Pharmacy Practice, College of Pharmacy, Purdue University, Heine Pharmacy Building, 575 Stadium Mall Drive, West Lafayette, IN 47907, USA*

Correspondence should be addressed to Aleda M. H. Chen; amchen@cedarville.edu

Academic Editor: Victoria Vaughan Dickson

Background. Inadequate health literacy may be a barrier to gaining knowledge about heart failure (HF) self-care expectations, strengthening self-efficacy for self-care behaviors, and adhering to self-care behaviors over time. *Objective.* To examine if health literacy is associated with HF knowledge, self-efficacy, and self-care adherence longitudinally. *Methods.* Prior to education, newly referred patients at three HF clinics ($N = 51$, age: 64.7 ± 13.0 years) completed assessments of health literacy, HF knowledge, self-efficacy, and adherence to self-care at baseline, 2, and 4 months. Repeated measures analysis of variance with Bonferroni-adjusted alpha levels was used to test longitudinal outcomes. *Results.* Health literacy was associated with HF knowledge longitudinally ($P < 0.001$) but was not associated with self-efficacy self-care adherence. In posthoc analyses, participants with inadequate health literacy had less HF knowledge than participants with adequate ($P < 0.001$) but not marginal ($P = 0.073$) health literacy. *Conclusions.* Adequate health literacy was associated with greater HF knowledge but not self-efficacy or adherence to self-care expectations over time. If nurses understand patients' health literacy level, they may educate patients using methods that promote understanding of concepts. Since interventions that promote self-efficacy and adherence to self-care were not associated with health literacy level, new approaches must be examined.

1. Introduction

Heart failure is identified as a leading cause of hospitalizations [1], morbidity, mortality, and rising healthcare costs for nearly six million Americans [2, 3]. After a diagnosis of heart failure, patients must perform self-care behaviors to reduce negative clinical outcomes [4, 5]. Self-care is a decision-making process, where patients perform activities to prevent symptoms (maintenance) and respond to symptoms as they occur (management) [4]. Self-care maintenance activities for heart failure patients include exercising daily, eating a low sodium diet, monitoring fluid intake, and monitoring weight. Patients may respond to symptoms by engaging in the following self-care management activities: consulting their healthcare provider, reducing fluid and sodium intake, and increasing the dose of a diuretic. However, patients' adherence to recommended self-care behaviors varies greatly and is generally poor [5–7].

Multiple factors may affect patients' adherence to heart failure self-care including heart failure knowledge. Patients may not have received recommended heart failure education [8, 9] if the heart failure diagnosis was secondary to another health problem, such as myocardial infarction, resulting in inadequate knowledge about heart failure [10]. Initial education about heart failure often occurs during hospitalization when the patient may be too ill or overwhelmed with acute care events, potentially reducing retention of information presented unless family members are available to be counseled [10]. Additional education occurs in the outpatient setting, but content variability can affect overall heart failure knowledge. Further, chronic heart failure is a complex condition to self-management. Patients must monitor their sodium intake, manage medications, manage fluids, perform physical activity, assess signs and symptoms of worsening condition, and follow up with healthcare providers [5, 8, 9]. Adherence to heart failure self-care regimens requires that patients apply heart failure knowledge and education principles when making decisions and managing situations [9]. Even when patients receive additional heart failure and self-care education in an outpatient setting based on clinical practice guidelines [8, 10], inadequate health literacy is a potential barrier that prevents knowledge and skills acquisition [5, 11–13].

Health literacy, defined as obtaining, understanding, and using health information, may impact knowledge gained during heart failure education and patient adherence to self-care in heart failure [13]. Prevalence of inadequate health literacy in patients with heart failure ranges from 17.5 to 41% [11, 14–16]. There is no consensus regarding the impact of health literacy on heart failure outcomes [13]. Patients with inadequate health literacy had less heart failure knowledge [17–19] and less adherence to heart failure related self-care regimen expectations [20, 21]; however, in a similarly designed, cross-sectional study, other researchers found no relationship between health literacy and self-care adherence [18].

Self-efficacy also may be influenced by health literacy. Self-efficacy, derived from Bandura's social cognitive theory, is defined as an individual's confidence in his or her ability to perform health behaviors [22, 23]. The level of self-efficacy an individual possesses influences adherence to goals and responses to challenges [22, 23]. Lack of disease-specific knowledge due to inadequate health literacy also may affect patients' self-efficacy regarding their ability to adhere to complex self-care regimens. If individuals lacked self-efficacy (i.e., confidence) regarding their decisions, they did not carry out appropriate self-care [18, 19]; however, in an other research, a lack of patient self-efficacy did not alter adherence to self-care regimens [20].

Educational interventions designed for patients with inadequate health literacy are thought to improve disease knowledge and self-care adherence. Although educational interventions for patients with heart failure and inadequate health literacy improved knowledge, self-efficacy, daily weight measurements [11], and medication adherence [15, 21], one group of researchers found that the effects of education did not last past the intervention [15]. Previously, much of the research on health literacy in heart failure was focused on the impact of inadequate health literacy. For different health literacy levels, little is known about their association with changes in heart failure knowledge, self-efficacy for self-care, and adherence to self-care over time.

2. Objectives

The objectives of this study were to examine associations between health literacy level (inadequate, marginal, and adequate) and heart failure knowledge, self-efficacy for self-care, and self-care adherence longitudinally over a four-month period in community-dwelling adults.

3. Methods

This multicenter study used a correlational, longitudinal design with three data collection periods; baseline, two, and four months. Institutional Review Board (IRB) approval was obtained from each clinical data collection site and Purdue University.

3.1. Participants and Procedures. Participants were recruited from 2009 to 2011 at three heart failure clinics: Cleveland Clinic in the Heart and Vascular Institute (Cleveland, OH, USA), Indiana University Health-Bloomington Hospital HEARTTEAM Cardiopulmonary Rehab and Congestive Heart Failure Center (Bloomington, IN, USA), and Community Health Network Indiana Heart Hospital Healthy Hearts Center (Indianapolis, IN, USA). At each site, heart failure patient education was provided as part of standard care procedures and typically completed in the first two months of care. Education in these clinics is provided primarily by advanced practice nurses (APNs) or registered nurses with consults from registered dieticians or other healthcare providers as applicable. Content is based on heart failure guidelines and includes heart failure diagnosis, self-care, medications, diet, and exercise. The settings differed in that the environments of care were urban, rural, and community based, respectively.

Nursing staff identified new clinic referrals who would meet study inclusion criteria, a new clinic referral, at least 18 years of age, able to read and speak English, and no cognitive impairment based on clinical judgment. Patients were excluded if they resided in a skilled nursing facility or received home healthcare services. Eligible adult patients with heart failure were invited to participate at the initial clinic appointment by researchers who were not involved in direct patient care.

Questionnaires were administered by trained researchers or research assistants; direct patient care providers were not involved in recruitment or data collection. At baseline, questionnaires were administered in private areas of each outpatient heart failure clinic before patients received education. At two, and four months, questionnaires were mailed to

Health Literacy Influences Heart Failure Knowledge Attainment but Not Self-Efficacy for Self-Care or Adherence to
Self-Care over Time

59

participants from the Bloomington Clinic and Community Health Network and were completed via telephone or by mail (at participant's request) at the Cleveland Clinic. The two-months data collection point was chosen as patients completed education by two months. This allowed for a two months period without scheduled education before the four-month assessment.

3.2. Measures. Health literacy was measured using the *Short-Form Test of Functional Health Literacy* (S-TOFHLA) [24]. The S-TOFHLA consists of 36 reading comprehension items, which contain examples of commonly used healthcare materials, and is required to be completed within a 7-minute time frame. Scores were categorized as recommended: inadequate (0–16 points), marginal (17–22 points), and adequate (23-36 points). The S-TOFHLA is a reliable and valid measure of health literacy, with Cronbach's alpha of 0.98 and established criterion validity [24].

Knowledge of heart failure was measured using the *Heart Failure Knowledge Questionnaire* (HFKQ). The HFKQ contains 14 close-ended items and one open-ended, item, and content includes heart failure pathology, symptoms, medications, and self-management. Scores range from 0 (lack of knowledge) to 15 (knowledgeable) and the previously reported Cronbach's alpha of 0.62 [6]. In this study, Cronbach's alpha at baseline assessment (n = 81) was similar at 0.66.

Self-efficacy for heart failure self-care and adherence to heart failure self-care behaviors were measured using the *Self-Care Heart Failure Index* v.6 (SCHFI) that assesses adherence to both self-care maintenance and management behaviors [4, 25]. Of 22 items, 6 items measure self-efficacy, 10 items measure self-care maintenance, and 6 items measure self-care management. Items were rated on a four-point response scale from 1 = never or rarely to 4 = always or daily for the maintenance subscale, from 1 = not confident to 4 = extremely confident for the confidence subscale, and 1 = not quickly, not likely, or not sure to 1 = very quickly, very likely, very sure for the management subscale; then each subscale score was standardized to 100 points [25]. In order to score subscale B (self-care management), patients must have experienced an exacerbation of heart failure within the past two months. A score of ≥70 was used as the cut-point to reflect self-care adequacy in each subscale. Psychometric performance of SCHFI was assessed previously and found to be valid and reliable (maintenance: alpha = 0.553, management: alpha = 0.597, confidence/self-efficacy: alpha = 0.827, and combined maintenance/management: alpha = 0.798) [4, 25, 26].

Patient characteristics were obtained at baseline and included gender, age, marital status, ethnicity/race, education, income, body mass index (BMI), and number of prescription medications.

3.3. Data Analysis. Descriptive statistics were calculated for patient characteristics and included frequencies and percentages for categorical variables and means and standard deviations for continuous variables. Associations between patient characteristics (age, education, BMI, and prescription medications) and study outcomes (heart failure knowledge,

self-efficacy for self-care, and self-care adherence) were examined using Pearson correlations. Difference in baseline patient characteristics and characteristics of patients who completed all follow-up evaluations were assessed using t-tests, Mann-Whitney tests, or One-Way Analysis of Variance (ANOVA) with Bonferroni corrections for multiple comparisons, as appropriate. Differences in characteristics of patients who completed all follow-up evaluations by health literacy level were assessed using t-, Chi-squared, or Kruskal-Wallis tests, as appropriate. Differences in characteristics of patients who completed all follow-up evaluations by study outcome (heart failure knowledge, self-efficacy for self-care, self-care maintenance, and self-care management) were assessed using Pearson correlations or One-Way Analysis of Variance (ANOVA) with Bonferroni corrections for multiple comparisons, as appropriate.

Means and standard deviations were calculated for health literacy at baseline and for knowledge, self-efficacy, and self-care at each assessment period. A power analysis was performed to with a power of 0.8, an alpha of 0.05, and a medium effect size. From that power analysis, a sample size of at least 36 participants was needed to perform the repeated measures ANOVA. Repeated measures ANOVA were performed to determine if differences existed over time, and when significant differences were found, Bonferroni corrections were used to perform multiple comparisons. Profile plots also were generated. An *a priori* level of 0.05 was used for statistical significance. All analyses were performed using IBM SPSS v. 19.0 for Windows (Armonk, NY, USA).

4. Results

4.1. Participant Characteristics. Eighty one participants completed baseline questionnaires; however, analyses were based on participants (n = 51) who completed two-month and/or four-month assessments. Participants were generally young compared to registry data on heart failure, white, graduated from high school, and took nearly 9 prescription medications on a regular basis. Compared to the 81 patients who enrolled in the study, those completing follow-up data collections (n = 51) were not significantly different (P > 0.05, data not shown). All results hereafter will include only patients who completed all follow-up data collections (N = 51). There were significant differences by age, BMI, recruitment site, and marital status by health literacy level (Table 1). Participants with inadequate health literacy were significantly older and were more likely to be recruited from the Bloomington Hospital site. Participants with marginal health literacy had significantly higher BMI than those with adequate health literacy.

Of participant characteristics, there were differences in heart failure knowledge by age, years of education, recruitment site, and marital status (Table 2). In Bonferroni-adjusted posthoc tests for recruitment site and marital status, participants at Cleveland Clinic had significantly more knowledge at baseline than Bloomington Hospital (P = 0.015) and CHN (P = 0.029). Participants who were married had significantly more knowledge than those who were widowed at baseline (P = 0.001), two (P = 0.002), and four months (P = 0.004).

TABLE 1: Demographic information.

Demographic characteristic	All participants $N = 51$	Inadequate health literacy $N = 10$	Marginal health literacy $N = 5$	Adequate health literacy $N = 36$	P value
Age, mean (SD), y	64.68 (13.04)	77.00 (11.79)*	69.20 (10.76)	60.97 (11.71)*	0.002
Years of education, mean (SD), y	13.72 (2.77)	11.89 (2.67)	13.2 (1.79)	14.27 (2.75)	0.061
BMI, mean (SD), kg/m^2	29.84 (8.14)	28.37 (5.59)	38.42 (13.74)*	29.06 (7.31)*	0.042
Prescription medications, mean (SD)	8.78 (4.28)	9.30 (3.53)	10.80 (1.79)	8.36 (4.66)	0.456
Recruitment site, N (%[a])					0.018
Bloomington hospital	19 (37.3)	7 (13.7)	3 (5.9)	9 (17.6)	
Community health network	4 (7.8)	1 (2.0)	0 (0.0)	3 (5.9)	
Cleveland clinic	28 (54.9)	2 (3.9)	2 (3.9)	24 (41.1)	
Male, N (%)	29 (56.9)	5 (9.8)	3 (5.69)	21 (41.2)	0.885
Marital status, N (%)					0.025
Unmarried	5 (9.8)	1 (2.0)	1 (2.0)	3 (5.9)	
Married	34 (66.7)	3 (5.9)	2 (3.9)	29 (56.9)	
Divorced/separated	3 (5.9)	0 (0.0)	1 (2.0)	2 (3.9)	
Widowed	9 (17.6)	6 (11.8)	1 (2.0)	2 (3.9)	
Ethnicity, N (%)					0.287
Black/African American	3 (5.9)	0 (0.0)	1 (2.0)	1 (2.0)	
White/Caucasian	45 (88.2)	9 (17.6)	4 (7.8)	32 (62.7)	
Hispanic/Latino	3 (5.9)	1 (2.0)	0 (0.0)	1 (2.0)	
Financial status, N (%)					0.379
More than enough to make ends meet	22 (43.1)	4 (7.8)	1 (2.0)	17 (33.3)	
Enough to make ends meet	20 (39.2)	5 (9.8)	2 (3.9)	13 (25.5)	
Not enough to make ends meet	9 (7.6)	1 (2.0)	2 (3.9)	6 (11.8)	

*Significant difference between groups in posthoc tests, $P < 0.05$.
[a]All % calculated with a denominator of $N = 51$.

TABLE 2: Participant characteristics and their significant associations or differences in study outcomes.

	Knowledge			Self-efficacy		Self-Care maintenance
	Baseline	2 months	4 months	Baseline	2 months	4 months
Age*						
r	−0.342	−0.482	−0.339	—	—	—
P	0.015	<0.001	<0.001	—	—	—
Years of education*						
r	0.364	0.299	—	—	—	—
P	0.010	0.037	—	—	—	—
BMI*						
r	—	—	—	−0.339	−0.322	—
P	—	—	—	0.017	0.028	—
Recruitment site**						
F	6.535	—	—	4.425	—	3.824
P	0.003	—	—	0.017	—	0.029
Marital status**						
F	5.779	5.169	4.789	—	—	—
P	0.002	0.004	0.005	—	—	—

*Assessed using Pearson correlations.
**Assessed using One-Way Analysis of Variance.

Health Literacy Influences Heart Failure Knowledge Attainment but Not Self-Efficacy for Self-Care or Adherence to
Self-Care over Time

61

TABLE 3: Health literacy, knowledge, self-efficacy, and self-care scores at baseline and followup overall and by health literacy level.

Group	Assessment	Heart failure knowledge[a]		Self-efficacy[b]		Self-care maintenance[b]		Self-care management[b]	
		Mean ± SD	Meaning	Mean ± SD	Meaning[c]	Mean ± SD	Meaning[c]	Mean ± SD	Meaning[c]
Overall	Baseline	8.2 ± 2.7	54.7% correct	69.6 ± 19.4	Not adequate	69.5 ± 16.9	Not adequate	64.3 ± 21.5	Not adequate
	2 months	9.3 ± 3.3	62.0% correct	72.2 ± 15.5	Adequate	76.3 ± 14.9	Adequate	73.4 ± 18.5	Adequate
	4 months	9.6 ± 2.4	64.0% correct	75.0 ± 16.0	Adequate	76.3 ± 14.5	Adequate	70.6 ± 19.7	Adequate
Inadequate health literacy	Baseline	5.3 ± 2.4	35.3% correct	64.2 ± 21.9	Not adequate	63.9 ± 21.7	Not adequate	52.9 ± 32.4	Not adequate
	2 months	5.9 ± 2.5	39.3% correct	72.3 ± 16.0	Adequate	69.7 ± 17.9	Not adequate	68.0 ± 20.2	Not adequate
	4 months	7.8 ± 1.7	52.0% correct	82.8 ± 19.4	Adequate	68.9 ± 15.2	Not adequate	68.6 ± 31.5	Not adequate
Marginal health literacy	Baseline	9.0 ± 1.6	60.0% correct	54.5 ± 10.0	Not adequate	63.3 ± 18.6	Not adequate	70.0 ± 22.0	Adequate
	2 months	9.0 ± 2.9	60.0% correct	67.8 ± 10.7	Not adequate	80.0 ± 13.3	Adequate	65.0 ± 35.4	Not adequate
	4 months	8.8 ± 3.8	58.7% correct	66.8 ± 6.7	Not adequate	76.7 ± 10.5	Adequate	62.5 ± 24.7	Not adequate
Adequate health literacy	Baseline	8.8 ± 2.3	58.7% correct	73.0 ± 18.8	Adequate	72.0 ± 15.1	Adequate	66.5 ± 17.8	Not adequate
	2 months	10.2 ± 3.0	68.0% correct	76.3 ± 16.2	Adequate	77.6 ± 14.1	Adequate	76.3 ± 16.6	Adequate
	4 months	10.3 ± 2.1	68.7% correct	74.3 ± 15.8	Adequate	76.3 ± 14.5	Adequate	72.4 ± 13.4	Adequate

[a]Possible range 0–15.
[b]Possible range 0–100.
[c]Adequacy, according to the SCHFI, is at scores ≥70.

TABLE 4: Longitudinal effects of health literacy on outcomes using repeated measures analysis of variance.

Effect	Knowledge		Self-efficacy		Self-care maintenance		Self-care management	
	F	P	F	P	F	P	F	P
Time	3.519	0.034	1.954	0.148	6.942	0.002	0.285	0.754
Health literacy	11.096	<0.001	1.364	0.267	1.682	0.197	0.307	0.741
Time*health literacy	1.189	0.131	1.037	0.393	0.707	0.589	1.376	0.269

There were differences in self-efficacy for self-care by recruitment site and BMI. In Bonferroni-adjusted posthoc tests, participants at Bloomington Hospital had significantly lower self-efficacy for self-care than participants at the CHN site ($P = 0.032$) at baseline. BMI was negatively associated with self-efficacy for self-care at baseline and two months.

There were differences in self-care maintenance by recruitment site. In Bonferroni-adjusted posthoc tests, participants at Cleveland Clinic had significantly higher self-care maintenance adherence than participants at the CHN site ($P = 0.026$) at 4 months. There were no other significant differences in or associations with outcomes based on participant characteristics.

4.2. Adequacy of Health Literacy and Outcomes. At baseline, mean health literacy was adequate, but heart failure knowledge was low (failing mean score by testing standards), and self-efficacy for self-care and adherence to self-care maintenance and management behaviors were below cut off scores, reflecting inadequacy (Table 3). Of participants, 41.2% had adequate self-efficacy for performing self-care at baseline.

By the four-month followup, knowledge level remained low but increased to 64% (equaling a "D grade" by testing standards), and self-efficacy for self-care behaviors and adherence to self-care increased to adequate levels. Patient knowledge and self-care maintenance significantly improved over time ($P = 0.012$ and $P = 0.002$, resp.), but patient

self-care management and self-efficacy did not significantly improve over time ($P = 0.754$ and $P = 0.148$, resp.).

4.3. Assessment of the Impact of Baseline Health Literacy over Time. Health literacy categories at baseline were used to assess outcomes over time (Table 4). There were significant effects of health literacy on heart failure knowledge over time, but no effects of health literacy on other outcomes (self-efficacy and self-care). There was a significant effect of time on heart failure knowledge. There was no time-health literacy interaction, as evidenced by a nonsignificant P value and the profile plot (Figure 1), which indicated significant effects of both time and health literacy.

To further examine the differences in knowledge by health literacy level, Bonferonni-adjusted posthoc tests were performed, and patients with inadequate health literacy had significantly less knowledge than those with adequate ($P < 0.001$) but not marginal ($P = 0.073$) health literacy, as seen in Figure 1. Although patients with inadequate health literacy had a larger rise in heart failure knowledge score at 4 months compared to those with marginal and adequate health literacy at baseline, heart failure knowledge levels remained below that of patients with adequate health literacy (Figure 1).

5. Discussion

In this study, the importance of health literacy on heart failure knowledge score, self-efficacy for heart failure self-care, and

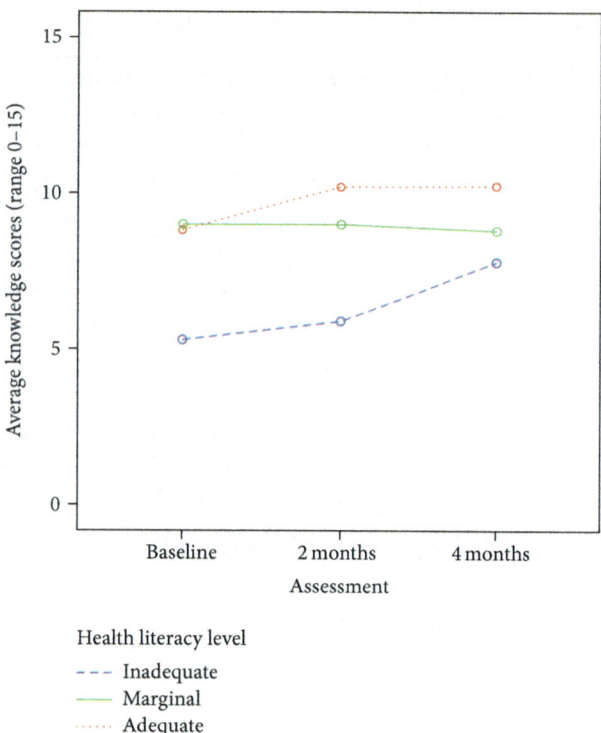

FIGURE 1: Changes in knowledge by health literacy level over time.

adherence to heart failure self-care was examined over a four-month period. There were positive, longitudinal associations between health literacy and knowledge (higher health literacy with greater knowledge) but not between health literacy and self-efficacy for self-care or self-care adherence. Traditional clinic-based education improved knowledge overall, but the knowledge level of individuals with inadequate health literacy never improved to the level of those with adequate health literacy. Therefore, traditional clinic-based education may not be the best method to improve heart failure knowledge gaps over time for patients with inadequate health literacy. Moreover, since adherence to heart failure self-care behaviors improves clinical outcomes in heart failure [5, 11, 27], determining reasons for nonadherence, beyond health literacy, may be a key element in promoting heart failure self-care maintenance and management.

Disease-specific education has been found to improve knowledge in heart failure [11, 28, 29]. In this study, patients with inadequate and adequate health literacy experienced gains in knowledge during traditional clinic-based education. DeWalt and colleagues found education for patients with inadequate health literacy improved heart failure knowledge [11]. Similarly, we found that patients with inadequate health literacy demonstrated improved heart failure knowledge over the course of traditional clinic-based education. Over time, patients with inadequate health literacy continued to experience knowledge gains but had less heart failure knowledge than patients with adequate health literacy across both assessments. Since the distribution of inadequate literacy patients in this study mirrors other research and the health

literacy levels are representative of the general heart failure population [11, 14, 15], the results of this study indicate that traditional education efforts may not reduce the knowledge disparity between patients with inadequate and adequate health literacy. Furthermore, researchers found in a diabetes educational intervention that although all patients gained considerable knowledge, patients with low health literacy did not gain as much as higher health-literate patients [30].

In three other studies, researchers consistently found that health literacy and patient heart failure knowledge are related [17–19]. Similar to our study, these studies used the TOFHLA [19] or the S-TOFHLA [17, 18] to measure health literacy, but each study utilized different measures of heart failure knowledge. Despite differences in measuring heart failure knowledge, other studies confirmed our findings that patients with inadequate health literacy had less heart failure knowledge. Furthermore, posthoc power analyses revealed that there was sufficient power to examine the difference (using repeated measures ANOVA) between health literacy categories with regard to knowledge (partial $\eta^2 = 0.316$, power = 0.988). Clinic-based education improves heart failure knowledge for patients with inadequate health literacy. However, further educational efforts for patients with inadequate health literacy are needed to reduce the disparity in knowledge between patients with inadequate and adequate health literacy.

Interestingly, patients with marginal health literacy did not improve over time. The relationship between marginal health literacy and heart failure knowledge is not a common focus of most research. Researchers in one study found no association between marginal health literacy and heart failure knowledge [17], although researchers in another study found that patients with marginal health literacy had significantly less knowledge than those with adequate health literacy [18]. Other researchers have taken the approach of collapsing the categories of inadequate and marginal health into one category of low health literacy. Further longitudinal research is needed to support our findings regarding marginal health literacy and heart failure knowledge.

We were surprised that over time, health literacy category was not associated with self-efficacy for heart failure self-care and self-care adherence in newly referred patients to a heart failure clinic. However, this could be due to a lack of power to detect differences. Posthoc power analyses revealed a lack of power in assessing self-efficacy (partial $\eta^2 = 0.062$, power = 0.277), self-care maintenance (partial $\eta^2 = 0.065$, power = 0.337), or self-care management (partial $\eta^2 = 0.045$, power = 0.089). Since the self-care management scale could only be scored if participants had symptoms in the prior two months, only 13 patients had scorable self-care management responses at all three assessments (participants with symptoms at baseline $N = 39$, two months $N = 23$, and four months $N = 26$) and were eligible for repeated measures ANOVA.

In prior literature, relationships between health literacy and heart failure self-efficacy for self-care and self-care adherence were measured at only one point in time, and results were inconsistent. In a small, cross-sectional pilot study, researchers found no relationship between health literacy and self-efficacy [20], similar to our results. In larger studies, relationships between health literacy and self-efficacy differed from ours. When 95 patients with chronic heart failure were assessed during hospital admission, a significant relationship between health literacy and self-efficacy was found on univariate analysis, but the sample was too small to complete multivariate analysis [18]. It is unknown if whether self-efficacy or patient characteristics (age, gender, etc.) would be mediators for the relationship between health literacy and self-care had further analyses been performed. In a large sample (N = 605), self-efficacy was a mediator between health literacy and self-care in a structural equation model [19]. To our knowledge, our research provides the first examination of health literacy and self-efficacy longitudinally. Further research with larger sample sizes and adequately powered to detect differences is needed to examine these relationships over time. With larger samples, significant baseline factors can be controlled for to learn the importance of health literacy on outcomes.

5.1. Limitations. Findings may be limited due to the majority of study participants having adequate health literacy scores. A new referral to a heart failure clinic may not necessarily mean a recent heart failure diagnosis. Patients may have had heart failure for some time and could have been treated elsewhere before referral. Previous heart failure education materials could have been developed based on low health literacy or reading levels, minimizing health literacy as an important factor in self-efficacy for self-care and self-care adherence. Prior education delivery and experiences in self-assessment and management of heart failure symptoms and outcomes of self-care behaviors could also have affected study findings, although heart failure knowledge, self-efficacy, and self-care adherence scores were below desired levels at baseline.

Participant recruitment and retention may impact study findings and contributed to a lack of statistical power to assess self-efficacy and self-care. A total of 80 participants were initially enrolled, but 51 completed the study. An attempt was made to minimize attrition by making multiple attempts for followup at each assessment, and there were no significant differences in demographic characteristics between those at baseline and those who completed the study. We found significant associations between several demographic characteristics and study outcomes. In particular, younger participant age and more years of formal education were associated with higher heart failure knowledge. However, due to attrition, multivariate regression between participant characteristics and outcomes (heart failure knowledge, self-efficacy for self-care, and self-care adherence) or between recruitment site (taking into account educational or patient differences) and outcomes was unable to be performed. Future work should include these characteristics and should be adequately powered to better assess self-efficacy, self-care maintenance, and self-care management.

Other limitations in this study include length of longitudinal assessment, potential of participants with mild cognitive dysfunction to be included, and the use of self-report measures that were valid and short but limited in scope. The four-month assessment (two months after education were completed) may not have been long enough to see the effects of health literacy on patient outcomes over time. However, Murray and colleagues [15] found that the effects of an educational intervention declined once the intervention ended, therefore, it is probable that the longitudinal effects could be seen at the four-month assessment. Future work should include a longer followup, such as six months or one year. While clinical judgment was utilized to exclude patients with cognitive impairment, some participants included in this study may have had undiagnosed mild cognitive impairment. Mild cognitive impairment has been found to lead to lower health literacy and poorer self-care and may have impacted results in this study.

6. Conclusions

Although health literacy was associated with patients' gain in heart failure knowledge over time, particularly in patients with low health literacy, health literacy was not associated with heart failure self-efficacy in performing self-care or self-care adherence. Examining the influence of health literacy on heart failure knowledge, self-efficacy for self-care, and self-care adherence over four months clarified some of the cross-sectional findings related to knowledge, self-efficacy, and self-care; however, these relationships are complex and merit further study. Investigators should examine approaches and work collaboratively with healthcare professionals to improve knowledge gains among inadequate health literacy patients during clinic-based education.

Acknowledgments

This work was supported by a seed grant from the Purdue University Regenstrief Center for Healthcare Engineering, the Clifford Kinley Trust (Purdue University), the American Association of Heart Failure Nurses Bernard Saperstein Grant, and the Delta Omicron Chapter of Sigma Theta Tau International. Support for Aleda Chen while a graduate student was provided by the National Institute on Aging (T32AG025671), the Purdue University Center on Aging and the Life Course, and from the American Foundation for Pharmaceutical Excellence. The authors would like to thank Susie Carter, RN, BC, FAACVPR, and AACC, Manager of Cardiopulmonary Rehab at the Advanced Heart Care Center, Indiana University Health Bloomington Hospital, Jennifer Forney, BSN, RN, Ellen Slifcak, BA, RN, and Susan Krajewski BSN, RN, and MPA, Cleveland Clinic for their assistance and support of this project. Thanks are due to Mary Kiersma, Pharm.D., Ph.D., Director of Assessment at Manchester College, for her review of this paper.

References

[1] L. Liu, "Changes in cardiovascular hospitalization and comorbidity of heart failure in the United States: findings from the National Hospital Discharge Surveys 1980–2006," *International Journal of Cardiology*, vol. 149, no. 1, pp. 39–45, 2011.

[2] P. A. Heidenreich, J. G. Trogdon, O. A. Khavjou et al., "Forecasting the future of cardiovascular disease in the United States:

a policy statement from the American Heart Association," *Circulation*, vol. 123, no. 8, pp. 933–944, 2011.

[3] A. S. Go, D. Mozaffarian, V. L. Roger et al., "Heart disease and stroke statistics—2013 update: a report from the American Heart Association," *Circulation*, vol. 127, no. 1, pp. e6–e245, 2013.

[4] B. Riegel, B. Carlson, D. K. Moser, M. Sebern, F. D. Hicks, and V. Roland, "Psychometric testing of the self-care of heart failure index," *Journal of Cardiac Failure*, vol. 10, no. 4, pp. 350–360, 2004.

[5] B. Riegel, D. K. Moser, S. D. Anker et al., "State of the science: promoting self-care in persons with heart failure: a scientific statement from the american heart association," *Circulation*, vol. 120, no. 12, pp. 1141–1163, 2009.

[6] N. T. Artinian, M. Magnan, M. Sloan, and M. P. Lange, "Self-care behaviors among patients with heart failure," *Heart and Lung: Journal of Acute and Critical Care*, vol. 31, no. 3, pp. 161–172, 2002.

[7] M. H. L. van der Wal, T. Jaarsma, D. K. Moser, N. J. G. M. Veeger, W. H. van Gilst, and D. J. van Veldhuisen, "Compliance in heart failure patients: the importance of knowledge and beliefs," *European Heart Journal*, vol. 27, no. 4, pp. 434–440, 2006.

[8] J. Lindenfeld, N. M. Albert, J. P. Boehmer et al., "HFSA 2010 comprehensive heart failure practice guideline," *Journal of Cardiac Failure*, vol. 16, no. 6, pp. e1–e194, 2010.

[9] N. M. Albert, "Promoting self-care in heart failure: state of clinical practice based on the perspectives of healthcare systems and providers," *Journal of Cardiovascular Nursing*, vol. 23, no. 3, pp. 277–284, 2008.

[10] D. G. Vreeland, R. E. Rea, and L. L. Montgomery, "A review of the literature on heart failure and discharge education," *Critical Care Nursing Quarterly*, vol. 34, no. 3, pp. 235–245, 2011.

[11] D. A. DeWalt, R. M. Malone, M. E. Bryant et al., "A heart failure self-management program for patients of all literacy levels: a randomized, controlled trial," *BMC Health Services Research*, vol. 6, article 30, 2006.

[12] L. S. Evangelista and M. A. Shinnick, "What do we know about adherence and self-care?" *Journal of Cardiovascular Nursing*, vol. 23, no. 3, pp. 250–257, 2008.

[13] N. D. Berkman, S. L. Sheridan, K. E. Donahue et al., "Health literacy interventions and outcomes: an updated systematic review," Evidence Report/Technology Assesment 199, Agency for Healthcare Research and Quality, Rockville, Md, USA, 2011, Prepared by RTI International—University of North Carolina Evidence-based Practice Center under contract no. 290-2007-10056-I, AHRQ Publication no. 11-E006.

[14] P. N. Peterson, S. M. Shetterly, C. L. Clarke et al., "Health literacy and outcomes among patients with heart failure," *Journal of the American Medical Association*, vol. 305, no. 16, pp. 1695–1701, 2011.

[15] M. D. Murray, J. Young, S. Hoke et al., "Pharmacist intervention to improve medication adherence in heart failure: a randomized trial," *Annals of Internal Medicine*, vol. 146, no. 10, pp. 714–725, 2007.

[16] D. Morrow, D. Clark, W. Tu et al., "Correlates of health literacy in patients with chronic heart failure," *Gerontologist*, vol. 46, no. 5, pp. 669–676, 2006.

[17] J. A. Gazmararian, M. V. Williams, J. Peel, and D. W. Baker, "Health literacy and knowledge of chronic disease," *Patient Education and Counseling*, vol. 51, no. 3, pp. 267–275, 2003.

[18] C. R. Dennison, M. L. McEntee, L. Samuel et al., "Adequate health literacy is associated with higher heart failure knowledge and self-care confidence in hospitalized patients," *Journal of Cardiovascular Nursing*, vol. 26, no. 5, pp. 359–367, 2011.

[19] A. MacAbasco-O'Connell, D. A. Dewalt, K. A. Broucksou et al., "Relationship between literacy, knowledge, self-care behaviors, and heart failure-related quality of life among patients with heart failure," *Journal of General Internal Medicine*, vol. 26, no. 9, pp. 979–986, 2011.

[20] A. M. H. Chen, K. S. Yehle, K. S. Plake, M. M. Murawski, and H. L. Mason, "Health literacy and self-care of patients with heart failure," *Journal of Cardiovascular Nursing*, vol. 26, no. 6, pp. 446–451, 2011.

[21] M. Noureldin, K. S. Plake, D. G. Morrow, W. Tu, J. Wu, and M. D. Murray, "of health literacy on drug adherence in patients with heart failure," *Pharmacotherapy*, vol. 32, no. 9, pp. 819–826, 2012.

[22] A. Bandura, "Self-efficacy: toward a unifying theory of behavioral change," *Psychological Review*, vol. 84, no. 2, pp. 191–215, 1977.

[23] K. S. Yehle and K. S. Plake, "Self-efficacy and educational interventions in heart failure: a review of the literature," *Journal of Cardiovascular Nursing*, vol. 25, no. 3, pp. 175–188, 2010.

[24] D. W. Baker, M. V. Williams, R. M. Parker, J. A. Gazmararian, and J. Nurss, "Development of a brief test to measure functional health literacy," *Patient Education and Counseling*, vol. 38, no. 1, pp. 33–42, 1999.

[25] B. Riegel, C. S. Lee, V. V. Dickson, and B. Carlson, "An update on the self-care of heart failure index," *Journal of Cardiovascular Nursing*, vol. 24, no. 6, pp. 485–497, 2009.

[26] K. S. Yehle, *A comparison of standard office visits and shared medical appointments in adults with heart failure [doctoral dissertation]*, Touro University International, Cypress, Calif, USA, 2007.

[27] F. A. McAlister, S. Stewart, S. Ferrua, and J. J. J. V. McMurray, "Multidisciplinary strategies for the management of heart failure patients at high risk for admission: a systematic review of randomized trials," *Journal of the American College of Cardiology*, vol. 44, no. 4, pp. 810–819, 2004.

[28] M. A. Caldwell, K. J. Peters, and K. A. Dracup, "A simplified education program improves knowledge, self-care behavior, and disease severity in heart failure patients in rural settings," *American Heart Journal*, vol. 150, no. 5, pp. 983.e7–983.e12, 2005.

[29] D. W. Baker, D. A. DeWalt, D. Schillinger et al., "The effect of progressive, reinforcing telephone education and counseling versus brief educational intervention on knowledge, self-care behaviors and heart failure symptoms," *Journal of Cardiac Failure*, vol. 17, no. 10, pp. 789–796, 2011.

[30] N. R. Kandula, P. A. Nsiah-Kumi, G. Makoul et al., "The relationship between health literacy and knowledge improvement after a multimedia type 2 diabetes education program," *Patient Education and Counseling*, vol. 75, no. 3, pp. 321–327, 2009.

9

Promoting Neonatal Staff Nurses' Comfort and Involvement in End of Life and Bereavement Care

Weihua Zhang[1] and Betty S. Lane[2]

[1] *Nell Hodgson Woodruff School of Nursing, Emory University, 1520 Clifton Road, Atlanta, GA 30322-4207, USA*
[2] *Clayton State University, 2000 Clayton State Boulevard, Morrow, GA 30260-0285, USA*

Correspondence should be addressed to Weihua Zhang; wzhang3@emory.edu

Academic Editor: Linda Moneyham

Background. Nurses who provide end of life and bereavement care to neonates and their families are potentially at risk for developing stress-related health problems. These health problems can negatively affect nurses' ability to care for their patients. *Purpose.* Nurses need to be knowledgeable about end of life and bereavement issues to provide quality care. This study sought to evaluate the effect of a bereavement seminar on the attitudes of nurses regarding end of life and palliative care of neonates. *Design.* A convenience sample of fourteen neonatal nurses completed a Bereavement/End of Life Attitudes about Care of Neonatal Nurses Scale after a bereavement seminar designed to provide information on end of life care. A pre- and posttest design with an intervention and control group was used to assess changes in nurse bereavement attitudes in relationship to comfort, role, and involvement. *Results.* After bereavement seminar, the seminar attendees had higher levels of comfort in providing end of life care than nurses in the control group ($t = -0.214$; $P = 0.04$). *Discussion.* Nurses' comfort levels can be improved by attending continuing education on end of life care and having their thoughts on ethical issues in end of life care acknowledged by their peers.

1. Introduction

Nurses who provide end of life and bereavement care to infants and their families are potentially at great risk for developing stress-related health problems. The emotional strain associated with end of life and bereavement care not only affects a nurse's health but can also affect relationships at home and with coworkers. The stress experienced by a nurse can even affect the quality of care provided to patients and parents [1, 2]. Moral distress is recognized as one of the major sources of stress for nurses who provide end of life care to infants. Factors that induce moral distress in nurses can result from providing care to infants who have withdrawal of treatment followed by death or extending futile treatment that induces unnecessary suffering [3]. There has been an increase in the proportion of deaths associated with decisions to forgo intensive care treatment from 23% in 1987 to 1988 to 64% in 1998 to 1999 [4]. More than half of neonatal deaths are associated with withdrawal of treatment [5], and treatment-related stressors to health care professionals have no doubt increased over the years as a result of advanced treatment options [6, 7].

Nurses need to be knowledgeable about bereavement and end of life issues and need to be comfortable in their interactions in order to provide quality bereavement and end of life care [8, 9]. It is a nurse's obligation to act on behalf of the patients and their families to ensure that the care provided is congruent with their preferences. A key to fulfilling this obligation is to cultivate relations with patients and their families [10]. The American Academy of Pediatrics committee on bioethics and its committee on hospital care stated in their integrated model of palliative care that palliative care should be offered at diagnosis and continued throughout the course of illness, whether care results in cure or death [11]. It is recommended that an uncertain prognosis should be a signal to initiate, rather than to delay, palliative care discussion [12]. Palliative care is not limited to end of life care; however, it ensures quality of end of life care. However, studies have indicated that neonatal nurses often are not comfortable with providing end of life care to infants. Some of the reasons associated with this discomfort are inadequate nursing education related to bereavement care in nursing school or in their place of employment [13, 14]. Other factors that may elevate the stress levels of nurses who provide end of life care to infants are provider's age, life experience, and clinical experiences that involve management of ethical dilemmas. It has been suggested that nurses' prior knowledge of end of life care is correlated with nurses' comfort in providing related care [15]. Nurses' moral distress can affect communication with parents, thus leading to changes in parents' perceptions of the quality of nursing care [16]. Nurses are viewed by families as being more supportive than physicians during grief. However, communication problems and a lack of awareness of cultural issues can serve as barrier that can cause parents to feel abandoned and that nurses lack sensitivity [17]. In addition, noneffective communication between health care professionals and infant's parents has been identified as one of the barriers that could cause unnecessary conflict in providing infant's care [18]. Issues related to the parents' cultural background can profoundly influence medical ethical decision making for infant's care [19, 20] and can result in moral distress in nurses.

The literature indicates that nurses experience stress and moral discomfort in the provision of end of life and bereavement care. Ethical issues related to withdrawal of treatment and futile treatments are major contributors to nursing stress. Nurses' personal characteristics and experiences can impact their response to bereavement stress. Communication and awareness of cultural needs are also recognized as important in the care of patients and families. This study contributes to the literature because it is an intervention study which evaluates nurses' perceptions about their role, comfort, and involvement in end of life and bereavement care following an educational seminar.

2. Purpose

In recognition of the stress experienced by nurses in providing end of life care to infants, the women's center of a level II hospital in the southeast offered a bereavement seminar to nurses who work in areas that experience infant deaths. The purpose of this study was to evaluate the effectiveness of the bereavement seminar on the attitudes of nurses regarding end of life care of neonates. The research questions were as follows: (1) what are the characteristics and attitudes of nurses who provide end of life/bereavement care to infants? (2) Is there a difference in nursing role, comfort, and involvement in providing end of life care between pre- and posttest scores of nurses who attended a bereavement seminar? (3) Will nurses who attend the educational seminar have higher scores in the domains of comfort, role, and involvement than the control group?

3. Design and Methods

A pre- and posttest design with a nonequivalent control group and intervention group was used to compare the effect of the bereavement seminar on role, comfort, and involvement. A convenience sample of nurses was drawn from a community hospital in the southeastern United States. Nurses were eligible to participate in the study if they worked in Labor and Delivery, NICU, Mother Baby, Pediatrics, or the Emergency Department and worked directly with patients and were not in an administrative position. Nurses who attended the one-day education program were enrolled in this study as the intervention group. The control group comprised those who did not attend the education program, but worked in areas that provide end of life or bereavement care to infants. Nurses voluntarily signed up to attend the bereavement seminar and participate in the study.

3.1. Instruments. Bereavement/End of life Attitudes About Care of Neonatal Nurses Scale (BEACONNS) was the instrument used for this study [21]. Permission to use the BEACONNS Scale was obtained from Engler and Associates, the researchers who had developed the instrument. Reliability for the instrument when used in a descriptive study ranged between 0.81 and 0.95 [21]; it has not yet been used in quasiexperimental design. There are three domains in the BEACONNS scale: (1) the comfort level of handling end of life and bereavement care, (2) role of propensity in providing end of life and bereavement care, (3) tendency of allowing family involvement in providing end of life care.

3.1.1. Comfort Scale. The comfort scale measures nurses' perceptions about the degree of comfort they felt with various aspects of bereavement/end of life care. There are 19 Likert-scale items in this subscale, with scores ranging from 1 (very uncomfortable) to 5 (very comfortable). The 19 items are summed for a total score. Higher total scores indicate greater comfort levels with providing end of life care. The reliability for the comfort scale Cronbach α is 0.95 [21].

3.1.2. Role Scale. The 18-item Likert-type role scale measures nurses' perceptions of their roles with families of critically ill and/or dying infants; scores range from 1 (strongly disagree) to 5 (strongly agree). Some items required reverse scoring. The 18 items are summed for a total score. Higher total scores indicate more supportive roles in facilitating families' involvement in end of life/bereavement care. The reliability of the role scale Cronbach α is 0.85 [21].

3.1.3. Involvement Scale. The 14-item involvement scale measures nurses' ratings of the importance of various factors relative to their involvement with patients and families. The Likert-type scale ranges from 1 (very unimportant) to 5 (very important), and the items are summed for a total score. The higher the total score, the more the involvement nurses thought they should have with their patients and families. The reliability for the involvement scale Cronbach α is 0.85 [21].

3.1.4. Other Demographic Variables. In the BEACONNS instrument, there are additional items that acquire information about a nurse's educational background, ethnicity, prior experience with infant death, and significant personal loss.

3.2. Procedure. Institutional approval for conducting the study was obtained prior to the study from the Professional Development Council from the institution where all nurses were recruited. Information obtained was confidential and findings were reported in group format. An eight-hour end of life/bereavement seminar was developed by a planning committee of staff representatives from the areas that experience fetal and infant deaths. The seminar was entitled "How do I make IT feel better?" "IT" refers to the physiological and psychological impact of loss on both family and staff. The objective of the seminar was to alleviate this impact and reduce staff's moral distress. The seminar focused on developing strategies to support the caregiver and family in dealing with their grief and to utilize support services in the community and hospital. It also focused on dealing with ethics issues and improving communication skills. Flyers and brochures were sent out to the Labor and Delivery, Mother-Baby, NICU, Pediatrics, and the Emergency Departments advertising the workshop.

Nurses who were direct patient care providers were invited to participate in the study through distribution of a flyer and communication at staff meetings. The morning of the bereavement seminar prior to the start of the program the nurses who wished to participate in the study signed a consent form and completed the BEACONNS survey. This group represented the intervention group and the survey completed before the seminar was the pretest survey. The BEACONNS survey and a consent form were also distributed to these selected departments and all staff nurses were invited to complete the survey as the control group. Two months after the bereavement program, the intervention group completed a second BEACONNS scale as the posttest survey.

4. Results

4.1. Characteristics of Sample. Data were analyzed using SPSS version 14. Descriptive statistics were performed to measure frequencies, means, and percentages. Independent and paired t-tests were conducted to test for statistical mean differences between the pre- and the posttest group. An independent t-test was used to compare the differences between the intervention and the control groups. A total of 63 nurses participated in the study. The majority was married (83%), Protestant (34.4%), and Caucasian (82.3%) and had children (84%). Most held a BSN (46.8%) or an ADN (41.9%) degree and worked in the NICU (38.7%). The average age of the nurses who participated in the study was 39.42 years (SD 10.5). The average years of working experience as a nurse were 5.29 years (SD 8.2). Nineteen percent had experienced a significant personal loss in the past year. Seventy-one percent had end of life/bereavement care in their basic nursing education. Less than half (43.5%) were satisfied or very satisfied with their prior end of life nursing education. Slightly more than a fourth (28.6%) had attended continuing education courses on end of life/bereavement care. Over three-fourths had cared for dying infants. When asked who was most important in providing support to families of critically ill infants on a daily basis participants indicated that

nurses (mean = 4.70) were most important (5 indicates the most important role, and 1 indicates the least important role), followed by physicians (mean = 4.43) and chaplains (mean = 4.05).

4.2. Data Analysis. To answer the research question "was there a difference between pre- and posttest scores of nurses who attended the bereavement seminar?", a paired t-test was used. Data from nurses prior to the seminar and two months after the seminar were compared. Nineteen participants completed the pretest questionnaire; only 14 participants returned the posttest questionnaire of nurses' comfort level with end of life/bereavement care being significantly increased ($t = -3.37$, $P = 0.01$).¡?ehlt?¿ However, postrole scores were not significantly different from the prerole scores ($t = 1.09$, $P = 0.30$). Likewise, postinvolvement scores were not significantly different from the preinvolvement scores ($t = -0.19$, $P = 0.84$). Boxplots and paired "ladder" plots were used to provide illustrative support for these findings.

An independent t-test was performed in order to answer the third research question, "is there a difference in the three domains between the nurse groups who attended the workshop and the group that had not attended the workshop?" The first survey prior to the seminar was used to analyze the difference. No differences were found between these two groups in comfort level ($t = 0.77$, $P = 0.44$), role ($t = 0.09$, $P = 0.92$), and involvement ($t = 0.24$, $P = 0.82$). Further, no difference was detected in those who signed up for the class and those who did not sign up for the class in whether they had previous training in end of life care/bereavement care. However, the difference in satisfaction with previous end of life/bereavement care training was significant in those who came to the workshop and those who did not come to the workshop. Those who came to the workshop were less satisfied with their previous end of life/bereavement care training than those who did not come ($t = -2.21$, $P = 0.03$).

5. Discussion and Conclusions

The majority of the sample was Caucasian, Christian, married, and had children. Slightly more of the staff was BSN prepared and the mean age was 39.42. These demographic characteristics were similar to the participants in a study by Engler et al. [21] that looked at neonatal staff and advanced practice nurses' perceptions of bereavement/end of life care. However, the nurses in Engler's study had worked on average over twice as long (16.4 versus 5.29 years) and had a greater percentage of nurses who had experienced a significant loss in the past year (31 versus 19 percent). The difference in the number of years worked may reflect the transient nature of the southeast population and the location of several nursing programs near the hospital. The greater percentage of nurses who had experienced loss in the Engler study may be due to that sample being slightly older than the nurses in the current study.

Most nurses had received end of life care in their basic nursing programs; interestingly, less than half were pleased with these offerings. Those who came to the workshop were less satisfied with their previous end of life nursing education training, which may have been a motivator for their attendance at the bereavement workshop. These nurses in the study have been working in areas that experience neonatal deaths; surprisingly only a third had attended continuing education on end of life/bereavement care.

Another important finding was that the intervention group's comfort level had increased at the posttest which was 2 months after the seminar. This supports the findings of Fredrickson et al. who found that a nurse's prior education about end of life care increases comfort and decreases moral distress. The comfort level increments could be the result of the seminar content as well as the interactions among nurses during the daylong seminar. A noticeable observation from this seminar is that nurses are gaining new knowledge while they were sharing their own experience and acknowledging their peers. There was not a significant difference in role perceptions between or among groups. The participants felt that their role in providing support to families of critically ill infants on a daily basis was more important than that provided by physicians. Involvement was not significantly different between the two groups. A lack of statistical difference between the control and intervention group may have been due to the small sample size. Also, nurses who did not attend the seminar may have already felt at ease in the areas of comfort, role, and involvement. In addition, the reliability of the involvement scale may have been affected by the phrasing of the directional stem on the Likert scale; many nurses found the involvement scale confusing.

The results of this study supported the use of a bereavement seminar to increase nurse comfort levels in the provision of end of life/bereavement care to infants and families in the intervention group. Nurses overall were not satisfied with the end of life/bereavement education they had received in their undergraduate nursing programs. This suggests a need for nursing schools to ensure their curricula should include content on caring for critically ill and dying neonates and their families. Nurses who work on units with neonates need supportive continuing education, since three-fourths of the nurses had experienced neonatal deaths, yet only one-fourth had attended continuing education on end of life/bereavement care. Future intervention studies are needed with larger nurse populations in order to evaluate the effectiveness of end of life/bereavement education on comfort and involvement in end of life care. Studies should also assess whether greater nurse comfort scores impact family satisfaction with end of life/bereavement of their neonate.

Acknowledgment

The authors wish to thank the nurses who participated in the bereavement workshop and study.

References

[1] M. C. Corley and P. Minick, "Moral distress or moral comfort," *Bioethics Forum*, vol. 18, no. 1-2, pp. 7–14, 2002.

[2] B. M. Yam, J. C. Rossiter, and K. Y. Cheung, "Caring for dying infants: experiences of neonatal intensive care nurses in Hong Kong," *Journal of Clinical Nursing*, vol. 10, no. 5, pp. 651–659, 2001.

[3] G. Gale and A. Brooks, "Implementing a palliative care program in a newborn intensive care unit," *Advances in Neonatal Care*, vol. 6, no. 1, pp. 37–53, 2006.

[4] C. M. Hagen and T. W. Hansen, "Deaths in a neonatal intensive care unit: a 10-year perspective," *Pediatric Critical Care Medicine*, vol. 5, no. 5, pp. 463–468, 2004.

[5] D. J. Wilkinson, J. J. Fitzsimons, P. A. Dargaville et al., "Death in the neonatal intensive care unit: changing patterns of end of life care over two decades," *Archives of Disease in Childhood*, vol. 91, no. 4, pp. F268–F271, 2006.

[6] C. A. Fajardo, S. Gonzalez, G. Zambosco et al., "End of life, death and dying in neonatal intensive care units in Latin America," *Acta Paediatrica*, vol. 101, no. 6, pp. 609–613, 2012.

[7] W. Meadow, "End-of-life: death and dying in neonatal intensive care units-a North American perspective," *Acta Paediatrica*, vol. 101, no. 6, pp. 550–551, 2012.

[8] M. F. Chan, F. L. Lou, F. L. Cao, P. Li, L. Liu, and L. H. Wu, "Investigating factors associated with nurses' attitudes towards perinatal bereavement care: a study in Shandong and Hong Kong," *Journal of Clinical Nursing*, vol. 18, no. 16, pp. 2344–2354, 2009.

[9] C. Moon Fai and D. Gordon Arthur, "Nurses' attitudes towards perinatal bereavement care," *Journal of Advanced Nursing*, vol. 65, no. 12, pp. 2532–2541, 2009.

[10] C. H. Rushton, B. D. Kaylor, and M. Christopher, "Twenty years since Cruzan and the patient self-determination act: opportunities for improving care at the end of life in critical care settings," *AACN Advanced Critical Care*, vol. 23, no. 1, pp. 99–106, 2012.

[11] American Academy of Pediatrics, "American academy of pediatrics. Committee on bioethics and committee on hospital care. Palliative care for children," *Pediatrics*, vol. 106, no. 2, part 1, pp. 351–357, 2000.

[12] B. Davies, S. A. Sehring, J. C. Partridge et al., "Barriers to palliative care for children: perceptions of pediatric health care providers," *Pediatrics*, vol. 121, no. 2, pp. 282–288, 2008.

[13] M. F. Chan, L. H. Wu, M. C. Day, and S. H. Chan, "Attitudes of nurses toward perinatal bereavement: findings from a study in Hong Kong," *Journal of Perinatal and Neonatal Nursing*, vol. 19, no. 3, pp. 240–252, 2005.

[14] B. Ferrell, M. Grant, and R. Virani, "Nurses urged to address improved end-of-life care in textbooks," *Oncology Nursing Forum*, vol. 28, no. 9, p. 1349, 2001.

[15] J. M. Fredrickson, W. Bauer, D. Arellano, and M. Davidson, "Emergency nurses' perceived knowledge and comfort levels regarding pediatric patients," *Journal of Emergency Nursing*, vol. 20, no. 1, pp. 13–17, 1994.

[16] C. H. Rushton, "Principled moral outrage: an antidote to moral distress?" *AACN Advanced Critical Care*, vol. 24, no. 1, pp. 82–89, 2013.

[17] K. J. Gold, "Navigating care after a baby dies: a systematic review of parent experiences with health providers," *Journal of Perinatology*, vol. 27, no. 4, pp. 230–237, 2007.

[18] A. E. Kopelman, "Understanding, avoiding, and resolving end-of-life conflicts in the NICU," *Mount Sinai Journal of Medicine*, vol. 73, no. 3, pp. 580–586, 2006.

[19] C. Hammerman, E. Kornbluth, O. Lavie, P. Zadka, Y. Aboulafia, and A. I. Eidelman, "Decision-making in the critically ill neonate: cultural background v individual life experiences," *Journal of Medical Ethics*, vol. 23, no. 3, pp. 164–169, 1997.

[20] K. L. Moseley, A. Church, B. Hempel, H. Yuan, S. D. Goold, and G. L. Freed, "End-of-life choices for African-American and white infants in a neonatal intensive-care unit: a pilot study," *Journal of the National Medical Association*, vol. 96, no. 7, pp. 933–937, 2004.

[21] A. J. Engler, R. M. Cusson, R. T. Brockett et al., "Neonatal staff and advanced practice nurses' perceptions of bereavement/end-of-life care of families of critically ill and/or dying infants," *American Journal of Critical Care*, vol. 13, no. 6, pp. 489–498, 2004.

10

Action Planning for Daily Mouth Care in Long-Term Care: The Brushing Up on Mouth Care Project

Mary E. McNally,[1,2] **Ruth Martin-Misener,**[3] **Christopher C. L. Wyatt,**[4] **Karen P. McNeil,**[2] **Sandra J. Crowell,**[2] **Debora C. Matthews,**[1] **and Joanne B. Clovis**[5]

[1] Faculty of Dentistry, Dalhousie University, P.O. Box 15000, Halifax, NS, Canada B3H 4R2
[2] Atlantic Health Promotion Research Centre, Dalhousie University, P.O. Box 15000, Halifax, NS, Canada B3H 4R2
[3] School of Nursing, Faculty of Health Professions, Dalhousie University, P.O. Box 15000, Halifax, NS, Canada B3H 4R2
[4] Faculty of Dentistry, University of British Columbia, 2329 West Mall, Vancouver, BC, Canada V6T 1Z4
[5] School of Dental Hygiene, Faculty of Dentistry, Dalhousie University, P.O. Box 15000, Halifax, NS, Canada B3H 4R2

Correspondence should be addressed to Mary E. McNally, mary.mcnally@dal.ca

Academic Editor: Rita Jablonski

Research focusing on the introduction of daily mouth care programs for dependent older adults in long-term care has met with limited success. There is a need for greater awareness about the importance of oral health, more education for those providing oral care, and organizational structures that provide policy and administrative support for daily mouth care. The purpose of this paper is to describe the establishment of an oral care action plan for long-term care using an interdisciplinary collaborative approach. *Methods.* Elements of a program planning cycle that includes assessment, planning, implementation, and evaluation guided this work and are described in this paper. Findings associated with assessment and planning are detailed. Assessment involved exploration of internal and external factors influencing oral care in long-term care and included document review, focus groups and one-on-one interviews with end-users. The planning phase brought care providers, stakeholders, and researchers together to design a set of actions to integrate oral care into the organizational policy and practice of the research settings. *Findings.* The establishment of a meaningful and productive collaboration was beneficial for developing realistic goals, understanding context and institutional culture, creating actions suitable and applicable for end-users, and laying a foundation for broader networking with relevant stakeholders and health policy makers.

1. Introduction

The last half-century has seen considerable improvements for dental health. Unlike previous generations, more and more older adults are maintaining their natural teeth into old age [1–3]. This is a welcome trend but results in new patterns of disease that become especially significant for those who are frail and who must depend on others for their personal care and hygiene [4–6]. Mouth care is an integral part of personal care yet it is inadequate [4, 6, 7] and given low priority for residents in long-term care [8, 9].

Poor oral hygiene resulting from inadequate mouth care causes considerable morbidity such as mucosal inflammation, caries (tooth decay), and periodontal disease (bone loss around teeth) [7, 10]. Evidence demonstrating links between dental disease and systemic conditions such as respiratory infections [11, 12], diabetes [13–16], and cardiovascular disease [17] also continues to emerge. Tooth loss, pain, and poorly functioning dentures result in problems chewing [18, 19] which is linked to poor nutrition, low body mass index [20], and involuntary weight loss [21]. Dental diseases and dysfunction impact quality of life are known to diminish the pleasures of eating, speaking and social interactions [12, 22]. Overall, the oral health status of residents in long-term care is poor [7, 10, 23–25] and those with dementia experience even higher rates of oral disease [26].

Oral care for dependent older adults in long-term care is becoming a challenge that is expected to grow in importance as our population ages [9]. Over the past several decades, research focusing on attitudes and behaviors of care providers; education and oral hygiene intervention programs; and more recently, environmental, organizational, or social influences on the delivery of care is shedding new light on the complexity of factors influencing the ability to provide adequate oral care.

Practical barriers to oral care include a perceived lack of time [27–29], inadequate staffing levels [27, 28], lack of readily available oral care equipment [30, 31], resistant behaviors by patients/residents [27, 28, 30, 31], and high care staff turnover rates that undermine oral care education programs [32, 33]. Social barriers include embarrassment and repulsion, lack of care staff confidence in their knowledge or ability to provide care [28, 34], a perception of oral care as invasive to the dignity and privacy of residents [35, 36] or unwanted by the resident [35], and the perception by nurses that oral care is professionally unrewarding [36]. Factors identified to facilitate care staff's ability and/or willingness to provide oral care include availability of oral health equipment [37], influence of and examples set by people seen as influential leaders [37], education and/or demonstration in oral health care procedures [27, 29, 35, 37], adequate time to provide care [29], and believing that oral health and oral care are important [28, 29].

Research involving staff education-based interventions directed toward improving oral health status of long-term care residents demonstrates conflicting results [38–40]. Some studies have demonstrated a decrease in disease indicators [32, 39] while others did not [40]. A similarly designed comprehensive personal mouth care program introduced in multiple facilities found different effects on oral hygiene practices and health status of residents of the different facilities [41]. In fact, structural variables expected to influence quality of care (e.g., on-site services, routines, and resources) explained very little of the difference between effective and ineffective programs [41, 42]. Rather, effectiveness appeared contingent upon the organizational context within facilities, comprised of both programmatic strategies and the organizational culture that supports or inhibits them [42].

Creating effective strategies to address the issue of oral health in long-term care is further complicated because oral health care has traditionally been peripheral to mainstream health considerations. The lack of interaction between dentistry and other domains of health care has fostered isolation in approaches for managing oral health. This has been recognized as a shortcoming and has resulted in a call for an interdisciplinary and collaborative approach to both research and practice [8, 9]. Our research attempts to address these shortcomings.

The purpose of this paper is to describe the experience of developing a meaningful interdisciplinary collaboration and to highlight the processes used to design a comprehensive set of actions to integrate oral care into organizational policy and practice within three long-term care facilities in rural Nova Scotia on the east coast of Canada. A collaborative approach is advantageous because the synergy created by the blending of perspectives, resources, and skills of various participants [43] enables the group to create something that is not attainable by single agents [44]. In this study, an interdisciplinary network of researchers and stakeholders were brought together with administrators and front-line care staff to think about the work in creative and practical ways; develop realistic goals; plan and carry out comprehensive interventions that connect multiple programs, services, and sectors; understand and document the impact of its actions; incorporate the perspectives and priorities of stakeholders including the target population; and communicate how actions will address problems [43].

2. Methods

2.1. The Collaboration. A common interest was established between the principal investigator (M. E. McNally) and a senior administrator of three long-term care facilities during a provincial oral health policy workshop. Over the course of a year, multiple face-to-face meetings, telephone, and email consultations were undertaken with administrative staff to: discuss the current level of oral care and associated challenges; develop realistic and practical research objectives; establish a formal commitment to the research; clarify roles and expectations; and establish mutual benefits. Through this process, a formal collaboration was established consisting of an interdisciplinary research team in partnership with Health Service Managers and Nurse Managers of the three facilities (i.e., the "site team"). All members of the collaboration were involved in establishing goals and strategies for the project. The Nurse Managers were further involved as direct liaisons to each of the sites and assisted with recruitment and data collection. To help focus the research goals and ongoing knowledge exchange, the site team identified training and resources as desired outcomes.

2.2. Research Site. Three long-term care facilities were the sites for this research. They are rurally situated within 1 hour of each other and are within 1-2-hour drive of a metropolitan area. The number of residents per site ranged from 25 to 40, which is typical of the majority of long-term care facilities found in rural settings in the region [45]. The three long-term care facilities are administered under the same health district where there is sharing of resources, budgets, and policy. Examining multiple sites within the same organizational structure was undertaken to provide a deeper understanding of how subcultures influence delivery of care at a micro-organizational level [46].

2.3. Study Design. A case study approach was used to explore the individual, organizational, and system factors associated with the integration of oral care in three long-term care settings. The unit of analysis was institutional [47]. The case study method was selected in order to gain a holistic understanding of "how" the development and implementation of actions may be influenced by the cultural systems of action that exist within each setting [48].

This research is consistent with the elements of a program planning cycle that include assessment, planning, implementation, and evaluation [49] of a set of actions to integrate oral care into both organizational policy and daily personal care practice. This paper describes details associated with the first two phases, assessment and action planning. *Assessment* involved an exploration of the internal and external factors that influence the provision of oral care and oral disease prevention and was undertaken through a document review, focus groups, and one-on-one interviews. The *action-planning* phase brought care providers and stakeholders (government representatives, educators, and dental professionals) together for a workshop to design a set of actions to integrate oral care into organizational policy and practice in each of the settings. The action plan is being *implemented* in each of the settings over a 12-month period and experiences of the health care team (front-line care staff and administrators) explored. The process and outcomes associated with the implementation of actions are being *evaluated* and are providing the basis of recommendations to revise organizational policy and oral care practice. The latter two phases of the project will be described in a subsequent manuscript at their completion.

A systematic analysis of multiple forms of evidence was used to enhance understanding of the context and the people within it [47]. Sources of triangulation [48] of data include multiple perspectives among investigators (i.e., dentistry, nursing, medicine, administration, policy decision-makers), multiple methods (i.e., document analysis, focus groups, interviews, journaling), multiple data sources (i.e., personal care providers, administrators, residents, and families), and multiple settings. It was also recognized that the term "oral care" connotes the broad spectrum of oral health care needs associated with both professional and personal care. This research is primarily concerned with the latter, "daily mouth care", for frail older adults. However, it was recognized that the scope of this work might also overlap with clinical and policy considerations of professional dentistry and public health. The term "oral care" is therefore used to encompass the broader range of considerations in the research.

2.4. Data Collection

2.4.1. Document Review. Document review was undertaken to provide an organizational and health system context [50]. Members of the collaboration determined the strategy and breadth of the review. Documents were selected on the basis of their topic relevance [51] and included those expected to inform the provision of oral care for long-term care in the region (e.g., job descriptions, clinical guidelines, health assessment tools, accreditation guidelines). Documents were collected directly from the site team, from government, academia, the health services and community college education sectors, and through internet searches of relevant government and education websites. They were individually read, coded, and organized according to four criteria: (1) general health terminology (that may or may not include oral care), (2) oral care (including terms "oral", "mouth", and "dental"), (3) foot care, and (4) wound care. References to foot care and wound care were included to provide a basis for comparing oral care to other aspects of care that may be similarly addressed through relevant documents.

Members of the collaboration suggested that it would be useful to examine oral care for consistency with existing and familiar clinical domains that may ultimately provide a useful framework for oral care.

2.4.2. Individual Interviews and Focus Groups. Experiential data were collected using a qualitative approach. This approach is constructivist and interpretivist [52, 53] seeking to distil from personal accounts the experiences and meaning behind oral health care for dependent older adults. Qualitative methods are particularly well suited to finding answers to "what" questions (what are people doing, what does it mean) and "how" questions (how are things done, how is meaning produced) [52]. Ethics approval was obtained from the Nova Scotia Capital District Health Authority (CDHA-RS/2009-033). Members of the site team identified potential participants who were invited by letter and a follow-up telephone call. One-on-one semistructured interviews were held with administrators and health professionals who provide a variety of health services to residents and clients associated with the three facilities. Two focus groups were held in each of the three facilities with (1) personal care providers (i.e., those who provide personal care within their job scope including personal care workers, continuing care assistants, and licensed practical nurses) and (2) residents and family members. Residents who had capacity to provide consent (as determined by the nurse manager) were invited to participate and family members were included to represent experiences of those not able to speak for themselves. One author (K. P. McNeil) facilitated focus groups and interviews.

Semistructured questions for both focus groups and individual interviews were designed to guide and generate discussion to elicit participants' description of practices associated with the provision of oral care, perceptions of barriers and facilitators to oral care in the care settings, attitudes toward oral health and oral health care, and relevant knowledge of formal oral health policies. Participants were also asked for suggestions that may improve or enhance oral care. This approach allowed for structure but was flexible enough for participants to raise issues not anticipated. Focus groups and interviews were audio-recorded and transcribed. Each verbatim interview underwent open coding to identify thematically group-related phrases and patterns arising from the data [54, 55] using HyperRESEARCH Qualitative Analysis Tool (Version 2.8.2).

2.4.3. Action Planning Workshop. A one-day interdisciplinary oral care action-planning workshop was held at a location central to the research sites. Members of the collaboration established workshop goals and identified invitees to ensure a broad range of relevant expertise and experience. The purpose of the workshop was to design a set of actions that would integrate oral care into organizational policy and personal care practices in each of the three long-term care settings. The two key goals were to: (1) identify and prioritize education, training, tools, and program strategies and (2) establish a detailed plan for implementing, tracking, and evaluating both professional and daily personal mouth care delivery.

The workshop was facilitated by the authors M. E. McNally and K. P. McNeil.

Forty-six invitees were contacted individually by M. E. McNally or K. P. McNeil. The workshop was attended by 34 participants: clinical researchers from dentistry, dental hygiene, nursing, and medicine ($n = 7$); researchers from health promotion and organizational management ($n = 4$); administrators ($n = 5$); nurse managers ($n = 2$); regulated and unregulated front line care staff ($n = 5$); policy makers in the health and continuing care sectors ($n = 3$); representatives of organized dentistry and dental hygiene ($n = 3$); community college educators ($n = 2$); speech language pathologist ($n = 1$); dietician ($n = 1$); as well as a representative from a seniors' government advisory organization. Findings from the document review and experiential data were presented to provide participants with an understanding of context. A review of current best practices [56] and a model of oral health care in long-term care [57] provided an evidence base to inform workshop discussion. Relevant topics identified through the document review, focus groups, and interviews were prioritized by the collaboration for discussion in one-hour breakout sessions and a discussion guide was developed for each topic (Table 1). Each session included 6–8 participants organized to ensure input from a variety of perspectives and disciplines [58].

Responses to the discussion questions were recorded by individual groups and reported back in a plenary session where further input was gathered from the larger group. At the plenary, the group was asked to consider the following: how to best synthesize the information to create a comprehensive "oral care action plan", how to best communicate the action plan to end users, and how to determine the biggest indicators of success over the next 18 months. Findings from the workshop were collated and synthesized into a draft "oral care action plan" for integration at each of the three long-term care sites. Strategies for implementing and evaluating actions were finalized as part of this process. Following the workshop, details of the action plan were prepared into a report and relevant materials circulated to the site team for final approval. The principal investigator and research coordinator met with both managers and front line care staff at each of the sites to ensure that the proposed action plan accommodated circumstances unique to each setting.

3. Results and Discussion

3.1. Document Review. Forty-two internal ($n = 28$) and external ($n = 14$) documents were collected and reviewed. Internal documents included information that was directly applicable to the sites (e.g., mission and values, job descriptions, accreditation standards) and external documents provided information on potentially influential outside factors (e.g., Continuing Care Provincial Policy, Professional Standards of Practice). Overall the document scan revealed a general lack of specific reference to oral health and oral care. Consistent with other findings [42], external documents clearly acknowledged a need for or commitment to whole body health and optimal well-being. However, internal documents reflected more direct activities of practice and referred

to general terms such as "personal care", "assessing all body systems", or "AM/PM care" without the specific mention of oral care. Where oral care was included ($n = 10$), terms such as "mouth/denture care" or "oral care" were used but not described. Overall, the scan revealed negligible references to oral or mouth care as an explicit domain of personal care. There are no government standards with specific reference to mouth or oral care in long-term care. Similar references and level of detail were provided for foot care ($n = 13$). Conversely, the five documents mentioning wound care included details regarding scopes of practice, an interdisciplinary clinic manual, a health services operational report, and a comprehensive manual developed by the provincial government [59]. Details provided for wound care were not surprising given its recognition as specialized care with established best practices for managing wound pathology [60]. This is informative for oral care where the consequences of unchecked oral disease have similar negative implications for health and quality of life.

3.2. Individual Interviews and Focus Groups. Thirteen one-on-one semistructured interviews ranging from 30 to 60 minutes were undertaken with administrators and health professionals who service the three facilities. Participants represented two distinct groups, 5 internal professionals who were involved with the day-to-day care of residents living in long-term care facilities (i.e., long-term care coordinators, nurse managers), and 8 external professionals who provided care to residents but who are not present on a daily basis (i.e., physician, dietitian, physiotherapist, occupational therapist, social worker, nurse practitioner, acute care coordinators). The former group was more involved in addressing and recognizing the needs of residents on a daily basis and their perspectives were very much aligned with those of front-line care staff described hereinafter. External professionals recognized the importance of oral care but generally felt removed from oral care and its implications. Neither group was aware of existing formal policies or supports related to oral care in long-term care. Some concerns raised by external participants centered on relevant health risks for residents. Regarding dysphagia, for example, "...we certainly have concerns about the people pocketing food, going to bed after lunch and that they could choke on that food". Lack of consideration for oral care in routine health assessments undertaken by the various professions was also identified as problematic: "...in a routine screening, I probably wouldn't ask about teeth unless I noticed something and that is probably not a good thing. It is probably something we should be asking about". Both groups acknowledged the importance of daily oral care: "[oral health is important] for overall general health, for nutrition status, for comfort, for self esteem. It's really important for basic health" and advocated for more educational opportunities for care staff: "I think that front line people need more education on oral health... I am not sure it is focused enough in the program they take... There doesn't seem to be a lot of emphasis on oral health and why it's important in what I see in the people who come here to work". All interviewees were generally aware of difficulties residents have in accessing professional dental services: "For a lot of our people, they find they can't do

TABLE 1: Action planning workshop break-out session guides.

Prioritized discussion topics	Questions for discussion guide
Education/training required to strengthen delivery of care	*Who needs to be involved?*
	What should they be doing (i.e., actions/activities)?
Planning and tracking oral care activities	*What will be required to make activities possible?*
	How will we measure/keep track of activities?
Special supports to manage residents with dementia	*Who will need to be involved in measuring/tracking progress?*
Access to professional dental services	*How will we know if activities are successful?*

anything. If they do have a problem with their dental or oral health, they can't really afford to do anything about it so they tend to leave it".

Focus groups held at each of the three sites included 17 residents and family members ($n = 8, 3, 6$) and 14 front-line personal care providers ($n = 5, 3, 6$). Sessions averaged 90 and 60 minutes, respectively. Residents and family members expressed feedback about availability of mouth care products and good communication between care staff and residents as being important features of mouth care. There was general satisfaction with care provided by personal care staff. Responses to direct questions about daily brushing and denture care met with positive responses by residents: *"They are a great bunch of girls".* Even with probing questions about daily hygiene care, residents and family members associated mouth care with professional dental care. There was deep concern about a lack of accessibility to professional services. Current residents who did have complaints about their teeth indicated that they would *"make do"* or *"put up"* with the discomfort: *"I'll put up with my teeth"; "I can't bite with [my dentures] like I used to with some things but I think they'll do me".* Access to professional services was limited by residents' mobility and funding issues associated with transportation costs to move residents off-site for professional care, costs that must be borne by residents themselves: *"It's really expensive to go to a dentist and get a cap or a filling, or even just to have your dentures fixed because some of the elderly, their dentures are loose and they can't afford a new set of dentures. Like who is going to pay for it?"* (Family member). Living in a rural area seemed to further complicate this issue: *"It's practically a whole day by the time you get to the dentist's and back again... Very draining. I get there but by the time I get home, I'm dead."* (Resident).

Not surprisingly, the most significant input came from front line care staff most involved with the day-to-day care of residents summarized in Table 2. They generally reported that they feel competent to provide mouth care. However, they identified numerous factors that either hindered or helped with carrying out these tasks that are consistent with other reported findings. For instance, although oral care is included in their personal care training, many felt a repulsion and lack of comfort (fear) when providing mouth care [28, 34]. This was intensified when residents exhibit resistant behavior as a result of dementia [28, 34] disability or indifference to the value of mouth care [35]. Participants acknowledged that the proportion of residents and clients with advanced frailty and dementia-related disease is increasing, placing greater demands for providing care [61]. The number of residents with natural teeth is also increasing and many enter long-term care with very poor oral health [1, 34]. In fact, the oral health status of residents was also seen to be an important factor influencing the quality of care they received especially if poor oral health is accompanied by sensitivity or pain. Constraints of resources and time for completing personal care tasks often leave mouth care low on care staff's list of priorities [31, 34]. Although one of the facilities did have a formal oral care protocol, it was acknowledged that there was little guidance for oral assessments, care planning, and accountability. Along with barriers, key facilitating influences were also identified and are consistent with the earlier findings [28, 34]. The level of residents' functional abilities and a good relationship with their care provider were seen as beneficial. Having a good routine, availability of mouth care products, and sufficient time were also identified as important for facilitating care. With respect to perspectives about education, there was a strong indication that standardized and in-depth oral health education during personal care and nursing training programs would be key to achieving improved and consistent daily oral care. Care staff were generally receptive to "in house" education and training opportunities as well. They suggested that "reminders" and "visuals" (such as those commonly posted for hand-washing) would be useful tools for raising awareness. They were unanimous in expressing a resistance to being monitored daily through check lists saying: *"Tick sheets are definitely not the answer".* Positive reinforcements, available resources, visual reminders, and education would be more readily accepted by care staff for enhancing mouth care.

Overall these findings provided a unique window into the continuing care environment and direct responsibilities of a range of front-line care staff, managers, and administrators working within the three facilities. This feedback, coupled with findings of the document analysis and input from the collaboration, provided the basis for establishing priorities for the action planning workshop, evaluation of prospective activities arising from the workshop, and planning next steps for introducing an oral care action plan.

3.3. Action Planning Workshop. As described previously, this one-day interdisciplinary workshop was held to develop an oral care action plan to be integrated into organizational policy and practice. Following formal presentations, significant contributions of the workshop were obtained through direct feedback from workshop participants' small group discussions. Topics and guiding questions are outlined in

TABLE 2: Personal care providers narrative findings—barriers, facilitators and education.

	Explanation of theme	Supporting quotes
Barrier themes		
Repulsion/fear	*Sometimes care providers are repulsed by certain aspects of oral care such as halitosis, or a resident spitting/coughing on them. Care staff are fearful of providing oral care for a variety of reasons (e.g., drop or break dentures, cause the resident to gag or aspirate, get bitten).*	"So I had to clean them; oh it was gross... I don't know how she even handled it but I guess it'd been like that and she had just gotten used to it." "You have to be careful because if you want to stick your finger in or anything close they can bite you."
Resident disability/ dementia/resistance	*Oral care provision is more complicated when a resident is disabled or has dementia. Often residents cannot express themselves when they are confused or suffering from oral pain or discomfort and this may be interpreted as resistant behaviour.*	"If you have a [resident with] dementia that might have some of their own teeth and can't tell you he's a got a toothache, you know what he's going to do... they're going to act out. ...They become agitated and they can't express it." "Sometimes it's hard to do oral care with people with dementia because they don't want you around their mouth; they don't know exactly what you're doing." "I mean somebody who's got advanced dementia there's no sense, just work with them and hope for the best."
Resident attitude/indifference	*Often residents appear to not care or are unaware of the importance of oral health. Many residents would not have gone to the dentist for regular check-ups throughout their lives and therefore oral care is not a priority for them.*	"People years ago didn't go to a dentist unless it really bothered them and they had an abscess and then they went to the family doctor and he gave them antibiotics and then he pulled the tooth out." "A lot of residents just don't want to be bothered [with oral care]... it's just not something that's important to them." "I think he wouldn't say a word if you didn't get to his teeth."
Current oral health status of resident	*If a resident comes into a facility with poor oral health, it is more difficult to provide them with adequate oral care, especially if they have sensitivity, discomfort, or pain.*	"[Resident Name] has very few teeth and has had over the years very poor mouth care, therefore he's got infections in his gums and his teeth are rotten." "Yes it makes you wonder if they have a bad history their whole life of bad mouth care. And that's why their teeth are so bad, or is this decline just recent, like within the last five years or whatever."
Lack of time	*"Visible" activities (dressing, combing hair, washing, etc.) take priority when there is a time crunch (e.g., in the morning). Staff indicated that if they had more time, oral care would likely get more attention.*	"If somebody's in a hurry... It's a wham, bam, thank you, ma'am, the teeth can be left." "I think the people that have their own teeth probably don't get the attention. Now as far as I'm concerned, they need more attention because they have their own teeth, but I think they're the ones that get neglected because of the fact that it takes longer to do natural teeth than it does dentures."
Facilitator themes		
Resident ability	*It can be helpful when residents are aware of their oral care and remind staff to brush their teeth. Having the resident provide the cue often ensures their teeth will be done.*	"We have two [residents] that will actually ask, will you brush my teeth?" "[Name of resident] is very insistent on having her teeth done after breakfast and before she goes to bed and her teeth are done faithfully."
Resident relationship with care provider	*Having a good relationship with a resident can make oral care provision easier. The care provider is familiar with likes/dislikes and routines and the resident is more comfortable around them.*	"You know what [the residents] want.... they sort of trust you... they feel, they don't care if you see them without their teeth [in]."

Table 2: Continued.

	Explanation of theme	Supporting quotes
Proper tools and products	*Oral care provision is easier when the necessary tools are available and on-hand. Using the proper tools for specific care needs is also important (e.g., denture brushes for dentures, child size toothbrushes for residents with small mouths).*	"Having everything there right where you can get it; you know your toothbrush, toothbrushes and things; just having it right close." "I wish we had those little toothbrushes back... [they] curved like this, so every time you used them it would get right in around their gums and everything else; it brought a lot of stuff out."
Education themes		
Oral health education	*Additional oral health care training may be beneficial for care providers who are currently in the workforce as well as family members or volunteers.*	"A lot of these [care providers] have been doing this for 25 years, they never took a course and were just grandfathered in... it's really hard for you to get across to them that just because you've been doing that that way doesn't mean you were doing it the right way. So a lot of people figure you're making waves if you say something." "Sometimes family members need to be educated; and just to be aware of what we're trying to do like promote good oral care; sometimes they say "If mom or dad won't open their mouth then don't make them". [Then] there's nothing I can do."
Education tools	*Tools suggested that would be helpful with oral health education and awareness (apart from formal education).*	"Well we have hand-washing posters all over the place, why not oral care posters?" "So if there was posters [about oral care] in each of the elders rooms, in their bathrooms, right by their sink then you're there with the teeth or with the elder, you're going to read it." "If this could be one of the subjects that is brought up at every care conference, also, every time we do rounds. Now, rounds is for a wing, a whole wing in general, so if oral care could be brought up then and discussed, just like I said, keep it fresh, keep it going, keep it on everybody's mind."
Care provider training programs	*Care providers should receive standardized, in-depth training on oral care provision.*	"So that's where the education has to come in—that everybody realizes what oral care is and what it entails." "It's always good when we have new young ones coming in because they're fresh out of the course and they've learned from the book the right way; so I always like to see them coming in."

Table 1. There was some overlap between topics but feedback was collated into the following summaries.

Education/Training Required to Strengthen the Delivery of Daily Oral Care. Education for residents may be important to heighten awareness regarding oral health. Strategies should be fun, with creative delivery. Laminated posters should be placed in residents' washrooms. These posters would be used as a visual reminder and would include information on the importance of proper oral care, steps outlining proper care, and so on. They should be bright and colorful and include a number of pictures. A "train the trainers" approach would be appropriate to enhance sustainability of the action plan. This would involve training nursing staff or a designate who would take a leadership role in providing ongoing oral health care support for personal care providers and other relevant staff within the facilities.

Planning and Tracking Daily Oral Care Activities (Daily and Professional). There is a need to change the built environment to provide appropriate space for oral health (i.e., designated space for oral care). To adequately plan and track oral care activities within long-term care, specific tools and resources were suggested. (i) Oral health kits should be created for each resident including the necessary tools to complete oral care such as toothbrushes, denture brushes, toothpaste, mouth rinses, and a towel to protect dentures in sink. The products in kits would be individualized depending on resident's oral care needs. (ii) Care cards should be developed and color coded according to tooth and denture status (i.e., natural teeth, dentures, partial dentures, no teeth) and would facilitate an individualized oral care plan for each resident. Cards could be used by care providers and, if residents go home for visits, by family members. (iii) A tool to enable personal care providers to conduct oral assessments as a part of providing oral care should be developed. The tool would provide guidance for a visual exam of the mouth and a record of any problems. Care providers would need to be educated on what to look for and recognized as being the "eyes of oral care" within the facility. They need to be involved in decision making about what they will be asked/required to do. (iv) A strategy for including oral care in dysphagia assessment that is performed by the Dysphagia Team should be developed. This would allow for a more formalized system of information sharing. By documenting issues related to oral care, it will increase the likelihood that something will be done about it.

Special Support Needed to Manage Resistant Residents/Residents with Dementia. A multidisciplinary approach to care planning is necessary. There is a need to raise the profile of oral care for these residents and look at preexisting tools, daily report sheets, and white boards to improve communication regarding oral care. Whatever is done, it needs to be practical for frontline workers. Role-playing may help to put care providers in the residents' shoes.

Access to Professional Dental Services. This is an issue that needs to involve everyone from frontline care staff, senior administration, to government. Funding for service is a key issue. Taking residents to a dentist requires funding for transportation in addition to the cost of service. Bringing a dentist to the residents requires funding for space, equipment, and costs of professional service. Ideally, hygienists could make regular visits to facilities. Oral care could be set up similar to foot care where a mobile unit makes site visits. Some mobile services exist but do not currently travel to the more rural areas. Good communication across silos of continuing care and professional dental services is required to improve resident care and potentially save money in the health care system. The value of professional dental care depends on the personal values of residents and their families. Participants recognized that access to professional dental services was an issue beyond the scope of the workshop and of the three facilities involved in the research.

3.4. Action Plan Implementation. The strategic action plan evolving from the workshop included each of the activities identified for action in the workshop. The plan emphasized targeted education and training for administrators, nursing staff, and daily personal care providers. The plan specified that oral health manuals should be developed for each site. The manuals would include education materials, pamphlets, and prepared forms to guide oral assessment, care planning, and intervention/referral documents, detailed work-plans, required oral hygiene products such as toothbrushes, toothpaste, denture care products, as well as individualized oral health toolkits for residents.

Proposed actions were implemented over a 12-month period. The site team liaison (or an appropriate designate) assumed responsibility for coordinating activities associated with the action plan. The research coordinator visited each of the three research sites at 6-week intervals to review progress, to provide support, and to gather data. Proposed hands-on education workshops were provided by qualified research team members at the outset of action plan intervention and during regularly scheduled visits. The site team liaison assumed responsibility for overseeing the care and reinforcing the skills with individual care providers as needed. Relevant research team members and the research coordinator provided ongoing support.

3.5. Evaluation of the Oral Care Action Plan. To ensure that proposed methods of collecting data to evaluate the action plan activities were relevant and acceptable, the draft evaluation framework was reviewed and refined by the research team based on feedback at the action-planning workshop (Table 3). According to Thorne et al. [42], success in oral health programs in long-term care is contingent upon effective programmatic strategies (e.g., routine oral hygiene, oral assessment, availability of professional dental services) as well as the organizational culture influencing them (e.g., administrative capacity to support and control a caring environment, the presence of "champions", organizational values) [42]. Recalling that the unit of analysis for this case study was institutional, the evaluation plan was designed to examine the institutional context and to consider both organizational culture and the programmatic strategies arising from the oral care action plan.

4. Conclusions

This paper highlights a variety of important considerations for developing meaningful collaborative and applied intervention research. A defining feature of the "Brushing Up on Mouth Care" project has been an enduring and positive collaboration with end-users. This has required careful attention to ongoing communication. It has also necessitated that frequent project updates and face-to-face meetings are balanced with ensuring that end-users do not become "burned out". Prior to the launch of this project, the collaboration (members of both the research and project site teams) invested time in getting to know each other and in coming to a common understanding of where the research should go. These early communications created a level of comfort and familiarity enabling all voices to be heard and respected. At the outset, this led to the development of realistic research goals about what could be achieved. It also laid the groundwork for the exploratory and planning phases of the project.

The document scan, focus groups, and interviews all contributed to our understanding of the institutional context and organizational culture influencing the delivery of mouth care. This directly informed the action plan that followed. The document scan revealed significant gaps in policy, education, and clinical standards available to guide oral care in long-term care. Our understanding of influences on the delivery of oral care was further informed through the workshop group discussions involving a broader stakeholder group. Here, mechanisms for addressing gaps were also identified and have become integrated into considerations for our ongoing work. One specific example has been the uptake of

TABLE 3: Evaluation Framework.

Outcome variables	Data source	Proposed metrics/indicators
Programmatic strategies		
Integration of individualized oral care plan	Focus group and key informant narratives Administrator diary studies Document review (e.g., policy)	Thematic analysis Proportion of residents in whom oral care is discussed during care planning meetings
Oral assessments	Oral care activities records	Summary data
Professional dental care	Oral care activities records	Use of referral systems (e.g., to dentist)
Daily mouth care protocol	Focus group and interview narratives Diary studies Oral care activity records	Thematic analysis Oral care product use
Material indicators of program uptake	Dental supply inventory Dental supply orders	Summary data
Nonmaterial indicators of program uptake (e.g., time allotment formal and informal practices)	Focus group and key informant narratives Diary studies Document review	Thematic analysis
Organizational culture		
Behavior/attitudes of staff toward delivery of oral care	Focus group and key informant narratives AWS Care provider and administrator diary studies	Thematic analysis Mean change in AWS scores
Satisfaction/acceptability of staff/residents/families	Focus group narratives and interviews	Pre/postintervention comparison of themes and patterns
Staff knowledge of oral health	Posteducation knowledge uptake questionnaires	Attendance at orientation and education in-service Pre/posteducation knowledge (scores)
Organizational values	Key informant narratives Document review	Pre/postcomparison of themes and patterns

the "Brushing Up on Mouth Care" action plan by local community colleges responsible for training relevant entry-level care staff. Engagement with government policy makers, directors of care, educators, health administrators, and a broad spectrum of health professionals has also been fruitful in creating awareness about the need for relevant policy as well as guidelines that consider the interdisciplinary nature of this realm of care. Finally, the creation of an oral care action plan that is suitable and applicable to end-users is benefiting both care staff and those who depend on them for care.

References

[1] D. C. Matthews, J. B. Clovis, M. G. S. Brillant et al., "Oral health status of long-term care residents—a vulnerable population," *Journal of the Canadian Dental Association*, vol. 78, article c3, 2012.

[2] P. E. Petersen and T. Yamamoto, "Improving the oral health of older people: the approach of the WHO Global Oral Health Programme," *Community Dentistry and Oral Epidemiology*, vol. 33, no. 2, pp. 81–92, 2005.

[3] R. J. Hawkins, "Oral health status and treatment needs of Canadian adults aged 85 years and over," *Special Care in Dentistry*, vol. 18, no. 4, pp. 164–169, 1998.

[4] C. C. L. Wyatt, F. H. C. So, P. M. Williams, A. Mithani, C. M. Zed, and E. H. K. Yen, "The development, implementation, utilization and outcomes of a comprehensive dental program for older adults residing in long-term care facilities," *Journal of the Canadian Dental Association*, vol. 72, no. 5, p. 419, 2006.

[5] J. Fitzpatrick, "Oral health care needs of dependent older people: responsibilities of nurses and care staff," *Journal of Advanced Nursing*, vol. 32, no. 6, pp. 1325–1332, 2000.

[6] M. I. MacEntee, "Oral care for successful aging in long-term care," *Journal of Public Health Dentistry*, vol. 60, no. 4, pp. 326–329, 2000.

[7] C. C. Wyatt, "Elderly Canadians residing in long-term care hospitals: part II. Dental caries status," *Journal of the Canadian Dental Association*, vol. 68, no. 6, pp. 359–363, 2002.

[8] P. Coleman, "Opportunities for nursing-dental collaboration: addressing oral health needs among the elderly," *Nursing Outlook*, vol. 53, no. 1, pp. 33–39, 2005.

[9] M. I. MacEntee, "Missing links in oral health care for frail elderly people," *Journal of the Canadian Dental Association*, vol. 72, no. 5, pp. 421–425, 2006.

[10] C. C. Wyatt, "Elderly Canadians residing in long-term care hospitals: part I. Medical and dental status," *Journal of the Canadian Dental Association*, vol. 68, no. 6, pp. 353–358, 2002.

[11] S. Awano, T. Ansai, Y. Takata et al., "Oral health and mortality risk from pneumonia in the elderly," *Journal of Dental Research*, vol. 87, no. 4, pp. 334–339, 2008.

[12] T. Yoneyama, M. Yoshida, T. Ohrui et al., "Oral care reduces pneumonia in older patients in nursing homes," *Journal of the American Geriatrics Society*, vol. 50, no. 3, pp. 430–433, 2002.

[13] S. G. Grossi and R. J. Genco, "Periodontal disease and diabetes mellitus: a two-way relationship," *Annals of Periodontology*, vol. 3, no. 1, pp. 51–61, 1998.

[14] T. Nakajima and K. Yamazaki, "Periodontal disease and risk of atherosclerotic coronary heart disease," *Odontology*, vol. 97, no. 2, pp. 84–91, 2009.

[15] G. E. Sandberg, H. E. Sundberg, C. A. Fjellstrom, and K. F. Wikblad, "Type 2 diabetes and oral health: a comparison between diabetic and non- diabetic subjects," *Diabetes Research and Clinical Practice*, vol. 50, no. 1, pp. 27–34, 2000.

[16] J. E. Stewart, K. A. Wager, A. H. Friedlander, and H. H. Zadeh, "The effect of periodontal treatment on glycemic control in patients with type 2 diabetes mellitus," *Journal of Clinical Periodontology*, vol. 28, no. 4, pp. 306–310, 2001.

[17] K. Joshipura, "The relationship between oral conditions and ischemic stroke and peripheral vascular disease," *The Journal of the American Dental Association*, vol. 133, pp. 235–305, 2002.

[18] J. M. Chalmers, K. D. Carter, and A. J. Spencer, "Caries incidence and increments in community-living older adults with and without dementia," *Gerodontology*, vol. 19, no. 2, pp. 80–94, 2002.

[19] D. Kandelman, P. E. Petersen, and H. Ueda, "Oral health, general health, and quality of life in older people," *Special Care in Dentistry*, vol. 28, no. 6, pp. 224–236, 2008.

[20] P. Mojon, E. Budtz-Jørgensen, and C. H. Rapin, "Relationship between oral health and nutrition in very old people," *Age and Ageing*, vol. 28, no. 5, pp. 463–468, 1999.

[21] D. H. Sullivan, W. Martin, N. Flaxman, and J. E. Hagen, "Oral health problems and involuntary weight loss in a population of frail elderly," *Journal of the American Geriatrics Society*, vol. 41, no. 7, pp. 725–731, 1993.

[22] M. I. Macentee, R. Hole, and E. Stolar, "The significance of the mouth in old age," *Social Science and Medicine*, vol. 45, no. 9, pp. 1449–1458, 1997.

[23] C. C. L. Wyatt, "A 5-year follow-up of older adults residing in long-term care facilities: utilisation of a comprehensive dental programme," *Gerodontology*, vol. 26, no. 4, pp. 282–290, 2009.

[24] J. Woo, S. C. Ho, A. L. M. Yu, and J. Lau, "An estimate of long-term care needs and identification of risk factors for institutionalization among Hong Kong Chinese aged 70 years and over," *Journals of Gerontology*, vol. 55, no. 2, pp. M64–M69, 2000.

[25] M. P. Sweeney, C. Williams, C. Kennedy, L. M. D. Macpherson, S. Turner, and J. Bagg, "Oral health care and status of elderly care home residents in Glasgow," *Community Dental Health*, vol. 24, no. 1, pp. 37–42, 2007.

[26] J. M. Chalmers, K. D. Carter, and A. J. Spencer, "Oral diseases and conditions in community-living older adults with and without dementia," *Special Care in Dentistry*, vol. 23, no. 1, pp. 7–17, 2003.

[27] B. Hijji, "Trained nurses' knowledge and practice of oral care on three wards in acute care hospital in Abu Dhabi, UAE," *Online Brazilian Journal of Nursing*, vol. 2, no. 3, 2003.

[28] J. M. Chalmers, S. M. Levy, K. C. Buckwalter, R. L. Ettinger, and P. P. Kambhu, "Factors influencing nurses' aides' provision of oral care for nursing facility residents," *Special Care in Dentistry*, vol. 16, no. 2, pp. 71–79, 1996.

[29] L. A. Furr, C. J. Binkley, C. McCurren, and R. Carrico, "Factors affecting quality of oral care in intensive care units," *Journal of Advanced Nursing*, vol. 48, no. 5, pp. 454–462, 2004.

[30] R. A. Jablonski, C. L. Munro, M. J. Grap, C. M. Schubert, M. Ligon, and P. Spigelmyer, "Mouth care in nursing homes: knowledge, beliefs, and practices of nursing assistants," *Geriatric Nursing*, vol. 30, no. 2, pp. 99–107, 2009.

[31] P. Coleman and N. M. Watson, "Oral care provided by certified nursing assistants in nursing homes," *Journal of the American Geriatrics Society*, vol. 54, no. 1, pp. 138–143, 2006.

[32] P. Glassman and C. E. Miller, "Effect of preventive dentistry training program for caregivers in community facilities on caregiver and client behavior and client oral hygiene," *The New York State Dental Journal*, vol. 72, no. 2, pp. 38–46, 2006.

[33] M. E. Kaz and L. Schuchman, "Oral health care attitudes of nursing assistants in long-term care facilities," *Special Care in Dentistry*, vol. 8, no. 5, pp. 228–231, 1988.

[34] S. Dharamsi, K. Jivani, C. Dean, and C. Wyatt, "Oral care for frail elders: knowledge, attitudes, and practices of long-term care staff," *Journal of Dental Education*, vol. 73, no. 5, pp. 581–588, 2009.

[35] I. Wårdh, L. Andersson, and S. Sörensen, "Staff attitudes to oral health care. A comparative study of registered nurses, nursing assistants and home care aides," *Gerodontology*, vol. 14, no. 1, pp. 28–32, 1997.

[36] D. R. Eadie and L. Schou, "An exploratory study of barriers to promoting oral hygiene through carers of elderly people," *Community Dental Health*, vol. 9, no. 4, pp. 343–348, 1992.

[37] K. Kite, "Changing mouth care practice in intensive care: implications of the clinical setting context," *Intensive and Critical Care Nursing*, vol. 11, no. 4, pp. 203–209, 1995.

[38] H. Frenkel, I. Harvey, and K. Needs, "Oral health care education and its effect on caregivers' knowledge and attitudes: a randomised controlled trial," *Community Dentistry and Oral Epidemiology*, vol. 30, no. 2, pp. 91–100, 2002.

[39] H. Frenkel, I. Harvey, and R. G. Newcombe, "Improving oral health in institutionalised elderly people by educating caregivers: a randomised controlled trial," *Community Dentistry and Oral Epidemiology*, vol. 29, no. 4, pp. 289–297, 2001.

[40] M. I. MacEntee, C. C. L. Wyatt, B. L. Beattie et al., "Provision of mouth-care in long-term care facilities: an educational trial," *Community Dentistry and Oral Epidemiology*, vol. 35, no. 1, pp. 25–34, 2007.

[41] M. I. MacEntee, "Conflicting priorities: oral health in long-term care," *Special Care in Dentistry*, vol. 19, no. 4, pp. 164–172, 1999.

[42] S. E. Thorne, A. Kazanjian, and M. I. MacEntee, "Oral health in long-term care the implications of organizational culture," *Journal of Aging Studies*, vol. 15, no. 3, pp. 271–283, 2001.

[43] R. D. Lasker, E. S. Weiss, and R. Miller, "Partnership synergy: a practical framework for studying and strengthening the collaborative advantage," *Milbank Quarterly*, vol. 79, no. 2, pp. 179–205, 2001.

[44] V. J. Shannon, "Partnerships: the foundation for future success," *Canadian Journal of Nursing Administration*, vol. 11, no. 3, pp. 61–76, 1998.

[45] Government of Nova Scotia Continuing Care Branch, "Nursing homes and homes for the aged: accurate bed count as of December, 2011," Department of Health, Nova Scotia, Canada, 2001, http://www.gov.ns.ca/health/ccs/pubs/approved_facilities/Dir_approved_facilities_NH.pdf.

[46] L. M. Franco, S. Bennett, and R. Kanfer, "Health sector reform and public sector health worker motivation: a conceptual framework," *Social Science and Medicine*, vol. 54, no. 8, pp. 1255–1266, 2002.

[47] J. E. Gangeness and E. Yurkovich, "Revisiting case study as a nursing research design," *Nurse Researcher*, vol. 13, no. 4, pp. 7–18, 2006.

[48] R. Yin, *Case Study Research: Design and Methods*, Sage Publications, Thousand Oaks, Calif, USA, 2003.

[49] C. Braden and N. Herban, *Community Health: A Systems Approach*, Appleton-Century-Crofts, New York, NY, USA, 1976.

[50] I. Hodder, "The interpretation of documents and material culture," in *Handbook of Qualitative Research*, N. Denzin and Y. Lincoln, Eds., pp. 703–715, Sage Publications, Thousand Oaks, Calif, USA, 2000.

[51] F. A. Miller and K. Alvarado, "Incorporating documents into qualitative nursing research," *Journal of Nursing Scholarship*, vol. 37, no. 4, pp. 348–353, 2005.

[52] J. Gubrium and J. Holstein, *The New Language of Qualitative Method*, Oxford University Press, New York, NY, USA, 1997.

[53] P. Mukerji, *Methodology in Social Research: Dilemmas and Perspectives, Essays in Honour of Ramkrishna Mukerjee*, Sage Publications, Thousand Oaks, Calif, USA, 2003.

[54] M. Lubrosky, "The identification and analysis of themes and patterns," in *Qualitative Methods in Aging Research*, J. Gubrium and A. Sankar, Eds., pp. 189–210, Sage Publications, Thousand Oaks, Calif, USA, 1994.

[55] P. Ulin, E. Robinson, and E. Tolley, *Qualitative Methods in Public Health: A Field Guide for Applied Research*, Wiley/Jossey-Bass, San Francisco, Calif, USA, 2004.

[56] Registered Nurses' Association of Ontario, Oral health: nursing assessment and interventions best practice guidelines, Registered Nurses' Association of Ontario, 2008.

[57] C. C. L. Wyatt and M. I. MacEntee, *Daily Oral Care for Persons in Residential Care*, Geriatric Dentistry Program Manual, The University of British Columbia, Vancouver, Canada, 2nd edition, 2007.

[58] A. Delbecq and A. Van de Ven, "A group process model for problem identification and program planning," *Journal of Applied Behavioral Science*, vol. 7, no. 4, pp. 466–492, 1971.

[59] Government of Nova Scotia, *Evidence Based Wound Management Protocol*, Department of Health—Community Care, Nova Scotia, Canada, 2000.

[60] F. Gottrup, "Optimizing wound treatment through health care structuring and professional education," *Wound Repair and Regeneration*, vol. 12, no. 2, pp. 129–133, 2004.

[61] D. P. Rice, H. M. Fillit, W. Max, D. S. Knopman, J. R. Lloyd, and S. Duttagupta, "Prevalence, costs, and treatment of Alzheimer's disease and related dementia: a managed care perspective," *American Journal of Managed Care*, vol. 7, no. 8, pp. 809–818, 2001.

11

Understanding Jordanian Psychiatric Nurses' Smoking Behaviors: A Grounded Theory Study

Khaldoun M. Aldiabat[1] and Michael Clinton[2]

[1] School of Nursing, University of Northern British Columbia, 3333 University Way, Prince George, BC, Canada V2N 4Z9
[2] Rafic Hariri School of Nursing, American University of Beirut, Riad El-Solh, Beirut 1107 2020, Lebanon

Correspondence should be addressed to Khaldoun M. Aldiabat; aldiabat@unbc.ca

Academic Editor: Maria Helena Palucci Marziale

Purpose. Smoking is prevalent in psychiatric facilities among staff and patients. However, there have been few studies of how contextual factors in specific cultures influence rates of smoking and the health promotion role of psychiatric nurses. This paper reports the findings of a classical grounded theory study conducted to understand how contextual factors in the workplace influences the smoking behaviors of Jordanian psychiatric nurses (JPNs). *Method.* Semi-structured individual interviews were conducted with a sample of eight male JPNs smokers at a psychiatric facility in Amman, Jordan. *Findings.* Constant comparative analysis identified *becoming a heavy smoker* as a psychosocial process characterized by four sub-categories: normalization of smoking; living in ambiguity; experiencing workplace conflict; and, facing up to workplace stressors. *Conclusion.* Specific contextual workplace factors require targeted smoking cessation interventions if JPNs are to receive the help they need to reduce health risks associated with heavy smoking.

1. Introduction

Smoking cigarettes is common practice among patients and staff in mental health services throughout the world [1]. Although few studies have assessed smoking behaviors among psychiatric nurses in different countries, their results reported indicate a high prevalence rates compared to those for nurses in other specialties. A literature review by Storr et al. [2] found that psychiatric nurses have higher smoking prevalence rates than nurses working in administration, emergency rooms, medical care, critical care, and gerontology. Psychiatric nurses in the United States are 2.4 times more likely to smoke cigarettes than nurses in other specialty areas [3]. The prevalence of smoking among mental health nurses in the United Kingdom was reported as 17.4% [4]. Two years later the reported prevalence rate was 35% [5] double that reported in the earlier investigation. in the 1980s the smoking the prevalence rates for psychiatric nurses in the United States was reported as 28.6% [6]; almost 14% less than that of 42.4% reported for Great Britain [7].

The high prevalence of smoking among psychiatric nurses threatens professional values (not to harm patients) and delivery of quality services, including patient education, if left unstudied. Furthermore, to neglect the high smoking prevalence rates among psychiatric nurses is to ignore an international agreement about the importance of a health promotion role for all health professionals [8] and to deny psychiatric nurses a legitimate role in health promotion [9]. The health promotion role fits well with the pride psychiatric nurses take in providing holistic care to meet patients' interrelated physical and mental health needs. However, psychiatric nurses who smoke have not yet acknowledged smoking reduction as one of their primary goals for patients, despite the opportunities they have for helping patients cut down on the number of cigarettes they smoke or to stop smoking altogether [9–12].

All the studies referred to in this introduction were conducted in Western countries. Hence, contextual workplace factors that influence smoking behaviors among psychiatric nurses in Arabic speaking countries, including in Jordan, have not been investigated or reported. Therefore, the purpose of this paper is to report the findings of a classical grounded theory study conducted to understand how contextual workplace factors influence the smoking behaviors of JPNs. We intend that our study will encourage other researchers to investigate the relationship between contextual workplace factors and the smoking behaviors of nurses in Arabic speaking countries. Such research is needed to better understand how to help nurses take better care of their health while addressing the smoking reduction and smoking cessation needs of their patients.

2. The Method

This section summarizes the research methods used in the study. A more detailed account can be found in Aldiabat and Clinton [13]. In essence, we used a classical grounded theory approach [14] to investigate how social, psychological, organizational, personal, and cultural factors influence JPNs to become heavy smokers. The study was conducted in Amman, Jordan between 2009 and 2010 following ethical committee approval in Canada and Jordan. Data were collected from a theoretical sample of eight male psychiatric nurses smokers at a psychiatric hospital. Semi-structured interviews, nonparticipant observation, sociometry and ethnographic field notes were used in the study. The constant comparative method of analysis was applied throughout the study. Thus, data collection, coding, and analysis occurred simultaneously. It was found that for JPNs, *becoming a heavy smoker* is a component of a longer process theorized as "*contextualizing smoking behavior over time.*" Four phases are fundamental to this process: (1) becoming a novice smoker; (2) becoming a regular smoker; (3) becoming a heavy smoker; (4) becoming an exhausted smoker. Throughout the study, care was taken to meet an acceptable standard of trustworthiness by fulfilling requirements for credibility, transferability, dependability, and confirmability [13].

3. Findings

3.1. Becoming a Heavy Smoker. This phase in the *contextualizing smoking behavior over time* psychosocial process explains how Jordanian psychiatric nurses transition from regular smoking to heavy smoking. The eight nurses in this study regarded themselves as regular smokers if the smoked 12–14 cigarettes on most days. They regarded themselves as heavy smokers if they smoked more than 14 cigarettes every day. The participants reported four contextual workplace factors that foster and maintain their habit of heavy smoking: (a) accommodating workplace challenges, (b) living in ambiguity, (c) experiencing workplace conflict, and (d) Facing up to workplace stressors.

3.2. Accommodating Workplace Challenges. The eight JPNs attributed heavy smoking to challenges in the workplace. The following verbatim statements describe challenges that influence their smoking.

3.2.1. Normalized Smoking. The participants regarding smoking in the psychiatric workplace as a normal and natural behavior. They distinguished between two kindes of normalization: institutionalized normalization and individualized normalization.

Organizational Normalization. According to the participants, organizational normalization of smoking has three salient characteristics:

(a) widespread tolerance of smoking in the organization: "As you see, smoking is not something strange in this organization" (Yasser);

(b) regular smoking among psychiatric patients and staff "Both patients and staff smoke freely in [name of psychiatric hospital] which means smoking is an acceptable behavior" (Osama);

(c) institutionalized availability of cigarettes: "Here, it is not uncommon to find cigarettes everywhere; (...). Sometimes, we miss some medications or equipment, but it is impossible to be without cigarettes" (Ismael).

Individualized Normalization. The three most salient charactristics of individualized normalization are:

(a) smokers and nonsmokers alike accept smoking as a common everyday activity: "I do not feel others [smokers and/or nonsmokers] perceive us differently (...). We are like other people who smoke in Jordan" (Mustafa);

(b) distributing cigarettes to patients is an integral part of the role of psychiatric nurses: "You know distributing cigarettes to patients is one of our roles, but accepting that role means we [nurses] normalize smoking..." (Kamal);

(c) none of the participants expressed dissonance associated with smoking. Smokers smoke freely in the presence of non-smoking friends and direct supervisors; although they know that is a clear contravention of Ministry of Health prohibitions.

3.2.2. Challenges That Encourage Smoking. JPNs offer several justifications smoking in the workplace: finding respite from work; managing self-perceptions, including shoring up self-esteem and promoting feelings of personal well being; making time at work go more quickly; rewarding oneself for small achievements; rewarding patients for good behavior; and, controlling them effectively.

Smoking promotes feelings of comfort and relaxation; I smoke at [name of psychiatric hospital] because smoking gives me more breaks. It helps me treat my negative self-perceptions and boosts my self-esteem. When I smoke I feel my personality becomes stronger (...). Actually, this workplace looks like a jail; smoking gives me the feeling that work time goes faster. Sometimes when I achieve something, I reward myself by smoking a cigarette. When patients behave well, I reward them with cigarettes. Smoking controls patients' behavior because there is nothing in this world more effective than a cigarette to control psychiatric patients who smoke. Yes, giving cigarettes to patients is used to prevent relapse and agitation (Aladdin).

At the same time, the nurses draw attention to perceived psychological and social benefits of smoking.

> The cigarette is part of my personality because I used to hold cigarettes between my fingers rather than smoke them. Now I just smoke them, which is why I smoke all the time. [A cigarette] helps my concentration during work tasks, improves my sense of freedom. I smoke to get enjoyment, to enhance my alertness, and to build a social relationship with others (...). From my perspective, smoking is necessary for psychiatric nurses because they spend the majority of their time observing patients; hence, they need to smoke to help focus their attention (Hassan).

3.3. Living in Ambiguity.

In this second subcategory, participants reported two kinds of ambiguity that increase smoking in the workplace: the role ambiguity and the task ambiguity associated with psychiatric nursing care.

3.3.1. Role Ambiguity.

One of the traditional roles of JPNs is to distribute cigarettes to psychiatric patients. When the participants were asked about this role, their answers divided them into two groups. The first group of five nurses said distributing cigarettes to patients is not part of the nurse's role. Furthermore, this group of JPNs did not regard assisting patients with smoking cessation as part of their role.

> Distributing cigarettes to patients is not an official job for nurses, but we [psychiatric nurses] give patients cigarettes to stop them getting agitated. we give out cigarettes because we do not want the patients to relapse, and we want to avoid administration accusing us of not controlling patients' behaviors. As smokers ourselves, we feel empathy towards patients who smoke and we put ourselves in their shoes. cutting down on smoking is not a priority for the psychiatric patients because they are here [name of psychiatric hospital] to receive treatment for mental illness, not to quit smoking. My role as psychiatric nurse is primarily to treat psychiatric disease. I do not think that teaching patients about smoking cessation is one of my nursing roles.

> I cannot quit smoking myself, so how can I encourage others to quit? As the proverb says; a gift cannot be made of something missing. (In other words, nurses who smoke cannot be role models for changing the smoking habits of patients) (Mohammed).

The remaining three nurses thought that distributing of cigarettes to patients is a psychiatric nursing role because "I perform what administrators expect me to do (...). So, I think it is a legal role and I believe it is my job; it is a customary nursing role in the psychiatric nursing field (...). Yes, yes, it is a nursing role and part of the treatment plan the patients" (Mustafa).

The eight JPNs were asked to describe their feelings after distributing cigarettes to patients. All eight reported ambivalent emotions in much the same way, for example:

> I feel happy because I see how patients enjoy smoking cigarettes... but at the same time, I feel guilty and disappointed because I offered them something harmful (...). Exactly what I feel, I do not know (...) I want them to smoke, but I do not like myself when give them cigarettes (...). When I distribute cigarettes I feel down because this is not my job. If there was someone else [non-nurse] to give them the cigarettes, I would be happy (Mohammed).

3.3.2. Task Ambiguity/Challenges in Providing Psychiatric Nursing Care.

The participants reported that the ambiguity due to the vagueness of psychiatric nursing is one of the commonest challenges they face on a daily basis. They categorized the sources of ambiguity into four levels: (1) ambiguity at the organizational and administrical level, (2) at the staff nurse level, (3) at the patient level, and (4) ambiguity of tasks at the family and societal level. These levels of ambiguity are italicized in the following participant statements.

> Psychiatric health care in Jordan is an undeveloped medical field. Much development is needed compared to other medical fields (...). Psychiatric settings in Jordan do not have a clearly organized working system (...). The big problem is that we have no multidisciplinary teams in the psychiatric field in Jordan (...). Psychiatric nurses receive low salary compared to nurses in other fields, and they have low job satisfaction (...). Indeed, in many cases, they have zero job satisfaction.... The big problem is the administrative corruption; there is cronyism and nepotism among administrators. In addition, there is an absence of trust between the administration and nurses, lack of transparency [*Ambiguity of the task at the organizational and administrational level*] (Kamal).

> Although nurses here were prepared through a Bachelor of Nursing program to provide comprehensive care, they are using the custodial model of care for psychiatric patients. They believe the patients will not respond to any treatment plan. They think that psychiatric diseases are incurable and they have accepted the role of distributing cigarettes to patients accordingly, which is completely against their health promotion role. I think all these circumstances increase my smoking rate here [name of psychiatric hospital] [*Ambiguity at the staff nurse level*] (Mohammed).

> It is horrible workload; we are two registered nurses, and three practical nurses to take care for 27 patients (...). You know, psychiatric patients often exhibit unexpected, aggressive and agitated behaviors (...). Nurses here are not sure if they can manage these behaviors (...). We are confused and upset

because psychiatric patients cannot communicate effectively with us (...); they often need around-the-clock observation to prevent self-harm or harm to others (...). I am not sure if I am a nurse or a guard [*Ambiguity at the patient care level*] (Aladdin).

Many reasons in [name of psychiatric hospital] force me to smoke more. For example, many Jordanians think that psychiatric nurses will be influenced by psychiatric patients and after a while, they [the nurses] will become crazy (...). They [Jordanians] think that mentally ill patients must always remain in hospital because mental diseases are long life and incurable. Thus, they [Jordanians] perceive psychiatric nurses as uneducated bodyguards, who protect patients from one another (...). Patients' families will do anything to keep their relatives in [name of psychiatrichospital] as long as possible (...). They [the families] do not want to take care of their relatives, but they still accuse nurses of lack of care [*Ambiguity of tasks at family and societal level*] (Hassan).

3.4. Experiencing Workplace Conflict. The third subcategory of *becoming a heavy smoker* is experiencing workplace conflict. This subcategory includes two conflicts reported by the participants to have increased their smoking rate: nursing-role conflict and interpersonal conflict.

3.4.1. Nursing-Role Conflict. The psychiatric nurses described nursing-role conflict in the following terms.

Nurses here [name of psychiatric hospital] are doing primarily custodial care (e.g., planning activities of daily living, administrating medications; adhering very closely to physician orders, and distributing cigarettes to patients). We do not have much authority to make decisions about treatment for the patients (...). Many of us [psychiatric nurses] reject the custodial nursing role and insist that psychiatric nursing care should be done differently based on international trends (...). I think that experiencing this conflict [in role] makes me to smoke more (Kamal).

3.4.2. Interpersonal Conflict. Interpersonal conflict in the study setting arises in a variety of ways. The italicized statements below indicate a conflict between male nurses and female supervisors, among nurse coworkers, and between nurses and physicians/psychiatrists.

I have a strongly conflicted relationship with her [a female supervisor]. The relationship can be described as fuel and fire (...) and very formal. A female leader evokes stress/creates conflicts for male followers [*Male nurses-female supervisor conflict*] (...). It is not uncommon to see some conflicts with co-workers; some of our nursing colleagues are just impossible to work with. We face difficulty and conflict when dealing with them because they are: arrogant, stubborn, sometimes abusive, slackers, spies, gossipers, and act

like they are right about almost everything [*Nurse-nursing co-workers' conflict*] (Yasser).

Physicians and nurses clash because nurses do not trust physicians and vice versa. Physicians create tensions to marginalize nurses and they ignore nursing knowledge (...). They [physicians] have misperceptions about nurses. They think nurses are not educated and they ignore nurses' requests for them [physicians] to see patients (...). They do not listen to nurses and they abuse them by shouting, by making accusations, and by blaming them [if anything goes wrong]. Nurse, use avoidance to cope with abusive physicians, thereby killing any opportunity for real communication [*Nurses-physicians conflict*] (Kamal).

3.5. Facing up to Workplace Stressors. This fourth subcategory of *becoming a heavy smoker* draws attention to stressors in the workplace that increase smoking among JPNs. The participants reported four sources of workplace stress: (a) the nurse does not control the steering wheel; (b) the power is within your "Wasta" (network); (c) living with negative feelings; (d) an unattractive career because due to stigmatization.

3.5.1. The Nurse Does Not Control the Steering Wheel. This subcategory is characterized by limited control over decision making. One participant reported that "Jordanian psychiatric nurses cannot make any administrative decisions. The decisions they can make regarding direct patient care are very limited (...). I think that making administrative decisions is the supervisor job (...). Nurses offer opinions more than making decisions" (Kamal).

Furthermore,

Administrators and physicians ask nurses to do only what they say and to obey their orders without question or discussion (...). They [administrators and physicians] want us to be good followers not autonomous nurses. We are here to follow orders and instructions, but we still dream to becoming decision makers in an independent profession (...). Smoking cigarettes is the most effective way to getting rid of these stressors (...) (Mohammed).

3.5.2. The Power Is within Your "Wasta"/Network. Wasta is a popular social phenomenon in Jordan and throughout the Arab world. It can be defined simply as cronyism and corruption, but such translations do not convey either its pervasiveness or the strength of its influence.

If anything serves as the symbol of corruption in Jordan, it is what is known as *Wasta*. Wasta literally means favouritism—the use of family, business or personal connections to advance personal interests. Although Wasta is culturally rooted, the vast majority of Jordanians believe that it is a prevalent form of corruption. At the same time, there is a public perception that citizens must have some sort of Wasta in order to run their day-to-day affairs smoothly, in a country largely ruled by bureaucracy" (Ma'ayeh, 2008) [15].

Participants reported two forms of Wasta that increases stress levels and smoking. Wasta or *cronyism at the administrational level* is manifested by "Administrators dealing with the employees on the basis of personal relationships and network ties. Feelings of injustice as a result of Wasta has increased my smoking rate (...). You know, some nurses use personal relationships to get benefits from the administrators" (Osama).

Cronyism at the nursing supervisor level was manifested by "Nursing supervisors deal with subordinates on the basis of personal and tribal relationships when allocating the more desired shifts [mornings] and when handling various promotions" (Aladdin).

3.5.3. Intense Negative Feelings. The participants identified three causes of intense negative feelings that increase workplace stress and smoking.

Increasing the Consumption of Cigarettes at Work. Brought out in statements of the following kind: "We, smokers and nurses are feeling very uncomfortable as our smoking habit becomes more uncontrollable (...). We feel like we have multiple-personalities because we are nurses who smoke. We blame ourselves for our smoking. We feel guilty because we smoke" (Mohammed).

Distributing Cigarettes to the Patients. "I am feeling like I am cheating because I provide patients a harmful product (...). I do not feel like a nurse when I do this and this feeling is punishing me. Smoking decreases this feeling temporarily" (Aladdin).

Lack of Control over Decision Making. "I am feeling hopeless about never being allowed to be a decision maker (...). I am feeling as if I will always be just a follower (...). Actually, I am feeling that I have no value and I am a useless employee (...). I feel upset, burnt-out, and exhausted because I have no decision making role" (Mohammed).

3.5.4. An Unattractive Career (Stigmatization). Jordanians have misconceptions and misperceptions about psychiatric nurses because of the negative ways they [the nurses] are portrayed in the Arabic media including on TV (...). I am too worried to tell others I am a psychiatric nurse. There are very few people that I talk to about my profession (...). I do not want to talk about it [my work] because I hate feeling stigmatized because of it. Stigmatization makes us perceive nursing as a service not a profession. The nursing profession has no respect from others and has low social status in comparison to other professions (...). The stigma makes us feel pain, grief, isolation, inferiority; low self-esteem and unappreciated in our role as psychiatric nurses (...). We look

at ourselves like we have limited power, knowledge, social status, and decision making (...). I smoke more and more to forget that I am working in psychiatric nursing—a low prestige profession (...). I have no job satisfaction at all and I blame myself for choosing this path (Kamal).

4. Discussion

Becoming a heavy smoker is the third and advanced phase in our contextualizing smoking behavior over time theory. It is a process that takes place in the work setting, a place where smoking is openly permitted and is considered to be a normal behavior. During this phase, JPNs integrate an increased rate of smoking behavior into their daily lives. This phase is similar to what DiClemente [16] called the "maintenance stage" of behavior change; it refers to when the individual becomes a fully addicted smoker, and thus smoking has become habitual and problematic. According to DiClemente [16], "the task for maintenance is to sustain and integrate the behavior change into the total life context so that it becomes normative, familiar, and integral" (page 30). A point to be emphasized regarding the difference between DiClemente's [16] "maintenance phase" and the current study is that JPNs do not "maintain" their smoking behaviors, but continue to increase their rate of smoking in the *becoming a heavy smoker* phase. Smoking behaviors are, therefore, not "maintained" but sustained at an increasingly higher rate.

4.1. Addiction Process. The addiction process is most commonly discussed from the perspective of two behavioral and learning theories: classical conditioning and schedules of reinforcement. From the perspective of classical conditioning, it is assumed that there is a strong relationship between smoking addictive behavior and associated stimuli [16, 17]. According to DiClemente [16], the conditioning process reaches its peak during the maintenance stage of smoking behavior. Similarly, the JPNs in out sample had many stimuli in their workplace that encouraged them to smoke with higher frequency.

As an addictive behavior, smoking is shaped by contingencies of positive and negative reinforcement [18]. JPNs who experience positive reinforcement from smoking (e.g., improved self-esteem and concentration) continue smoking to maintain positive feelings and experience other rewards as described above. However, for the nurses in out sample, the frequency of smoking is increased by negative reinforcement as well. Negative reinforcement derived from satisfying the withdrawal symptoms associated with craving more cigarettes, but it occurs also through the stress reduction that occurs as a result by smoking to escape the workplace challenges we have described.

4.2. Heavy Smoking in Context. JPNs report contextual factors that influence them to become heavy smokers. The use of the constant comparison method [14] revealed that some of the findings reported here are similar to those reported in the literature, while others are unique to the current study.

The nursing profession is distinguished from other professions by its high degree of work-related stress [19–21]. A literature review of stress among nurses showed that psychiatric nurses have a higher level of work related stresscompared with nurses in general [22]. Work-related stress occurs when the physical or psychological demands exceed the ability of employees to control their workload [23, 24]. Nursing is a stressful profession not only because it is a demanding one, but also because nurses are exposed to numerous social, physical, and environmental stressors [25]. The sources of these stressors have been identified as follows: low job control and excessive job demands [26], low control over decisions [27], and the negative leadership style of supervisors [28, 29].

Work-related stress can affect human health directly by disturbing physiological processes and indirectly through risky health behaviors such as smoking [30, 31]. Moreover, work stress affects a multitude of non-health promoting behaviors such as smoking, drinking, or weight gain more than a single unhealthy behavior [32, 33]. Previous studies indicate that many workers smoke to reduce and manage work-related stress [34–37]. For example, psychiatric nurses in the United Kingdom used smoking and alcohol to adapt to high levels of work-related stress [38].

Job satisfaction is strongly related to work-related stress. Much of the literature indicates a strong inverse relationship between job stress and job satisfaction [39–41]. For example, psychiatric nurses in the United Kingdom who had experienced a high level of stress showed low levels of job satisfaction [42]. An Australian study showed that high job satisfaction among nurses buffers and lowers work-related stress [43]. A study of the relationship between the smoking behaviors of military nurses and social support, stress, and job satisfaction found that nurses who smoked experienced a high level of work-related stress and had both low social support and low job satisfaction [44].

4.3. Unique Contextual Factors. In our study, JPNs reported unique contextual factors that increased their smoking rate: normalization of smoking (at nurse and organizational levels), living in ambiguity, experiencing workplace conflict, and facing up to workplace stressors, including the pernicious effect of Wasta and job stigmatization.

5. Conclusion

Specific workplace contextual factors require targeted smoking reduction and smoking cessation interventions if male JPNs are to receive the help they need to reduce the health risks associated with heavy smoking for both themselves and the patients in their care.

Nurses and other decision makers can use these insights to guide culturally sensitive smoking reduction and cessation programs to benefit those male Jordanian psychiatric nurses who want to reduce their smoking or stop smoking completely.

However, smoking reduction and cessation programs are likely to be more successful in those work settings in which psychiatric nurses are encouraged to work to the full scope of their professional role.

References

[1] P. Reilly, L. Murphy, and D. Alderton, "Challenging the smoking culture within a mental health service supportively," *International Journal of Mental Health Nursing*, vol. 15, no. 4, pp. 272–278, 2006.

[2] C. L. Storr, A. M. Trinkoff, and P. Hughes, "Similarities of substance use between medical and nursing specialties," *Substance Use and Misuse*, vol. 35, no. 10, pp. 1443–1469, 2000.

[3] A. M. Trinkoff and C. L. Storr, "Substance use among nurses: differences between specialties," *American Journal of Public Health*, vol. 88, no. 4, pp. 581–585, 1998.

[4] G. L. Dickens, J. H. Stubbs, and C. M. Haw, "Smoking and mental health nurses: a survey of clinical staff in a psychiatric hospital," *Journal of Psychiatric and Mental Health Nursing*, vol. 11, no. 4, pp. 445–451, 2004.

[5] R. N. Bloor, L. Meeson, and I. B. Crome, "The effects of a non-smoking policy on nursing staff smoking behavior and attitudes in a psychiatric hospital," *Journal of Psychiatric and Mental Health Nursing*, vol. 13, no. 2, pp. 188–196, 2006.

[6] R. Tagliacozzo and S. Vaughn, "Stress and smoking in hospital nurses," *American Journal of Public Health*, vol. 72, no. 5, pp. 441–448, 1982.

[7] L. Hawkins, M. White, and L. Morris, "Smoking, stress and nurses," *Nursing Mirror*, vol. 155, no. 15, pp. 18–22, 1982.

[8] World Health Organization, "Health professionals to promote a new code of conduct on tobacco control," 2003, http://www.who.int/en/.

[9] B. Hancock and D. Hancock, "Registered mental nurses' perceived role in health education about smoking," *Health Education Journal*, vol. 52, no. 2, pp. 85–90, 1993.

[10] J. K. Cataldo, "The role of advanced practice psychiatric nurses in treating tobacco use and dependence," *Archives of Psychiatric Nursing*, vol. 15, no. 3, pp. 107–119, 2001.

[11] A. McCloughen, "The association between schizophrenia and cigarette smoking: a review of the literature and implications for mental health nursing practice," *International Journal of Mental Health Nursing*, vol. 12, no. 2, pp. 119–129, 2003.

[12] C. J. Van Dongen, "Smoking and persistent mental illness: an exploratory study," *Journal of Psychosocial Nursing and Mental Health Services*, vol. 37, no. 11, pp. 26–34, 1999.

[13] K. Aldiabat and M. Clinton, "Contextualizing smoking behavior over time: a smoking journey from pleasuring to suffering," *Turkish Online Journal of Qualitative Inquiry*, vol. 3, no. 1, pp. 1–19, 2012.

[14] B. Glaser and A. Strauss, *The Discovery of Grounded Theory: Strategies for Qualitative Research*, Aldine, Chicago, Ill, USA, 1967.

[15] S. Ma'ayeh, Call your Wasta, 2008, http://commons.global-integrity.org/2008/06/jordan-call-your-wasta.html.

[16] C. DiClemente, *Addiction and Change: How Addictions Develop and Addicted People Recover*, Guilford Press, New York, NY, USA, 2003.

[17] T. J. Payne, M. Etscheidt, and S. A. Corrigan, "Conditioning arbitrary stimuli to cigarette smoke intake: a preliminary study," *Journal of Substance Abuse*, vol. 2, no. 1, pp. 113–119, 1990.

[18] L. M. Cohen, D. M. McCarthy, S. A. Brown, and M. G. Myers, "Negative affect combines with smoking outcome expectancies

to predict smoking behavior over time," *Psychology of Addictive Behaviors*, vol. 16, no. 2, pp. 91–97, 2002.

[19] M. J. Foxall, L. Zimmerman, R. Standley, and B. Bené, "A comparison of frequency and sources of nursing job stress perceived by intensive care, hospice and medical-surgical nurses," *Journal of Advanced Nursing*, vol. 15, no. 5, pp. 577–584, 1990.

[20] P. Hingley, "The humane face of nursing," *Nursing Mirror*, vol. 159, no. 21, pp. 19–22, 1984.

[21] E. D. Ogus, "Burnout and coping strategies: a comparative study of ward nurses," in *Occupational Stress: A Handbook*, R. Crandall and P. L. Perrewe, Eds., pp. 249–261, Taylor & Francis, Washington, DC, USA, 1995.

[22] D. Edwards, P. Burnard, D. Coyle, A. Fothergill, and B. Hannigan, "Stressors, moderators and stress outcomes: findings from the All-Wales Community Mental Health Nurse Study," *Journal of Psychiatric and Mental Health Nursing*, vol. 7, no. 6, pp. 529–537, 2000.

[23] R. A. Karasek Jr., "Job demands, job decision latitude and mental strain: implications for job redesign," *Administrative Science Quarterly*, vol. 24, pp. 285–308, 1979.

[24] R. Karasek, C. Brisson, N. Kawakami, I. Houtman, P. Bongers, and B. Amick, "The Job Content Questionnaire (JCQ): an instrument for internationally comparative assessments of psychosocial job characteristics," *Journal of Occupational Health Psychology*, vol. 3, no. 4, pp. 322–355, 1998.

[25] S. Uğur, A. Acuner, B. Göktaş, and B. Şenoğlu, "Effects of physical environment on the stress levels of hemodialysis nurses in Ankara Turkey," *Journal of Medical System*, vol. 31, no. 4, pp. 283–287, 2007.

[26] R. A. Karasek, "Lower health risk with increased job control among white collar workers," *Journal of Organizational Behavior*, vol. 11, no. 3, pp. 171–185, 1990.

[27] M. Elovainio, M. Kivimäki, and J. Vahtera, "Organizational justice: evidence of a new psychosocial predictor of health," *American Journal of Public Health*, vol. 92, no. 1, pp. 105–108, 2002.

[28] J. Seltzer, R. E. Numerof, and B. M. Bass, "Transformational leadership: is it a source of more burnout and stress?" *Journal of Health and Human Resources Administration*, vol. 12, no. 2, pp. 174–185, 1989.

[29] S. Stordeur, W. D'hoore, and C. Vandenberghe, "Leadership, organizational stress, and emotional exhaustion among hospital nursing staff," *Journal of Advanced Nursing*, vol. 35, no. 4, pp. 533–542, 2001.

[30] E. Brunner and M. Marmot, "Social organization, stress, and health," in *Social Determinants of Health*, M. Marmot and R. G. Wilkinson, Eds., pp. 17–43, Oxford University Press, Oxford, UK, 1999.

[31] T. Theorell, "To be able to exert control over one's own situation: a necessary condition for coping with stressors," in *Handbook of Occupational Health Psychology*, C. J. Quick and L. E. Tetrick, Eds., pp. 201–219, American Psychological Association, Washington, DC, USA, 2003.

[32] M. Kivimäki, J. Head, J. E. Ferrie et al., "Work stress, weight gain and weight loss: evidence for bidirectional effects of job strain on body mass index in the Whitehall II study," *International Journal of Obesity*, vol. 30, pp. 982–987, 2006.

[33] A. Kouvonen, J. Vahtera, M. Elovainio et al., "Organisational justice and smoking: the Finnish public sector study," *Journal of Epidemiology and Community Health*, vol. 61, no. 5, pp. 427–433, 2007.

[34] M. Bobak, H. Pikhart, C. Hertzman, R. Rose, and M. Marmot, "Socioeconomic factors, perceived control and self-reported health in Russia. A cross-sectional survey," *Social Science and Medicine*, vol. 47, no. 2, pp. 269–279, 1998.

[35] H. Graham, "Women's smoking and family health," *Social Science and Medicine*, vol. 25, no. 1, pp. 47–56, 1987.

[36] C. G. Healton and K. Nelson, "Reversal of misfortune: viewing tobacco as a social justice issue," *American Journal of Public Health*, vol. 94, no. 2, pp. 186–191, 2004.

[37] R. Niaura, W. G. Shadel, D. M. Britt, and D. B. Abrams, "Response to social stress, urge to smoke, and smoking cessation," *Addictive Behaviors*, vol. 27, no. 2, pp. 241–250, 2002.

[38] M. Coffey and M. Coleman, "The relationship between support and stress in forensic community mental health nursing," *Journal of Advanced Nursing*, vol. 34, no. 3, pp. 397–407, 2001.

[39] A. Adams and S. Bond, "Hospital nurses, job satisfaction, individual and organizational characteristics," *Journal of Advanced Nursing*, vol. 32, no. 3, pp. 536–543, 2000.

[40] R. Knoop, "Relationship among job involvement, job satisfaction, and organizational commitment for nurses," *Journal of Psychology*, vol. 129, no. 6, pp. 643–649, 1995.

[41] S. E. Sullivan and R. S. Bhagat, "Organizational stress, job satisfaction and job performance: where do we go from here?" *Journal of Management*, vol. 18, no. 2, pp. 353–374, 1992.

[42] B. Parry-Jones, G. Grant, M. McGrath, K. Caldock, P. Ramcharan, and C. A. Robinson, "Stress and job satisfaction among social workers, community nurses and community psychiatric nurses: implications for the care management model," *Health and Social Care in the Community*, vol. 6, no. 4, pp. 271–285, 1998.

[43] C. M. Healy and M. F. McKay, "Nursing stress: the effects of coping strategies and job satisfaction in a sample of Australian nurses," *Journal of Advanced Nursing*, vol. 31, no. 3, pp. 681–688, 2000.

[44] L. L. Alexander and K. Beck, "The smoking behavior of military nurses: the relationship to job stress, job satisfaction and social support," *Journal of Advanced Nursing*, vol. 15, no. 7, pp. 843–849, 1990.

12

Oral Health and Hygiene Content in Nursing Fundamentals Textbooks

Rita A. Jablonski

School of Nursing, The Pennsylvania State University, 201 Health and Human Development East, University Park, PA 16802, USA

Correspondence should be addressed to Rita A. Jablonski, raj16@psu.edu

Academic Editor: Mary George

The purpose of this paper is to describe the quantity and quality of oral hygiene content in a representative sample of before-licensure nursing fundamentals textbooks. Seven textbooks were examined. Quantity was operationalized as the actual page count and percentage of content devoted to oral health and hygiene. Quality of content was operationalized as congruency with best mouth care practices. Best mouth care practices included evidence-based and consensus-based practices as published primarily by the American Dental Association and supported by both published nursing research and review articles specific to mouth care and published dental research and review articles specific to mouth care. Content devoted to oral health and hygiene averaged 0.6%. Although the quality of the content was highly variable, nearly every textbook contained some erroneous or outdated information. The most common areas for inaccuracy included the use of foam sponges for mouth care in dentate persons instead of soft toothbrushes and improper denture removal.

1. Introduction

Oral hygiene is vitally important because oral health is directly related to systemic health [1–3]. Poor oral health results in plaque buildup and inflammation of the gingiva. Plaque harbors pathogens associated with pneumonia [4]. In fact, poor oral hygiene has been linked to ventilator-associated pneumonia across the lifespan [5, 6]. Inflammation of the gingival tissues, either with or without periodontal disease, has been related to adverse outcomes in pregnancy, such as premature-birth and low-birth-weight infants [7]. Other systemic diseases associated with inadequate oral hygiene and resulting poor oral health include diabetes [8–10] and coronary artery disease [11]. Inadequate oral health negatively impacts quality of life and mortality, as well [12].

In 1986, Jones et al. surveyed nursing schools in the New England region to determine the quantity of oral health in both undergraduate and graduate curricula [13]. At the undergraduate level, Jones et al. reported an hour or less of overall oral health content in the entire curricula for 50% of the surveyed schools [13]. Fourteen percent of the undergraduate programs included 2 to 3 hours of oral

health content specific to older adults; the remaining schools reported zero to 1 hour [13]. More recent reports of oral health content in undergraduate/predoctoral nursing, medical, and pharmacy schools show little, if any, improvement. Nearly 60 percent of educators in nursing, medicine, and pharmacology in English-speaking universities around the world currently describe their curricula in oral health as insufficient [14].

In 2009, at the request of the Department of Health and Human Services (DHHS), the Institute of Medicine convened an oral health panel. The panel, The Committee on an Oral Health Initiative, was charged with "assessing the current oral health care system, reviewing the elements of an HHS Oral Health Initiative, and exploring ways to promote the use of preventive oral health interventions and improve oral health literacy [15, page vii]. Members of the committee invited experts to share their experiences and perspectives during public meetings held across the United States. One area that members of the committee explored was the important contributions nondental clinicians make to the prevention, diagnosis, and treatment of oral diseases [15]. The committee-desired information regarding the quantity and quality of oral health content in nursing education because nurses are responsible for either providing oral hygiene for their patients or supervising and delegating this task to unlicensed personnel [16]. This author was invited to address the committee and discuss the quantity and quality of oral health content in nursing education. In order to substantiate the content of the presentation, a search of nursing fundamentals textbooks was conducted in order to describe both the quantity and quality of oral hygiene content. Thus, the purpose of this paper is to describe the quantity and quality of oral hygiene content in before-licensure nursing fundamentals textbooks.

2. Materials and Methods

2.1. Search Description. The purpose of this search was to obtain a representative sample of nursing fundamental textbooks in order to describe the quantity and quality of oral hygiene content. The Google search engine was used to conduct the textbook search because it interfaced with content found in the Google Book Projects. In 2007, Google and the Committee on Institutional Cooperation (CIC), a consortium of 12 universities, entered into a partnership that would allow Google to convert the millions of books owned by CIC libraries to electronic formats [17]. The goal was to digitize 10 million volumes. Many textbooks were not fully digitized due to copyright restraints, but the titles, table of contents, and other information are available for searching [17]. The search terms "nursing," "fundamentals," and "textbook" were used in the search. Only textbooks in English published from 2006 through 2010 were included; when multiple editions were identified, only the most recent edition was included in the sample. The intended audience for the textbooks was before-licensure registered nursing students; textbooks for before-licensure practical nursing students or nursing assistants were excluded. Study guides or companion books to the primary textbooks were excluded. Additionally, the same search terms and criteria were used to search Amazon and Barnes & Noble websites. No additional textbooks were identified. Finally, if a publisher of any nursing textbooks did not appear in these searches (such as SAGE), the website was searched as well. Seven fundamental textbooks were identified using these criteria.

The textbooks were obtained via interlibrary loan. Quantity was operationalized as the actual page count and percentage of content devoted to oral health and hygiene in order to determine the quantity of oral hygiene content. Percentages were obtained by dividing the actual page count by the total pages of content and multiplying by 100. Total page count was determined by the last page of actual content, excluding indices, appendices, glossaries, and bibliographies. Quality of content was operationalized as congruency with best mouth care practices. Best mouth care practices included evidence-based and consensus-based practices as published primarily by the American Dental Association [18, 19] and supported by both published nursing research and review articles specific to mouth care and published dental research and review articles specific to mouth care [5, 6, 16, 20–28]. For example, nurse researchers have demonstrated the efficacy of specific oral health protocols, such as the use of

soft toothbrushes instead of foam swabs for both dentate and edentate persons [27, 29–32]. Chalmers et al. [22] published a comprehensive evidence-based protocol for oral hygiene care targeting older adults with functional and cognitive impairments. Thus, contents in the nursing fundamental textbooks were examined for content congruent with oral hygiene practices tested and endorsed by nurses, dental hygienists, and dentists.

3. Results and Discussion

Seven textbooks meeting the search criteria were obtained and are listed in Table 1. The percentage of oral health and hygiene content ranged from 0.27% [33] to 1.10% [34] with an average of 0.6%. Assessment of the oral cavity ranged from a few sentences [35] to 3.3 pages [34]. The assessment content in three textbooks [33, 35, 36] contained no information about assessing dentures for fit, integrity, or plaque. Potter and Perry [37] and Wilkinson and Van Leuven [34] offered the most complete information pertinent to oral health assessment. Potter and Perry [37] alone clearly articulated the oral-systemic link. This textbook also provided the clearest instructions for oral care with an unconscious or mechanically ventilated patient, for example, instructing the nurse to use an oral airway to keep the mouth of an unconscious or debilitated patient open. Three textbooks suggested using a tongue blade wrapped in gauze, which is not the safest or most comfortable approach [33, 35, 38]. Wilkinson and Van Leuven [34], on the other hand, recommended either the use of a tongue blade wrapped in gauze or a bite block.

One textbook contained no information on how to correctly floss or brush teeth [36] such as brush at a 45 degree angle and use short strokes [19]. The same textbook, however, offered a recipe for toothpaste (2 parts baking soda, one part salt) without referencing the source of this information. The remaining six textbooks provided information on correct brushing techniques. On the other hand, content about flossing was problematic. The American Dental Association [19] recommends using 18 inches of string floss, winding the bulk of the floss around a finger of the nondominant hand, and using the dominant hand to spool the floss and take up the soiled sections as different teeth are flossed. While string floss is acceptable when assisting a cognitively intact patient with mouth care, floss holders and interdentate brushes are better choices when providing mouth care to dependent patients or those with cognitive impairments. In fact, the American Dental Association [19] does suggest floss holders and interdentate brushes for persons who have difficulty using string floss. Interdentate brushes, also called proximal brushes, resemble plastic toothpicks but with spiral shaped brushes on the end. These brushes are also perfect for nurses providing mouth care to fully dependent patients because the brushes allow the nurse to floss if the patient is unable or unwilling to open his or her mouth [40]. Furthermore, the use of interdentate brushes prevents bite injuries because the nurses' fingers are not in patients' mouths. In spite of these considerations, the authors of one textbook directed nurses to use string floss,

Table 1: Summary of Results.

Bibliographic data	Pages devoted to oral health and hhygiene	Total Pages*	Percent of oral health and hygiene content	Significant findings
Craven and Hirnle [35]	4.5	1408	0.32%	(i) Assessment was 0.25 page. (ii) Recommended cleaning dentures with soft-bristled toothbrush "because hard-bristled brushes can produce grooves in dentures" (page 722). Although this sentence is congruent with the American Dental Association guidelines [18, 19], it could be misconstrued as advising against using denture brushes, which tend to have firmer bristles than soft toothbrushes. (iii) Directed nursing student to use string floss, not floss heads or interdentate sticks. (iv) Suggested the use of a padded tongue blade oral to keep the mouth of an unconscious patient open. (v) Recommended either a soft toothbrush or foam swabs to brush teeth. (vi) Denture removal incongruent with published dental research.
Delaune and Ladner [36]	8.5 with pictures	1391	0.61%	(i) Oral health assessment content did not address checking dentures for fit, integrity, or plaque. (ii) Recommended the use of foam swabs for "clients with impaired physical mobility or who are unconscious (comatose)" (page 759). (iii) No information on how to correctly floss or brush teeth, although the text provided a recipe for toothpaste: 2 parts salt and 1 part baking soda, no citations for this recipe. (iv) Recommended brushing dentures with toothpaste. (v) Did not direct nurses to brush the bums of edentate patients with soft toothbrushes. (vi) Simultaneously recommended the use of foam sponges with toothpaste or toothbrushes with toothpaste. (vii) Confusing content in the area of flossing. For generic mouth care, solely advised the use of string floss for flossing. For patients who were comatose, directed the use of floss holders BUT also recommended against flossing teeth for patients fully dependent on nurses for care. (viii) Denture removal incongruent with published dental research.
Lynn [38]	10	1042	0.96%	(i) Assessment content focused on the oral cavity (10 lines) but did not address normal versus abnormal findings. (ii) Included content specific to oral hygiene and persons with cognitive impairments consistent with published articles in this area by Chalmers [20–23]. (iii) No mention of soft toothbrush, simply "toothbrush." (iv) For assisting the patient, did recommend flossing, but technique was incorrect—recommended that the nurse use 6 inches of floss. Did recommend "a plastic floss holder" (page 338). (v) Mouthwash is presented a simply a mechanism for "leaving a pleasant taste in the mouth" (page 338) instead as an adjuvant to prevent caries and gingivitis. (vi) Recommended use of a padded tongue blade to prop open the mouth of a "dependent" patient (page 341). (vii) For a dependent patient, recommended use of toothpaste and toothbrush. (viii) For a dependent patient, Remove dentures if present and use a foam swab or gauze-padded tongue blade "moistened with water or dilute mouthwash to gently clean gums, mucous membranes, and tongue." (page 341). (ix) Denture removal incongruent with published dental research. (x) No direction about need to remove dentures overnight. (xi) Recommended toothpaste to brush dentures.

TABLE 1: Continued.

Bibliographic data	Pages devoted to oral health and hhygiene	Total Pages*	Percent of oral health and hygiene content	Significant findings
Potter and Perry [37]	7.5	1408	0.53%	(i) Out of all 7 textbooks, best description of oral health assessment (defined and described caries, periodontal disease, gingivitis; also addressed the components of an oral health assessment such as presence/absence of plaque quality of saliva and integrity of buccal mucosa). (ii) Oral-systemic link clearly articulated. (iii) Recommended brushing 4x/day. (iv) Stated that foam swabs) are ineffective and should not be used—but then, in procedure section, recommended foam swabs for unconscious or debilitated patients (page 889) and showed them in pictures. (v) Provided clearest instructions for oral care on an unconscious/mechanically ventilated patient. (vi) Recommended oral airway to keep mouth open for unconscious/debilitated patient. (vii) Foam swabs recommended for patients without teeth. (viii) Best description of oral health assessment, defined and described caries, periodontal disease, gingivitis. (ix) No mention of using toothpaste to clean dentures, but picture on page 891 shows toothpaste being used. (x) Denture removal and insertion directions simplistic too and incongruent with published dental research. (xi) No recommendation to use interdentate sticks or floss heads for flossing.
Taylor et al. [33]	4.75	1742	0.27%	(i) The oral health assessment was limited to 3 paragraphs in one health assessment chapter. There was no information on checking dentures for fit, integrity, or plaque. (ii) Provided overall correct mouth care techniques, including tongue brushing. (iii) Gave detailed directions for flossing using string floss; nothing about alternatives. (iv) For dependent patient, advised the use of padded tongue depressor to prop mouth open instead of a bite block. (v) Advised using toothpaste for dentures. (vi) No content on removing dentures from patient's mouth. (vii) Recommended mouth care every 1-2 hours, especially for persons who were not able to take anything by mouth.
Wilkinson and Leuven [39]	4.5	1089	0.41%	(i) Erroneously instructs patients in "Teaching Your Client About Oral Hygiene" to use regular toothpaste when brushing dentures. (ii) Also included a recipe for toothpaste, 1 part baking soda, 2 parts salt. (iii) Did not recommend removing and leaving dentures out overnight.
Wilkinson and Leuven [34]	11.3	1026	1.10%	(i) Included 3.3 pages about assessing the oral cavity; one of the most comprehensive. (ii) Included the use of foam swabs for mouth care, although the authors stated that toothbrushes better remove plaque and debris. (iii) Included content on the use of a floss holder. (iv) Recommended dilute hydrogen peroxide as a mouth wash. (v) Recommended toothpaste for cleaning dentures. (vi) Denture removal incongruent with published dental research. (vii) No indication for leaving dentures out overnight. (viii) For providing mouth care to an unconscious patient, recommended using a bite block or a padded tongue depressor.

instead of floss holders or interdentate brushes, when caring for a dependent patient [33]. The use of floss heads was recommended by Lynn [38] and Wilkinson and Van Leuven [34]. No textbooks contained recommendations for the use of interdentate brushes. Lynn [38] erroneously advised nurses to use 6 inches of string floss instead of the 18 inches as advised by the American Dental Association [18]. Flossing information provided by Delaune and Ladner [36] appeared contradictory. In one section of the textbook, nurses were advised to refrain from flossing the teeth of patients who were fully dependent on others for care. In another section, nurses were instructed to use floss holders when flossing the teeth of comatose patients.

Another problematic content area was the use of foam sponges in lieu of soft toothbrushes. Foam sponges do not remove plaque and debris as efficiently or completely as soft toothbrushes. Soft toothbrushes can be safely used for dentate patients, even unconscious ones [27]. In spite of the availability of this information since the mid-seventies [22], the use of foam sponges to provide oral hygiene was endorsed in some of the textbooks. Craven and Hirnle [35] and DeLaune and Ladner [36] advocated the use of a foam sponge to clean the teeth of dependent or unconscious patients. Wilkinson and Van Leuven [34] and Potter and Perry [37] explicitly stated that soft toothbrushes were superior to foam sponges but still recommended their usage.

Regular toothpaste can contain particles that scratch acrylic denture material; the American Dental Association [18] recommends that regular toothpaste be avoided and suggests the use of household dish cleaning liquid for cleaning dentures. The authors of five textbooks promoted the use of toothpaste for denture cleaning [33, 34, 36, 38, 39]. Taylor et al. [33] provided no information on denture removal; the remaining six textbooks recommended the removal of top dentures first, followed by bottom dentures. In the dental and nursing literature, clinicians recommend removing the bottom denture first because it is easier to remove and minimizes bite risk for the caregiver [20, 22, 23]. Dentures also must be removed overnight to avoid damage to gingival surfaces and to prevent the growth of thrush on the hard palate. Yet, this important information was missing from two of the seven textbooks [34, 38].

Only one textbook, Lynn [38], included content about oral hygiene and cognitively impaired older adults, but was vague regarding the best way to address care-resistant behavior. Given the aging of the American population [15, 41], registered nurses will find themselves caring for greater numbers of older adults and, very likely, older adults with cognitive impairments. All seven of the reviewed textbooks directed nurses to refer any dental problems, such as broken and loose teeth or poorly fitting dentures, to a dental professional.

This review was an attempt to systematically describe the quantity and quality of oral hygiene content in a representative sample of before-licensure nursing fundamentals textbooks. A strength of the search strategy was the use of identical search terms within multiple sources, which should have resulted in a representative sample of nursing fundamentals textbooks meeting the inclusion criteria. On the other hand, there is no primary database from which to identify nursing fundamentals textbooks. In spite of searching in a methodical manner and replicating the search within several sources, there exists the possibility that textbooks meeting the inclusion criteria may have been overlooked. Another limitation of this paper was the use of textbook titles and descriptions, and not the actual textbooks, in order to determine if the textbooks met the inclusion criteria before being obtained via interlibrary loan. It is possible that textbooks meeting the inclusion criteria may have been inadvertently excluded if the available title and description did not fully convey the intended audience or content.

4. Conclusion and Recommendations

In conclusion, the oral health and hygiene content in these seven nursing fundamental textbooks were highly variable in quantity and quality. One challenge faced, by nurse authors writing the chapters and by nurse educators evaluating the content in the textbooks, was the lack of evidence-based guidelines addressing oral health and hygiene. For example, the sole evidence-based guidelines regarding the care and maintenance of dentures became available in 2011 [42]. These guidelines, however, do not provide concrete directives for the length of time dentures should be daily removed "While existing studies provide conflicting results, it is not recommended that dentures should be worn continuously (24 hours per day) in an effort to reduce or minimize denture stomatitis" [42, page S3]. Given the difficulty of obtaining accurate oral health and hygiene information without systematically poring through the dental and nursing literature, nurse educators are encouraged to engage in partnerships with dental professionals, especially those teaching in dental hygiene programs. In one such partnership, for example, dental hygiene faculty and students provided expertise in oral health assessments, while the nursing faculty and students shared their geriatric expertise with the entire team [31]. Nurse educators are also encouraged to incorporate the use of current clinical practice guidelines if the available textbooks do not contain the appropriate oral health content. Finally, it is imperative for nurse researchers involved in oral health and hygiene activities to actively engage in the dissemination of accurate information through publication and presentations. One such venue is the Oral Health Nursing Education & Practice Initiative within the New York University's College of Nursing at the College of Dentistry. This initiative was launched in April, 2011, and one of its goals includes disseminating best oral care practices to nurse educators [43].

Oral health and hygiene has been an area overlooked in overall nursing education, but the growing body of research linking poor oral health to systemic diseases merits the need for added emphasis on the provision of oral hygiene [1–3]. In clinical practice, registered nurses provide oral hygiene either directly or supervise the provision of oral hygiene by others. Registered nurses who were not taught best mouth care practices may be providing inadequate mouth care as well as inadvertently promoting poor mouth care by unlicensed care personnel, who are dependent upon the knowledge and direction of registered nurses. It is important, therefore, for registered nurses to use current clinical mouth care practice guidelines.

Acknowledgments

This study was supported by the Brookdale Foundation and the National Institutes of Health/National Institute of Nursing Research (NIH/NINR) 1R01NR012737-01.

References

[1] M. P. Cullinan, P. J. Ford, and G. J. Seymour, "Periodontal disease and systemic health: current status," *Australian Dental Journal*, vol. 54, supplement 1, pp. S62–S69, 2009.

[2] P. J. Ford, S. L. Raphael, M. P. Cullinan, A. J. Jenkins, M. J. West, and G. J. Seymour, "Why should a doctor be interested in oral disease?" *Expert Review of Cardiovascular Therapy*, vol. 8, no. 10, pp. 1483–1493, 2010.

[3] J. R. Gurenlian, "Inflammation: the relationship between oral health and systemic disease," *Dental Assistant*, vol. 78, no. 2, pp. 8–43, 2009.

[4] A. Azarpazhooh and J. L. Leake, "Systematic review of the association between respiratory diseases and oral health," *Journal of Periodontology*, vol. 77, no. 9, pp. 1465–1482, 2006.

[5] K. Hutchins, G. Karras, J. Erwin, and K. L. Sullivan, "Ventilator-associated pneumonia and oral care: a successful quality improvement project," *American Journal of Infection Control*, vol. 37, no. 7, pp. 590–597, 2009.

[6] L. Johnstone, D. Spence, and J. Koziol-McClain, "Oral hygiene care in the pediatric intensive care unit: practice recommendations," *Pediatric Nursing*, vol. 36, no. 2, pp. 85–97, 2010.

[7] Y. W. Han, "Oral health and adverse pregnancy outcomes—what's next?" *Journal of Dental Research*, vol. 90, no. 3, pp. 289–293, 2011.

[8] S. Bakhshandeh, H. Murtomaa, R. Mofid, M. M. Vehkalahti, and K. Suomalainen, "Periodontal treatment needs of diabetic adults," *Journal of Clinical Periodontology*, vol. 34, no. 1, pp. 53–57, 2007.

[9] L. N. Borrell and S. P. Joseph, "Periodontal treatment may control glycemic status among diabetic patients," *Journal of Evidence-Based Dental Practice*, vol. 11, no. 2, pp. 92–94, 2011.

[10] W. J. Teeuw, V. E. A. Gerdes, and B. G. Loos, "Effect of periodontal treatment on glycemic control of diabetic patients: a systematic review and meta-analysis," *Diabetes Care*, vol. 33, no. 2, pp. 421–427, 2010.

[11] N. Kurihara, Y. Inoue, T. Iwai et al., "Oral bacteria are a possible risk factor for valvular incompetence in primary varicose veins," *European Journal of Vascular and Endovascular Surgery*, vol. 34, no. 1, pp. 102–106, 2007.

[12] D. M. P. Padilha, J. B. Hilgert, F. N. Hugo, A. J. Bos, and L. Ferrucci, "Number of teeth and mortality risk in the Baltimore Longitudinal Study of Aging," *Journals of Gerontology*, vol. 63, no. 7, pp. 739–744, 2008.

[13] J. A. Jones, T. Fulmer, and T. Wetle, "Oral health content in nursing school curricula," *Gerontology and Geriatrics Education*, vol. 8, no. 3-4, pp. 95–101, 1988.

[14] C. Hein, D. J. Schönwetter, and A. M. Iacopino, "Inclusion of oral-systemic health in predoctoral/undergraduate curricula of pharmacy, nursing, and medical schools around the world: a preliminary study," *Journal of Dental Education*, vol. 75, no. 9, pp. 1187–1199, 2011.

[15] Institute of Medicine, *Advancing Oral Health in America*, The National Academies Press, Washington, DC, USA, 2011.

[16] A. M. Berry, P. M. Davidson, J. Masters, and K. Rolls, "Systematic literature review of oral hygiene practices for intensive care patients receiving mechanical ventilation," *American Journal of Critical Care*, vol. 16, no. 6, pp. 552–563, 2007.

[17] Google Book Project at Penn State, http://www.libraries.psu.edu/psul/googlebooksproject/faq.html.

[18] Oral health topics: dentures, http://www.ada.org/2648.aspx?currentTab=2.

[19] Oral Health Topics: Cleaning Your Teeth & Gums, http://www.ada.org/2624.aspx?currentTab=2.

[20] J. Chalmers and A. Pearson, "Oral hygiene care for residents with dementia: a literature review," *Journal of Advanced Nursing*, vol. 52, no. 4, pp. 410–419, 2005.

[21] J. M. Chalmers and A. Pearson, "A systematic review of oral health assessment by nurses and carers for residents with dementia in residential care facilities," *Special Care in Dentistry*, vol. 25, no. 5, pp. 227–233, 2005.

[22] J. Chalmers, V. Johnson, J. H. Tang, and M. G. Titler, "Evidence-based protocol: oral hygiene care for functionally dependent and cognitively impaired older adults," *Journal of Gerontological Nursing*, vol. 30, no. 11, pp. 5–12, 2004.

[23] J. M. Chalmers, "Behavior management and communication strategies for dental professionals when caring for patients with dementia," *Special Care in Dentistry*, vol. 20, no. 4, pp. 147–154, 2000.

[24] D. A. Clemmens and A. R. Kerr, "Improving oral health in women:nurses' call to action," *The American Journal of Maternal Child Nursing*, vol. 33, no. 1, pp. 10–16, 2008.

[25] J. A. Fitch, C. L. Munro, C. A. Glass, and J. M. Pellegrini, "Oral care in the adult intensive care unit," *American Journal of Critical Care*, vol. 8, no. 5, pp. 314–318, 1999.

[26] J. A. Gil-Montoya, A. L. F. de Mello, C. B. Cardenas, and I. G. Lopez, "Oral health protocol for the dependent institutionalized elderly," *Geriatric Nursing*, vol. 27, no. 2, pp. 95–101, 2006.

[27] M. J. Grap, C. L. Munro, B. Ashtiani, and S. Bryant, "Oral care interventions in critical care: frequency and documentation," *American Journal of Critical Care*, vol. 12, no. 2, pp. 113–118, 2003.

[28] D. J. Jones, C. L. Munro, M. J. Grap, T. Kitten, and M. Edmond, "Oral care and bacteremia risk in mechanically ventilated adults," *Heart and Lung*, vol. 39, supplement 6, pp. S57–S65, 2010.

[29] R. A. Jablonski, "Examining oral health in nursing home residents and overcoming mouth care-resistive behaviors," *Annals of Long-Term Care*, vol. 18, no. 1, pp. 21–26, 2010.

[30] R. A. Jablonski, C. L. Munro, M. J. Grap, C. M. Schubert, M. Ligon, and P. Spigelmyer, "Mouth care in nursing homes: knowledge, beliefs, and practices of nursing assistants," *Geriatric Nursing*, vol. 30, no. 2, pp. 99–107, 2009.

[31] R. A. Jablonski, T. Swecker, C. Munro, M. J. Grap, and M. Ligon, "Measuring the oral health of nursing home elders," *Clinical Nursing Research*, vol. 18, no. 3, pp. 200–217, 2009.

[32] C. L. Munro, M. J. Grap, R. Jablonski, and A. Boyle, "Oral health measurement in nursing research: state of the science," *Biological Research for Nursing*, vol. 8, no. 1, pp. 35–42, 2006.

[33] C. R. Taylor, C. Lillis, P. LeMone, and P. Lynn, *Fundamentals of Nursing: The Art and Science of Nursing Care*, Lippincott Williams & Wilkins, Philadelphia, Pa, USA, 6th edition, 2008.

[34] J. M. Wilkinson and K. Van Leuven, *Fundamentals of Nursing: Theory, Concepts, & Applications*, vol. 2, FA Davis, Philadelphia, Pa, USA, 2007.

[35] R. F. Craven and C. J. Hirnle, *Fundamentals of Nursing: Human Health and Function*, Wolters Kluwer Health/Lippincott Williams & Wilkins, Philadelphia, Pa, USA, 6th edition, 2009.

[36] S. C. Delaune and P. K. Ladner, *Fundamentals of Nursing: Standards and Practice*, Thomson Delmar, New York, NY, USA, 3rd edition, 2006.

[37] P. A. Potter and A. G. Perry, *Fundamentals of Nursing*, Mosby Elsevier, St. Louis, Mo, USA, 7th edition, 2009.

[38] P. Lynn, *Taylor's Clinical Nursing Skills: A Nursing Process Approach*, Wolters Kluwer Health/Lippincott Williams & Wilkins, Philadelphia, Pa, USA, 2nd edition, 2008.

[39] J. M. Wilkinson and K. Van Leuven, *Fundamentals of Nursing: Theory, Concepts, & Applications*, vol. 1, FA Davis, Philadephia, Pa, USA, 2007.

[40] R. A. Jablonski, B. Therrien, E. K. Mahoney, A. Kolanowski, M. Gabello, and A. Brock, "An intervention to reduce care-resistant behavior in persons with dementia during oral hygiene: a pilot study," *Special Care in Dentistry*, vol. 31, no. 3, pp. 77–87, 2011.

[41] Institute of Medicine, *Retooling for an Aging America: Building the Health Care Workforce*, National Academy Press, Washington, DC, USA, 2008.

[42] D. Felton, L. Cooper, I. Duqum et al., "Evidence-based guidelines for the care and maintenance of complete dentures: a publication of the American college of Prosthodontists," *Journal of Prosthodontics*, vol. 20, supplement 1, pp. S1–S12, 2011.

[43] NYUCN Launches Oral Health Nursing Education Program, http://www.nyu.edu/about/news-publications/news/2011/04/26/nyucn-launches-oral-health-nursing-education-and-practice- program.html.

13

A Concept Analysis of Attitude toward Getting Vaccinated against Human Papillomavirus

Nop T. Ratanasiripong and Kathleen T. Chai

School of Nursing, California State University, Dominguez Hills, CA 90747, USA

Correspondence should be addressed to Nop T. Ratanasiripong; nratanasiripong@csudh.edu

Academic Editor: Maria Helena Palucci Marziale

In the research literature, the concept of attitude has been used and presented widely. However, attitude has been inconsistently defined and measured in various terms. This paper presents a concept analysis, using the Wilsonian methods modified by Walker and Avant (2004), to define and clarify the concept of attitude in order to provide an operationalized definition for a research study on attitudes toward a behavior: getting vaccinated against HPV. While the finding is not conclusive, three attributes of attitude: belief, affection, and evaluation are described. A theoretical definition and sample cases are constructed to illustrate the concept further. Antecedents, consequences, and empirical referents are discussed. Recommendations regarding the use of the concept of attitude in research, nursing practice, and nursing education are also made.

1. Introduction

The concept of "attitude" has been used widely in daily living communication and in science. As of the end of 2012, when entering the term "attitude" as a keyword in the "title search" on the Medline and PubMed databases for biomedical and life science publications, over 6,400 articles have been identified on each database. On Cumulative Index to Nursing and Allied Health Care Literature (CINAHL), there are 2,041 articles with the word attitude as a part of the title. In the nursing discipline, nurse scholars have used the attitude concept in conducting research studies in various populations including nursing staff, nursing students, and patients or clients (EBSCO Publishing, 2012). Nurses may use / refer to the term "attitude" as a part of patient assessment or explaining a patient's character. Although the concept of attitude (toward an object, person, thing, issue, event, and behavior) has been commonly used in the nursing literature, the abstract concept of attitude has not been clearly defined [1, 2].

In the beginning steps of developing a research study, it is important that the concepts of the study are reviewed, defined, and provided operational definitions. "Concept" is a major component of theory and conveys the abstract ideas within theory [3]. Concept provides us with a concise summary of thoughts related to a phenomenon or a group of phenomena [4]. The nursing discipline has traditionally valued the concept analysis process to help identify appropriate terms to use in subsequent research and as a means to determine the suitable methodology for investigating the concept of interest [5]. Walker and Avant (2004) describe concept analysis as a process of examining the basic elements of a concept [6]. The analysis process allows us to distinguish similar concepts and the similarity and differences between concepts. It also helps simplify, clarify, refine, and determine the concept's internal structure.

This paper aims to clarify the concept of "attitude" to facilitate the development of a research study of attitudes toward a behavior: obtaining the human papillomavirus (HPV) vaccine. However, the authors also believe that this analysis may be beneficial for other nurse scholars who consider examining the attitude concept in other behavioral aspects.

2. Materials and Methods

In the analysis of the concept of attitude toward a behavior, the Wilsonian methods of concept analysis modified by Walker and Avant are used [6]. Walker and Avant were among the first to bring Wilson's techniques of concept analysis into nursing [7]. They modified Wilson's 11 techniques into eight steps for beginners to use. Even though this method is criticized for its lack of the intellectual rigor, the method is easy to use [8] and seems to be very appropriate for novice researchers by providing a structural guideline to conduct a concept analysis. The concept analysis steps used in this paper are as follows: (1) selecting a concept, (2) determining the aims or purposes of analysis, (3) identifying all uses of the concept that can be discovered, (4) determining the defining attributes, (5) identifying a model case, (6) identifying borderline, related, invented, contrary, or illegitimate cases, (7) identifying antecedents and consequences, and (8) defining empirical referents [6].

3. Results and Discussion

3.1. Uses of the Concept. As the literature is being used as data in the analysis of a concept, adequacy and appropriateness of the chosen sample are important evaluative criteria [9]. This literature review methodology includes reviewing definitions of "attitude" in various dictionaries, searching through "Google" by using attitude as a keyword, reading attitude-related theories from various textbooks, and reviewing research abstracts or articles found on PubMed, Medline, and CINAHL. The findings from the literature review are discussed in the following section.

3.1.1. General Definitions of Attitude. The term "attitude" is a French term, originated from the Italian word "attitudine" and originally from the late Latin "aptitudinis" and "aptitude" [10]. An internet search for the "attitude" term by using the Google search engine resulted in over 340 million citations in various websites such as medical/health education, psychosocial test, quotes, magazine, movie/music entertainment, and aviation. The term "attitude" is most often defined or referred to as a noun. Based on Webster's New World Dictionary of the American Language [10], the definitions of attitude are

(1) the position or posture assumed by the body in connection with an action, feeling, mood, and so forth (to kneel in attitude of prayer);

(2) a manner of acting, feeling, or thinking that shows one's disposition, opinion, and so forth (a friendly attitude);

(3) one's disposition, opinion, mental set, and so forth;

(4) the position of an aircraft or spacecraft in relation to a given line or plane, as the horizon.

The following definitions are also found in various dictionaries. The American Heritage Dictionary of the English Language [11] offers the following. (1a) A state of mind or a feeling; disposition. (1b) An arrogant or hostile state of mind or disposition. (2) A position of the body or manner of carrying oneself. See synonyms at posture. (3) The orientation of an aircraft's axes relative to a reference line or plane, such as the horizon. (4) The orientation of a spacecraft relative to its direction of motion. (5) A position similar to an arabesque in which a ballet dancer stands on one leg with the other raised either in front or in back and bent at the knee. Merriam-Webster [12] supplies the following. (1a) A mental position with regard to a fact or state (a helpful attitude). (1b) A feeling or emotion toward a fact or state. (2) The arrangement of the parts of a body or figure: posture. (3) A position assumed for a specific purpose (a threatening attitude). (4) A ballet position similar to the arabesque in which the raised leg is bent at the knee. (5) The position of an aircraft or spacecraft determined by the relationship between its axes and a reference datum (as the horizon or a particular star). (6) An organismic state of readiness to respond in a characteristic way to a stimulus (as an object, concept, or situation). (7a) A negative or hostile state of mind. (7b) "A cool, cocky, defiant, or arrogant manner" and "predisposition or a tendency to respond positively or negatively towards a certain idea, object, person, or situation." The Business Dictionary adds "attitude influences an individual's choice of action and responses to challenges, incentives, and rewards" [13].

From the definitions described in dictionaries and thesauri, the definitions related to physical and aircraft positions are omitted from analysis as they are not pertinent to the psychosocial use and these definitions are out of the authors' research interest context. With those definitions being excluded, the remaining definitions of attitude seem to be within the research context and these definitions are repeatedly mentioned in similar ways. Those meanings involve the position of feeling or affection, thinking, or acting that shows one's belief and/or opinion.

3.1.2. Theoretical Definitions of Attitude. In the psychosocial discipline, the attitude concept received its first attention from Darwin in 1872. Darwin defined attitude as a motoric (behavioral) concept or physical expression of an emotion [14]. In the 1930s, psychologists agreed that all attitudes contain an evaluative component. They also viewed that attitude has both affective and belief components and that attitude and behavior should be consistent. "Attitude toward a behavior" is constructed by beliefs about engaging in the behavior and the associated evaluation of that belief [14]. Crano and Prislin viewed attitude as the evaluative judgment that integrates and summarizes cognitive and affective reactions [15].

According to the theory of planned behavior, if behavior is under volitional control, the intention to perform an action will highly correlate with the action itself [16]. The theory refers to "attitude toward the behavior" as "the degree to which a person has favorable or unfavorable evaluation or appraisal of the behavior in question" [16]. Attitudes are made up of the beliefs people hold about the object and the associated evaluation of that belief. The theory posits that attitude is usually assumed to form a bipolar continuum, from a negative evaluation on one end to a positive evaluation on the other [16].

Another model related to attitude is the attitude accessibility theory. The theory defines attitude as a learned association between a concept and an evaluation [17]. The theory indicates that the more rapidly an attitude can be expressed, the greater its strength. The stronger the attitude, the more accessible it is. Highly accessible attitudes are more difficult to change. Attitudes that are highly accessible from memory are more likely to guide behavior than less accessible attitudes [17].

From selected psychosocial theory perspectives above, the attitude concept is described as evaluation or appraisal of an object/issue/behavior after a person learns or acquires the information about the object/issue/behavior. How a person evaluates the issue may depend on what the person believes. The personal evaluation may result in a bipolar continuum of attitude. The attitude is then demonstrated through a physical or emotional expression. Attitude also can lead to behavioral intention and action.

3.1.3. Research Definitions of Attitude.

The literature searches in PubMed were conducted with the keyword "attitude." There were over 250,000 articles shown. To narrow down the finding, "HPV" keyword was added and the publication year was limited to five years. Out of 527 articles shown, 70 research studies indicated the attitude term on the titles. However, 52 studies conducted outside the United States were excluded due to the assumption that the attitude concept might be defined, understood, and utilized differently in various cultures and languages, leaving 17 studies for further review. After reviewing the abstracts, seven studies with attitudes related to HPV vaccination or getting vaccinated against HPV were chosen for the review.

Out of these seven studies, five studies included the term "attitude" as a part of their study aims or objectives [18–22]. One study stated the study objective as to "identify psychosocial factors correlated to HPV vaccination intention" [23] and another study used the word vaccine "acceptability" instead of attitude as a part of the study objective [24]. Six studies quantitatively measured the attitude concept by using a questionnaire [18–20, 22–24]. Out of these, one study measured the attitude concept by asking the participants what they thought about HPV vaccination, using a semantic differential scale (i.e., harmful/beneficial, bad/good). However, the definition of attitude is not specifically presented [23]. The attitude toward HPV vaccine or vaccination was interchangeably referred to and expressed through the verbs such as want, desire, feel, concern, accept, and support [18–20, 22, 24] and through the nouns such as belief, opinion, and willingness [19, 22, 23]. One study qualitatively explored attitude toward the vaccine by using a semistructure interview [21]. The study reported that the participants were "positive about the HPV vaccine" and often used the words such as belief, view, thinking, risk determination perception, and acceptance in order to present the attitude concept [21].

The literature review of attitude-related studies obviously showed that the definitions of attitude are not directly presented and often measured under various terms or concepts such as belief, feeling/desire, opinion, concern, and acceptance. However, the reviewed articles showed one common theme of referring to attitude with the spectrum from positive to negative.

3.2. Working Definition and Defining Attributes.

Walker and Avant stated that determining the defining attribute is the most critical part of concept analysis [6]. Defining the attributes can be done by searching for the cluster of attributes that are the most frequently associated with the concept. When analyzing the findings from various perspectives, the authors somewhat agree with Altmann's conclusion that attitude has cognitive and affective components [1]. However, the authors believe that a behavioral component is not an attribute, but a consequence of attitude. The authors propose three characteristics that have repeatedly appeared or been used to describe the concept of attitude: belief, feeling, and evaluation.

Based on the above defining attributes of attitude, it is possible to theoretically define attitude toward a behavior as a feeling response toward the behavior once the person has evaluated the behavior based on the person's belief. The attitude can be physically or verbally expressed in a negative to positive continuum. In addition, because the attitude concept is sometimes used interchangeably with the "opinion" concept in the literature review, it is important to differentiate these two concepts to confirm that the attitude concept's definition and attributes are properly established.

"Opinion" is described as "(1) a belief not based on absolute certainty or positive knowledge but on what seems true, valid, or probable to one's own mind, judgment; (2) an evaluation, impression, or estimation of the quality or worth of a person or thing; (3) the formal judgment of an expert on a matter in which his advice is sought; (4) law, the formal statement by a judge, court referee, and so forth of the law bearing on a case" [10]. The authors believe that the opinion concept may have shared belief and evaluation attributes with attitude concept. However, opinion may not contain the feeling attribute.

3.3. Antecedents.

Walker and Avant [6] posited that identifying antecedents and consequences is helpful in further refining the defining attributes. Antecedents are events that must take place before the attitude concept. A defining attribute cannot be either an antecedent or a consequence.

In the case of attitude concept, attitude theorists believe that the attitude is acquired through cognitive learning experiences [15, 25]. Past experiences and informational influences contribute to the attitude at the time it occurs. Attitude is the result of sequential and information integration processes. Altmann [1] provided an example of a child who was born with no past experiences and free from ideas. After gathering information and gaining more life experiences, the child then developed his/her attitude. In the authors' own words, attitude required ability to think and make a decision. Attitude develops over years when the person acquires more knowledge and experience in life. Attitude can be influenced by culture and can be changed through time and space.

3.4. Consequences. Consequences are the incident or events that happen as a result of the occurrence of the concept [6]. Based on theory of reasoned action and theory of planned behaviors, attitude toward a certain behavior is a strong predictor of intention to perform that specific behavior [2, 16]. Attitude is also a good prediction of behavior [2, 16, 17]. Altmann [1] noted that, while people do not always act according to an attitude, they are predisposed to behave in a certain manner. In summary, the authors believe that the consequences of attitude are behavioral intention, maintenance, or change, which in turn, can result either in positive or negative health outcomes.

3.5. Cases. Identifying a model case and additional cases help define and refine the attributes of the concept [6]. The following cases are created in order to find the best fit attributes.

3.5.1. Model Case. A female college student attends a sexual health workshop and learns about HPV and HPV vaccine. She believes that getting the HPV vaccine and using safe sexual practices will be beneficial to prevent HPV. She desires to obtain the vaccine and decides to do so. This model case illustrates a real life example and demonstrates all the defining attributes: belief, feeling, and evaluation of the attitude concept.

3.5.2. Borderline Case. A teenage girl starts having sexual intercourse with her boyfriend. When the mother of the girl knows about this, she decides to talk about sexually transmitted infections (STIs) and HPV vaccination. The girl then decides to get an HPV vaccine for her mother's "peace of mind." This example is considered as a borderline case because it contains most of the attributes of the attitude concept but not all of them. In this case, the girl may believe that HPV vaccine protects against cervical cancer and is safe. Nevertheless, she may not favor the idea of getting vaccinated (feeling). Her decision to obtain the vaccine is because of her mother not because how she believes, evaluates, and feels about getting vaccinated against HPV.

3.5.3. Related Case. A nursing student studies about HPV and other STIs for her final examination. She memorizes the cause and consequences of each STI. Then, she takes the test. She is glad that she passes the examination. This related case example shows a knowledge or cognition concept that is related to the attitude concept but does not contain all the defining attributes of attitude.

3.5.4. Contrary Case. A baby is in a pediatrician office's waiting room for an annual checkup. There are posters about HPV vaccine posted on the wall. The baby is smiling when looking at the bright colorful posters. This case clearly demonstrates what the attitude concept is not. This case does not meet any criteria of attitude attributes. The baby has not gained a set of beliefs to evaluate the vaccine. The baby's smile is not related to HPV issue but to the colorful pictures.

3.5.5. Illegitimate Case. At a theater, many young women are practicing standing on one leg with the other raised either in front or in back and bent at the knee. They try to make their attitudes balanced and perfectly synchronous. This case example demonstrates the attitude concept term entirely used out of the authors' research context.

3.6. Empirical Referents. Empirical referents are "classes or categories of actual phenomena that by their existence or presence demonstrate the occurrence of the concept itself" [6, Page 46]. Empirical referents are very useful in instrument development because they are clearly linked to the theoretical base of the concept, thus contributing to both the content and construct validity of the instrument. Since attitude cannot be measured directly, measuring attitude may be more appropriately done by correlating and combining the findings from defined attributes of attitude. This method may more accurately support the inferences made regarding an attitude [1].

Since the authors are planning to conduct a cross sectional survey, observation of "attitude" through behaviors or actions (e.g., talking positively about obtaining the vaccine) will not be included. The expression of attitude will be measured by asking the research participants to complete an attitude survey toward getting vaccinated against HPV. The attitude questionnaire will be built by combining the attitude attributes of belief, evaluation, feeling, and bipolarity into the questions.

3.7. Discussion. In the process of reviewing the current literature, the attitude concept has been inconsistently defined and measured in various terms (i.e., belief, opinion, acceptance, and perception). When thinking about the model and additional cases, the authors realized that it was difficult to create true borderline and related cases in order to differentiate the attitude concept from the opinion concept. It seemed that the scopes of these concepts are overlapping. These findings confirmed that the attitude concept is indeed very abstract and may not be directly measured. While there is no current solution to measure the attitude more clearly, the authors suggest that researchers interested in measuring the attitude concept should consider building a research tool based on belief, feeling, and evaluation as the attributes of the concept. In addition, while opinion may be assessed by using "agree-disagree" questions, attitude may be assessed by using "desirable-undesirable, valuable-worthless, pleasant-unpleasant, interesting-boring, positive-negative, good-bad, like-dislike" questions which show the affection and evaluation attributes in a bipolar spectrum [2, 16]. Once the tool is tested and used, additional concept reviews and revisions of the tool may be necessary to improve attitude concept measurement.

4. Conclusion and Recommendations

The authors' philosophical belief toward getting to the truth is to seek an answer from one perspective and then seek answers from various perspectives. Although the authors may not be able to get the truth/answer of the real meaning of "attitude," they believe they can come close to it. In order to do so, more research studies can be conducted to test and refine the attitude definition and attributes. For nursing practice, the attitude concept can be continually used as a part of patient assessment. As described above, attitude can influence behavior. Nurses may understand patient's particular behaviors when they also assess and are aware of certain attitudes toward the behavior in question. Nurses can also create an intervention focusing specifically on changing attitude to influence changing such behavior. Finally, in nursing education, while nursing organizations have suggested that nursing programs need to assess not only knowledge and competency but also attitude in nursing students, the measurement of attitude is not clear and is not standardized [26]. To ensure that conducting an attitude assessment in nursing students is useful, nursing organizations should define the attitude concept, tailor, and standardize the attitude assessment tool that can be used across the board. Otherwise, having attitude as a part of the program assessment may not be useful for benchmarking results.

References

[1] T. K. Altmann, "Attitude: a concept analysis," *Nursing Forum*, vol. 43, no. 3, pp. 144–150, 2008.

[2] P. Zhang, "Roles of attitude in initial and continued ICT use: a longitudinal study," 2007, http://melody.syr.edu/pzhang/publications/AMCIS_07_Zhang_Attitude_Longitudinal.pdf.

[3] P. L. Chinn and M. K. Kramer, *Integrated Theory and Knowledge Development in Nursing*, Mosby, St. Louis, Mo, USA, 2nd edition, 2008.

[4] A. I. Meleis, *Theoretical Nursing Development & Progress*, Lippincott Williams & Wilkins, Philadelphia, Pa, USA, 4th edition, 2007.

[5] J. Penrod and J. E. Hupcey, "Enhancing methodological clarity: principle-based concept analysis," *Journal of Advanced Nursing*, vol. 50, no. 4, pp. 403–409, 2005.

[6] L. O. Walker and K. C. Avant, *Strategies For Theory Construction in Nursing*, Pearson Education, Upper Saddle River, NJ, USA, 4th edition, 2004.

[7] J. E. Hupcey, J. M. Morse, E. R. Lenz, and M. C. Tasón, "Wilsonian methods of concept analysis: a critique," *Scholarly Inquiry for Nursing Practice*, vol. 10, no. 3, pp. 185–210, 1996.

[8] J. M. Morse, J. E. Hupcey, C. Mitcham, and E. R. Lenz, "Concept analysis in nursing research: a critical appraisal," *Scholarly Inquiry for Nursing Practice*, vol. 10, no. 3, pp. 253–277, 1996.

[9] J. M. Morse, "Exploring pragmatic utility: concept analysis by critically appraising the literature," in *Concept Development in Nursing: Foundations, Techniques, and Applications*, W.B. Saunders, Philadelphia, Pa, USA, 2nd edition, 2000.

[10] D. B. Guralnik, *Webster's New World Dictionary of the American Language*, Prentice Hall, New York, NY, USA, 2nd edition, 1986.

[11] *The American Heritage Dictionary of the English Language*, 2000, http://www.thefreedictionary.com/attitude.

[12] Merriam-Webster, *Merriam-Webster's Online Dictionary*, 2012, http://www.merriam-webster.com/dictionary/attitude.

[13] *Business Dictionary Attitude*, 2012, http://www.businessdictionary.com/definition/attitude.html.

[14] B. H. Kantowitz, J. D. Lee, C. A. Becker et al., *Development of Human Factors Guidelines for Advanced Traveler information System and Commercial Vehicle Operations: Exploring Driver Acceptance of in-Vehicle information Systems*, Office of Safety and Traffic Operations, Seattle, Wash, USA, 1997.

[15] W. D. Crano and R. Prislin, *Attitude and Persuasion*, 2006, http://www.psychology.sdsu.edu/new-web/facultystaff/Prislin_pdfs/annurev.psych.57.102904.pdf.

[16] I. Ajzen, "The theory of planned behavior," *Organizational Behavior and Human Decision Processes*, vol. 50, no. 2, pp. 179–211, 1991.

[17] R. H. Fazio and C. J. Williams, "Attitude accessibility as a moderator of the attitude-perception and attitude-behavior relations: an investigation of the 1984 presidential election," *Journal of Personality and Social Psychology*, vol. 51, no. 3, pp. 505–514, 1986.

[18] D. G. Ferris, J. L. Waller, J. Miller et al., "Men's attitudes toward receiving the human papillomavirus vaccine," *Journal of Lower Genital Tract Disease*, vol. 12, no. 4, pp. 276–281, 2008.

[19] C. Flaherty, G. E. Ely, L. S. Akers, M. Dignan, and T. B. Noland, "Social work student attitudes toward contraception and the HPV vaccine," *Social Work in Health Care*, vol. 51, pp. 361–381, 2012.

[20] C. Han, D. G. Ferris, J. Waller, P. Tharp, J. Walter, and L. Allmond, "Comparison of knowledge and attitudes toward Human papillomavirus, HPV vaccine, Pap tests, and cervical cancer between US and Peruvian women," *Journal of Lower Genital Tract Disease*, vol. 16, no. 2, pp. 121–126, 2012.

[21] M. B. Short, S. L. Rosenthal, L. Sturm et al., "Adult women's attitudes toward the HPV vaccine," *Journal of Women's Health*, vol. 19, no. 7, pp. 1305–1311, 2010.

[22] L. A. Watts, N. Joseph, M. Wallace et al., "HPV vaccine: a comparison of attitudes and behavioral perspectives between Latino and non-Latino women," *Gynecologic Oncology*, vol. 112, no. 3, pp. 577–582, 2009.

[23] C. W. Wheldon, E. M. Daley, E. R. Buhi, A. G. Nyitray, and A. R. Giuliano, "Health beliefs and attitudes associated with HPV vaccine intention among young gay and bisexual men in the southeastern United States," *Vaccine*, vol. 29, pp. 8060–8065, 2011.

[24] V. L. Sanders-Thompson, L. D. Arnold, and S. R. Notaro, "African-American parents' attitudes toward HPV vaccination," *Ethnicity & Disease*, vol. 21, pp. 335–341, 2011.

[25] W. E. Craighead and C. B. Nemeroff, *The Corsini Encyclopedia of Psychology and Behavioral Science*, vol. 1, John Wiley & Sons, New York, NY, USA, 3rd edition, 2001.

[26] K. P. Dawson, "Attitude and assessment in nurse education," *Journal of Advanced Nursing*, vol. 17, no. 4, pp. 473–479, 1992.

14

Assessment of Ethical Ideals and Ethical Manners in Care of Older People

Marianne Frilund,[1,2] **Lisbeth Fagerström,**[1,3] **Katie Eriksson,**[4,5] **and Patrik Eklund**[6]

[1] *Åbo Akademi University, Vaasa, Finland*
[2] *Novia University of Applied Sciences, Vaasa, Finland*
[3] *Buskerud University College, Drammen, Norway*
[4] *Department of Caring Science, Åbo Akademi University, Vaasa, Finland*
[5] *Helsinki Hospital District of Helsinki and Uusimaa, Finland*
[6] *Department of Computing Science, Umeå University, Umeå, Sweden*

Correspondence should be addressed to Marianne Frilund; marianne.frilund@novia.fi

Academic Editor: Pirkko Routasalo

The aim of this study is to establish structured clusters and well-defined ontological entities (nodes) describing ethical values as both ideal and opportunity for ethical manner as perceived by the caregiver. In this study, we use Bayesian Belief Networks (BBNs) to analyse ethical values (ethos) and ethical manners in daily work with older people. Material is based on questionnaire data collected by the instrument for the self-assessment of individual ethos in the care of older people (ISAEC) in spring 2007 in a municipality in Western Finland. This study is unique in its kind, both concerning the selected approach and methodological questions. BBNs have not been used significantly in nursing research, nor are there any studies that examine the ethical possibilities with focus on the probable effects upon changing conditions.

1. Introduction

Ethical discussions between caregivers affect the quality of the older person's care, and Ågren Bolmsjö et al. [1] have found that ethical decision-making supports ethically good care of patients. Berggren et al. [2] associate the discussion of ethical values with a deeper level of communication, and in order to achieve depth in such a dialogue, an ethical code and a set of ethical values which penetrate caring are needed. Awareness of such ethical values equips caregivers with a freedom and strength to make conscious decisions to do well and to do right in a given care situation. A caregiver's ability to do well and do right is strengthened in the dialogue between caregivers and other health care professionals [3].

In this study, we use Bayesian Belief Networks [4, 5] (BBNs) to analyse ethical values (ethos) and ethical manners in daily work with older people. The advantage with BBNs is the possibility to use and compute with symbolic (symbolic data has no per se measurable or comparable values), as opposed to numeric or nominal (. . . 1, 2, 3, 4, 5 are nominal not to be seen as numerical . . .), data. Linear regression and comparable methods require numeric data for its computations. Data used in this study are nominal in the answers to questions in the questionnaire, but inherently symbolic when arriving at ethical data and classifications of ethical manner. Further, BBNs are able to manage stochasticity and uncertainty and can work simultaneously with objective and subjective probabilities in one and the same model.

Material is based on questionnaire data collected by the instrument for the self-assessment of individual ethos in the care of older people (ISAEC) in spring 2007 in a municipality in Western Finland [6]. The study is based on a caring science perspective, and caregivers' ethical values and ethical manner which are evaluated in the study have been interpreted to the theory of caritative caring ethics [7] and to previous research on ethics in the care of older people [8–13]. The caring science perspective appears in the statements of the questionnaire, and in the concept, which are given the clusters and nodes, generated with BBN.

Biostatistics or, generally speaking, statistics as used in the care domain is indeed strictly statistics. "Statistic inference" is not logic inference but ad hoc conclusions derived from statistical observations and analysis. Such conclusions are not expressed in any logical language but still within the statistical machinery. However, health and social care involving observations, assessments, and decision-making mean that somewhere along the line *statistics moves over to logics*.

Logical entailment ⊢ is a relation between premises and conclusions. It is syntactic reasoning as related to its semantic counterpart, namely, logical satisfaction ⊨. We will illuminate our epistemology with syntactic entailments, where the choice of a specific logic, first-order or otherwise, is not relevant as we are providing a complete ethical ontology in this paper.

1.1. Theoretical Framework. In the theory of caritative caring ethics [14] and in the previous research on ethics in caring, related to the care of older people can we see, among other, values as dignity, [10, 15–17] integrity, [11, 16, 18–20] autonomy and participation, [10, 16, 17, 21], respect and safety [13, 20, 22, 23]. We can also find different explanations about caregivers' possibilities to act in an ethical manner in the daily work with the older persons. It is not self-evident that ethical values of the caregivers turn into ethical manners in the daily work, and we have to state that *a good intention goes wrong* [11], and the caregiver encounters different ethical problems and challenges that need to be resolved. Often there is not one solution to the problem, rather, many different solutions. The essence of caring is to alleviate the patient's suffering and promote health and wellbeing. Eriksson [24] described caring ethics in terms like love and mercy, caring relationship, human dignity and respect, which accordingly affects human beings' decisions and choices in a specific manner [7, 24–26]. The *caring communion* is the deepest motive for every kind of caring. A professional caring relationship implies a responsibility of caregiver vis-à-vis the patient he/she takes care of.

An ethically aware caregiver strives to invite the patient into a caring relation that mediates strength as well as respect for the integrity and wholeness of the human being [15]. An ethically aware caregiver also strives to "do well," "do right," and "take responsibility," and he/she wanted to show the patient respect [9].

To act ethically in an ontological sense is not always related to time. Acting ethically exists in the moment when goodness becomes a conscious choice for the caregiver. To act ethically in the daily work requires a professional freedom, enabling caregiver to choose and decide just in the moment when caregiver and patient meet each other. This kind of freedom goes behind routines and stereotypical behaviours and thereby promotes unique meetings.

1.2. Aim. The aim of this study is to establish structured clusters and well-defined ontological entities (nodes) describing

ethical values as both ideal and opportunity for ethical manner as perceived by the caregiver. This additionally provides an enlargement and enrichment of the underlying ethical assumptions about ethical values and the dynamics in spectra of caregiver ethical manner. An additional objective is to evaluate the effect of fixing nodes to certain assessments levels, in order to see how other nodes are affected in themselves and from the viewpoint of the entire cluster. This in turn contributes to knowledge elicitation and epistemological enhancement with respect to the ontological framework.

This paper focuses on the following questions:

(1) (ontological question) which are the main patterns involving ethical value and ethical manner emerging from this study, given the underlying structural entities and dynamical ethical values and manners?

(2) (complementary epistemological question) which are the various types of conditional changes of ethical values and their related ethical manners that appear when fixing nodes to particular values and thereby clusters to specific characters?

(3) (societal impact) how will this elicited knowledge in the end affect daily care of older people and as viewed from an ethical perspective?

2. Method

2.1. Participants. Caregivers from 10 units in the care of older persons were invited to participate in the study. Three units represented Home Care, four units Nursing Home Care, and three units Long-Term Care. A majority ($n = 80$) of the informants worked within Nursing Home Care or within Long-Term Care, whereas the remaining informants ($n = 25$) worked within Home Care.

A majority of the informants had a vocational degree, for instance, registered nurses and practical nurses. Totally, 24 caregivers had attended shorter courses according to older educational programs, such as courses for care assistants, and six of the informants lacked formal competence for their work.

2.2. Data Collection. Data were collected with an instrument called "*the instrument for self-assessment of individual ethos in care of older persons*" and redact ISAEC. Totally, the instrument consists of 58 statements. Twenty-eight statements refer to ethical values as ideals, and 30 statements refer to the possibilities to act in an ethical manner, in the daily work with the older person. A total of 110 questionnaires were handed out by leaders from each unit. Totally, 105 questionnaires were returned, which gives a response rate on 95%.

Total data consist of 6900 observations. Statements in ISAEC instruments were allocated into five groups, as follows: Group I = individual care, Group II = dignified care, Group III = safety care, Group IV = caring communion, and Group V = closeness or/and distance.

The participants were asked to answer the questionnaires by choosing the alternative which best responded to their opinion. The alternatives were stated as follows: not at all agree = 1, partly agree = 2, sometimes = 3, nearly agree = 4, and totally agree = 5 (ethical values as ideals) and never = 1, nearly never = 2, sometimes = 3, mostly = 4, and always = 5 (ethical manners).

These alternatives were textually presented so that the attached numbering was only intended as an index for that particular alternative and not a gradation. In other words, the instrument aims at presenting the alternatives as symbols and not as numerical values. However, as numbers 1–5 were visible in the instrument, it can be expected that the set of alternatives was seen as an ordinal scale, so that, for example, "sometimes" is *before* "mostly," but there is no distance measure between the two. This is indeed the main reason why we cannot compute with 1–5 as numbers, but rather as symbols in an ordinal scale, and this is why computing with conditional probabilities in Bayesian networks is very suitable.

2.3. Data Analysis

2.3.1. Conditional Probabilities and Bayesian Networks. We use Hugin as our tool for Bayesian network generation based on data. Learning from data by Hugin creates a network of nodes connected according to respective conditionalities between nodes. For a higher level of information, clusters of nodes can be created. Clustered nodes are then also linked by conditionalities between nodes.

The structure learning algorithms in Hugin are based on making dependence tests that calculate a test statistic which is asymptotically chi-squared distributed assuming (conditional) independence. If the test statistic is large for a given independence hypothesis, the hypothesis is rejected; otherwise, it is accepted. The probability of rejecting a true independence hypothesis is given by the level of significance, which was selected to be 0.05.

Several methods, including numerical, logical, and probabilistic ones, have been proposed to manage uncertainty in decision-support systems. The probabilistic approach with Bayesian networks are appealing as they capture a computational view of conditional probabilities, which is particularly useful in presence of questionnaires with interdependent questions and using symbolic or ordinal values.

Let $P(A, B)$ be the joint probability for A and B. Then, the conditional probability is defined as $P(A \mid B) = P(A, B)/P(B)$. This then gives the expression $P(A, B) = P(A \mid B)P(B)$ for joint probabilities with dependent variables.

The event A is said to be *conditionally independent* of event B if $P(A \mid B) = P(A)$, that is, whenever $P(A, B) = P(A)P(B)$.

The previous formulas are used to arrive at Bayes' rule $P(A \mid B) = P(B \mid A)P(A)/P(B)$ which is the most important rule used and manipulated in Bayesian networks. Bayes' rule makes it possible to calculate conditional probabilities $P(A \mid B)$, once the opposite conditional probability $P(B \mid A)$ is known together with the probabilities for the individual events A and B.

The Bayesian network notation for the probability situation $P(A, B) = P(A \mid B)P(B)$ is depicted as

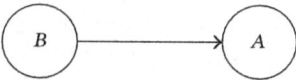

indicating that B is conditional to A. Similarly, $P(A, B) = P(B \mid A)P(A)$ is depicted as

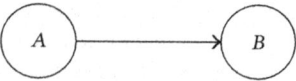

indicating A conditional to B. Given Bayes' rule, it is then clear that the direction of the arrow is interchangeable depending on the conditional context.

For several nodes, we then need to consider all pairs of conditional probabilities, that is, for the joint probability

$$P(A, B, C, D) = P(A) P(B \mid A) P(C \mid A, B) P(D \mid A, B, C). \tag{1}$$

We have the depiction

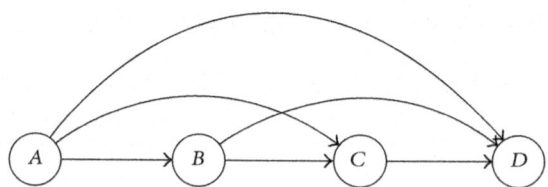

In the most simple cases, events are two valued, and we may, for example, write either $A = 0$ or $A = 1$. A probability like $P(C = 1)$ is then computed as

$$P(C = 1)$$
$$= \sum_{a \in \{0,1\}} \sum_{b \in \{0,1\}} \sum_{d \in \{0,1\}} P(A = a, B = b, C = 1, D = d), \tag{2}$$

and a conditional probability like $P(A = 1 \mid C = 1)$ is computed as

$$P(A = 1 \mid C = 1)$$
$$= \frac{P(A = 1, C = 1)}{P(C = 1)} \tag{3}$$
$$= \frac{\sum_{b \in \{0,1\}} \sum_{d \in \{0,1\}} P(A = 1, B = b, C = 1, D = d)}{P(C = 1)}.$$

In the aforementioned we depict the use of binary data only. Clearly, we can work with more than just two classes of events. In this study, we work mainly with the alternative set $\{0, 1, 2, 3, 4, 5\}$, and conditionalities like $P(A \in \{3, 4, 5\} \mid B = 4)$ can be computed for tables in the Results section.

The learning algorithm, as implemented in Hugin, finds the appropriate and correct conditionalities given data. This then creates the Bayesian Belief Network (BBN), where the interconnection defines the structure of the network. This structure and network identification capability is one of the significant advantages of BBN developments. A *cluster* is

TABLE 1: Cluster I: Dignity.

		Distribution function for Cluster I (percent)					
		5	4	3	2	1	Missing
F4	Human love and mercy	*88,2*	*9*	*2,9*			
C5	Moments of peace	94,3	5,7				
E2	To see the needs of the older person	85,7	10,5	1			2,9
B1	Respect the needs and wishes of the older person	87,6	8,6	1,9			1,9
E4	Caring community	87,1	12,4	0,5			
C2	Encourage the older persons to utilize their own resources	85,7	10,5	2,9			1
A2	To respect the equal value of each older person	94,3	2,9	1			1,9

a subset of entities, so that, on the one hand, no entity in this subset is conditionally dependent with any other entity outside that cluster, and, on the other hand, there are no further subclusters within that cluster. We may also speak of *independent* clusters, to further underline that such clusters with no conditional dependency to their outside world are *molecular*.

2.4. Findings. Results are polarized, on the one hand, by *ethical values in the daily care with older people*, and, on the other hand, by *possibilities to act in an ethical manner in the daily care with older people*. However, ethical value and possibility are not complementary or mutually exclusive but rather appear as valuation domains for enabling projection and transformation of given value criteria.

From ethical point of view, good care refers in particular to *dignity, participation, safety, caring community*, and *closeness and distance*, where the latter is concerned mostly with aspects of possibility and the others project to both ethical value and possibilities. This enables, for example, the concept of dignity to be seen as fundamentally ethical at the same time as consideration of dignity becomes a possibility. Similar multimodality with respect to ethical value and possibility can be said about the other concepts, respectively, participation and safety and caring community.

Concepts for ethical value and possibility are further characterized by underlying nodes or entities in clusters related to these concepts, thereby also the entities being members of specific clusters, and conditionalities between these entities.

Among all 58 statements, it turned out that ten statements became one-node clusters; that is, these statements did not show any conditionality with any other statements. These statements were left out of further analysis, since no matter how the dynamics within such a statement is further analysed, it has no effect on any other statement. Indeed, a main objective of this paper is to analyse situations within clusters, where fixation of particular ordinal values for one statement may affect dynamics concerning sibling statements in that cluster. Note that we may speak of sibling nodes, even if it is seldom clear where parent nodes reside in clusters. This is given by the fact that conditionality is really not "directed," and "changing directions" of conditionalities is done by Bayes' rules.

Structure identification by Hugin also resulted in a number of two-node clusters. Interesting among these clusters were that clashing and enforcing them into one node and restructuring all the remaining nodes provided such two-node clusters to became singleton clusters, in all cases expect for one case where that singleton node become integrated into a larger cluster. This is a motivation for leaving also two-node clusters outside further analysis.

The number of remaining clusters is 9, and the number of nodes in those respective clusters varies from 3 to 7. Among these 9 clusters, 4 clusters contain ethical value statements, and 5 clusters contain possibility statements. The interesting next step is now the semantics of these 9 clusters and their nodes. What is the *name* of the cluster, and what is the *interpretation* of that name? A major part of this Results section is to analyse what happens when certain nodes in clusters are frozen to particular ordinal values. The Bayesian network then recomputes the distribution functions for the other nodes, and the recomputation is enabled by the conditional probabilities. This enables a number of interesting what-if analyses, like if E2, E4, and C2 are fixed at 4, that is, the distribution functions for all these nodes become 100% at ordinal value 4, how does the "move" or "shift" of the function is dynamic for the other nodes?

2.5. Ethical Values in the Daily Care with Older People

2.5.1. Cluster I: Dignity. The cluster *dignity* consists of seven nodes or entities. There are small differences between the agreement levels of respective informants. About 85–94 percent of the informants totally agree with all seven statements. In Table 1, we have the distribution function for the cluster *dignity*.

Nodes where level "4" responses in percentage exceed 10 are selected for fixation to a response rate of 100%. These respective fixations are then compared with the shift in response rates for the other nodes, as well as the way they shift in response rates according to the underlying conditional probabilities model of the network.

In order to see this more precisely, let node E2, *to see the needs of the older person*, be fixed at response level "4" = 100%. The influence on node E4, *caring community*, is a 17% shift of level "5" responses to level "4" responses, and on node C2,

TABLE 2: Effects on distribution function when E4 fixed to "4" = 100%.

		5	4	3	2	1	Missing
F4	Human love and mercy	−11,51	1,91	9,59			
C2	Encourage the older persons to utilize their own resources	−10,5	−8,06	12,1			6,46
A2	To respect the equal value of each older person	−19,3	4,84	1,35			13,11

TABLE 3: Effects on distribution function when C2 fixed to "4" = 100%.

		5	4	3	2	1	Missing
F4	Human love and mercy	−9,03	11,32	−2,3			
E4	Caring community	8,15	−9,5	1,36			

TABLE 4: Cluster II: Community.

		Distribution function for Cluster II (percent)					
		5	4	3	2	1	Missing
A4	Caring community	94,3	5,7				
B3	Listen to the wishes of the older person	85,7	10,5	1			2,9

TABLE 5: Cluster III: Safety.

		Distribution function for Cluster III (percent)					
		5	4	3	2	1	Missing
A3	The experience of confidence	99					
E3	Professionally caregivers make safety	96	3		1		
D3	Knowledge make safety	79	13				2

encourage the older persons to utilize their own resources, the effect is an increase of level "4" responses by 18% and level "3" responses by 16%.

Further, for node E4, *caring community*, fixed at level "4" = 100%, node F4, *human love and mercy*, decreases at level "5" by 10% to level "3," node C2, *encourage the older persons to utilize their own resources*, decreases at level "5" by 10% and at level "4" by 8% with an increase at level "3" by 12% and increase on missing data, that is, "cannot say" data, by 6%, and for A2, *to respect the equal value of each older person*, there is decrease of 13% from level "5," and as this node had a rather low occurrence of missing data, it is notable how the portion of missing data increases as much as 13% (see Table 2).

Concerning node C2, *encourage the older persons to utilize their own resources*, changes due to conditionalities for node F4 and E4 are seen in Table 3.

2.5.2. Clusters II–IV. The following clusters are named *community* (cluster II), *safety* (cluster III), and *integrity* (cluster IV). In Table 6, we find the clusters and the named nodes for each cluster. We did not find any dynamical shift in the distribution functions after conditionalities for the nodes had been fixed in level "4" to 100%.

Based on these results, we can state that caregivers, participating in the study, agree that dignity, community, safety, and integrity are important ethical values, in order to guarantee an ethically defensible care, in care with older people.

The last cluster of ethical ideal was named integrity. The distribution function for this cluster is explained in Table 6.

2.6. Possibilities to Act in an Ethical Manner in the Daily Care with Older People. Five clusters describe the caregivers' possibilities to act in an ethical manner, within their daily work with the older persons. The clusters are named as follows: *possibility for closeness and distance, community, dignity, safety,* and *participation.* The degree of coherence between the statements and the own opinions varies significantly between the informants.

A dynamical shift in the distribution functions, when conditionalities for respective node have been changed, can be found within all clusters. It is apparent that the shape of the clusters is affected as the underlying conditions and properties change, for example, with respect to change of caregivers,

as new personnel enter the unit, and the condition spectra change at the unit either for particular individuals or by individuals leaving and new patients entering. The changes obviously affect care intensity as a whole. Further, organizational and administrative aspects and/or changes may also have effect on ethical manner.

2.6.1. Cluster V: Possibility for Closeness and Distance. Cluster V consists of three nodes: *sensitivity, professional approach,* and *a genuine interest in the quality of life of the older person.* The nodes are closely intertwined, and dynamics of the conditionality in respective nodes affects each other within the cluster. Fixation in one node implies adjustments of frequencies in the other nodes. Thereby changes like fixations at level "4" will imply downshifts in the other nodes towards levels "4" and "3." Thereby, ethical manners, as caregivers' *professional approach* and *interest for the older person,* will be important entities for upholding closeness and/or distance in the daily work with the older person (Table 7).

2.6.2. Cluster VI: Possibilities for Dignified Care. Cluster VI consists of six nodes (the nodes and the distribution function for the cluster are presented in Table 8).

For upholding dignified care, entities as *respecting the philosophy of life, creating a meaningful life,* and *continuously keeping the older patients informed on the phenomena of significance* for their health and wellbeing, will be of most

TABLE 6: Cluster IV: integrity.

| | | Distribution function for Cluster IV (percent) | | | | | |
		5	4	3	2	1	Missing
D1	The older person is unique with unique needs	84	13	1			2
B4	Inviolability	88	9	3			
C3	Be responsible for the safety of the older person	89	6	2	2		1
C4	Respectfully done nursing	95	4	1			

TABLE 7: Cluster V: Possibilities for closeness and distance.

| | | Distribution function for Cluster V (percent) | | | | | |
		5	4	3	2	1	Missing
B51	Sensitivity	48	39	8	3		2
E51	Professional approach	47	38	10	2		3
C51	A genuine interest in the quality of life of the older person	34	45	14	3		4

TABLE 8: Cluster VI: Possibilities for dignified care.

| | | Distribution function for Cluster VI (percent) | | | | | |
		1	2	3	4	5	Missing
C21	Respecting the philosophy of live of the older person	52,4	31,4	10,5	1,9	1	2,9
A21	Observing the older person's dignity	55,2	39,1	3,8	1,9		
B21	Treating the older person as an adult person	63,1	32,2	3,7			1
E21	Creating a meaningful life for the older person	41,9	41,9	10,5		1	4,8
F21	Continuously informing the older person	27,6	44,8	18,1	3,8		5,7

importance. As many as 18 percent feel that their possibilities to continuously inform the older about their health situation remain at level "3," and 10 percent of the informants state that they "sometimes" have possibilities to respect *the philosophy of life* of the older person. About 16 percent of the informants feel they have limited possibilities to create a meaningful life for the older patients.

We shall see what most likely happens inside the cluster if we fix some of the entities at level "4" to be 100 percent. A dignified care seems to be dependent on caregivers' attitude to the older patients. A fixation at level "4" for node B21 (*treating the older as an adult person*) will imply downshifts in nodes F21 (*to continuously inform the older person*), C21 (*to respect the philosophy of the life of the older*), and E21 (*to create a meaningful life for the older*).

The following example also reinforces the attitude of the caregivers as an important factor for opportunities to enable dignified care for the older persons. A fixation at level "4" for node E21 (*to create a meaningful life for the older*) downshifted nodes D21, A21, and B21, at level "3" about 4–19 percent (Table 10).

These two examples show how the attitude of caregivers makes distinctions about upholding the dignity of the older person in the daily work, and we can see the same tendencies with fixation at level "3" or "4" for the other nodes within the cluster.

2.6.3. Cluster VII: Possibilities for Participation. The cluster consists of seven nodes, where the nodes including *freedom* and *believing* the older person are entities that informants perceive as important entities to facilitate patient involvement in their own care. The distribution functions show that *ability for the patients to participate* in their own care is limited. The *caregivers' desire to care for the same patient during a longer period, sharing moods with the older,* and *being humble when facing the older person* provide further dimensions for evaluations and enrichment as related to patients themselves given possibilities for participation. Making use of the older person's resources and capacities is a real challenge, and on the basis of the results, it appears that caring is more about doing *for* than doing *with* the patient, that is, indeed being participative in these respects.

What happens within the cluster if a fixation at level "4" to 100% is done for some of the nodes in the cluster? Nodes A41 (*promote continuity and preservation in the care process as a whole*), F41 (*being emphatic and sharing the moods with the older person*), A11 (*support resources of the older patient*), G41 (*being humble while caring for the older person*), and D41 (*encourage participation*) being affected both upwards and downwards in the set of alternatives, as well as participation of the patient, are dependent on caregiver attitudes. The effects on distributions for respective nodes are described in Tables 11, 12, 13, and 14.

TABLE 9: Effects on distribution function when B21 fixed to "4" = 100%.

		5	4	13	2	1	Missing
D21	The older person is treated respectfully regardless of health status	−2,2	3,21	0,28			−1,29
C21	Respecting the philosophy of life of the older person	−6,53	8,63	0,63	2,05	−0,26	−2,61
A21	Observing the older person's dignity	−5,2	6,14	0,5			−1,44
E21	Creating a meaningful life for the older person	−9,93	11,4	2,55		0,53	−3,6
F21	Continuously informing the older person	−16,06	24,67	−5,03	1,62		−5,2

TABLE 10: Effects on distribution function when E21 fixed to "4" = 100%.

		5	4	3	2	1	Missing
D21	The older person is treated respectfully regardless of health	−20,91	15,54	4,47			
A21	Observing the older person's dignity	−36,37	20,45	15,91			
B21	Treating the older person as an adult person	−36,46	15,51	18,57			

The node with the strongest effect on the nodes within the cluster is D41. The way caregivers feel about *encourage participation* has effect on each of the nodes within Table 12.

2.6.4. Cluster VIII: Possibilities for Safety Care. Cluster VIII consists of three nodes, respectively, to *be responsible for the inner safety of older persons, to create a safe situation for the older person,* and *protect against mistreatment of the older person* (see Table 16).

2.6.5. Cluster IX: Possibilities to Create a Caring Communion. The final cluster, *caring communion,* contains seven nodes, which are described in Table 15. A caring communion will be established when the older person is in charge of his/her own life. In these situations, caregivers really want to fulfil the needs of the older person and thereby also show respect for the older person, that is, *show respect for the older person, be flexible,* and *encourage participation* (Table 17).

The potential for a caring communion to reach care relationships is dependent on the *desire to listen* to the older person, *monitoring of older person's satisfaction about care, flexibility,* and *respect for the older person's own decisions.* Node C11 (flexibility) has the greatest ability to affect other nodes within the cluster. Fixing node C11 level to "4," corresponding to an improvement of the original result, the number of observations for each node increases (Table 18).

3. Discussion

In the study of ethical values and ethical manners, the Bayesian approach, represented by the use of Bayesian Belief Networks (BBNs), has been a useful method, because of the ability to compute with symbolic data. In particular, the ability to show the effects of using extended conditionalities, involving both original nodes as well as clusters of nodes,

has been a useful insight. The computing process, as enabled by the structure identification capability of BBNs, generated clusters of network structures and ended up in a total of nine clusters. Four clusters described ethical values (ethos), and five clusters explained possibilities as experienced by caregivers and how to act in an ethical manner in the daily work with the older people.

Clusters consist of a BBN of nodes (three to seven nodes per cluster), and the relation between nodes within a cluster forms the specific character of the cluster. The comprehension of clusters is therefore given by the statements, in form of conditional probabilities, within that specific BNN. We can state that the Bayesian approach had possibilities to generate clusters and underlying structural entities of relevance for the aim of the study. The structure identification capabilities enabled to find distinct dynamics within the clusters, as soon as the conditions of individual nodes were changed from the initial conditions.

Our intension was to find "what-if questions," like *"what happens if the conditions of one or several specified nodes within a cluster are changed?,"* in order to prevent irregularities in the area of ethics. The dynamics of fixation of one or more entities to a given level can be seen in the cluster *dignity* consists of seven nodes or entities. There are small differences between the agreement levels of respective informants. About 85–94 percent of the informants totally agree with all seven statements. In Table 1, we have the distribution function for the cluster *dignity*.

Tables 1, 4, 5, and 6 represent changes between different assessment levels. We have to note that the material for the study was limited, and far-reaching conclusions cannot be made, but the results of the study point at entities possess power to change ethical ideals and manners in a remarkable way. This insight is of vital importance for the development of ethical manners in daily nursing care. Ethical values (ideals) such as integrity, dignity, safety, and caring community are embraced by the majority of respondents. However, we still have to note that cluster *dignity* has three percent ($n = 735$) of the observations at level "3" (sometimes) or lower, while within cluster *integrity* four percent ($n = 315$). Within this group of clusters, *dignity* was the only cluster which showed significant effects when the conditions for any of the nodes were changed.

Clusters describing ethical manners were the following: *closeness, distance, dignity, safety, participation,* and *caring communion.* Within these clusters, we can see numbers of significant effects if the conditionalities for given node were changed (Tables 9, 10, 12, and 15). Powerful negative effects on the entities probably change the opportunities for the older

TABLE 11: Cluster VII: Possibilities for participation.

| | | Distribution function for Cluster VII (percent) | | | | | |
		5	4	3	2	1	Missing
C1	Freedom for the older person	77,14	18,1	1,9			2,86
E1	To believe in the older person	89,52	8,57	0,95			0,95
D41	Encourage participation	33,43	42,65	14,45	6,09		3,38
A41	Promote continuity and preservation in the care process as a whole	23,81	42,86	24,76	3,81	0,95	3,81
F41	Being emphatic and sharing the moods with the older person	29,5	40	24,76	2,86		2,86
A11	Support resources of the older person	15,24	57,14	24,76	1,9		0,95
G41	Being humble while caring for the older person	42,8	36,84	13,52	5,36		1,47

TABLE 12: Effects on distribution function when D41 fixed to "3" = 100%.

		5	4	3	2	1	Missing
C1	Freedom for the older person	−4,4	6,36	−1,14			−0,82
E1	To believe in the older person	−0,48	1,33	−0,6			−0,27
A41	Promote continuity and preservation in the care process	−2,61	13,24	−7,06	−0,57	−0,52	−2,48
F41	Being emphatic and sharing the moods with the older person	−10,87	6,27	7,99	−1,79		−1,57
A11	Support resources of the older person	−3,31	−0,17	2,87	0,46		0,15
G41	Being humble while caring for the older person	−1,9	−2,43	3,61	1,57		−0,83

TABLE 13: Effects on distribution function when A41 fixed to "4" = 100%.

		5	4	3	2	1	Missing
D41	Encourage participation	−6,8	13,18	−2,87	−2,16		−1,36
G41	Being humble while caring for the older person	5,26	6,57	−10.89	−0,04		−0,9

TABLE 14: Effects on distribution function when F41 fixed to "4" = 100%.

		5	4	3	2	1	Missing
D41	Encourage participation	−2,73	6,68	1,68	−4,18		−1,47
A11	Support resources of the older person	−10,48	9,53	−0,95	0,48		1,43
G41	Being humble while caring for the older person	6,08	5,55	−6,69	−4,41		−0,52

person to have good ethical care. However, earlier studies highlight the importance to develop an ethical culture at the unit. Without ethical discussions and models, the way to act in ethically critical situations, each caregiver acts in their own way, and it will not be possible to guarantee the older person ethical good care, because the quality of the care is depending on the individual caregiver's attitudes and manners [27, 28]. Promoting ethical good care is the responsibility of the whole work team.

Caregivers participating in the study indeed approved ethos as it was expressed in the clusters of dignity, community, security, and integrity. A certain dynamics can be seen within cluster dignity, that is, coherence between the statement and the opinion of the informant. This was clear particularly in relation to basic care needs and in care situations with older people who generally suffer from frailty and increasing degree of cognitive decline.

The study shows that the caregivers' attitudes to entities like compassion and mercy, moments of calm, respect, and compliance with the wishes and needs of the older person are of major importance in maintaining a dignified care. The perception and comprehension of the older person, as a person who lived a rich and meaningful life and where disease and illness changed that person's life, is important for the formation of ethical manner. Positive approaches to the older person, seeing the person behind the illness and suffering, are basic prerequisites for ethical manners in the daily care. Based on earlier research and results from this study, we know that the view of the older person and knowledge about ageing processes are some of the most important entities in the daily care of older persons [29–31]. Respect and dignity of the older person were also in earlier research proven to constitute one of the major caring challenges. The views of the older person link to numerous ethical challenges, and therefore greater attention should be considered in both education and training of caregivers.

Tornstam shows in his theory of gerotranscendence how the ageing process results in a value of displacement in the elderly [29, 32]. The older persons experience about their life as meaningful, having the right to control their lives

TABLE 15: Effects on distribution function when A11 fixed to "4" = 100%.

		5	4	3	2	1	Missing
D41	Encourage participation	−0,65	−0,13	0,31	0,04		0,42
F41	Being emphatic and sharing the moods with the older	−4,5	6,67	−4,76	0,47		2,14
G41	Being humble while caring for the older person	0,12	0,48	−0,86	−0,26		0,54

TABLE 16: Cluster VIII: possibilities for safety care.

		Distribution function for Cluster VIII (percent)					
		5	4	3	2	1	Missing
D31	Be responsible for the inner safety of older person	66,7	26,6	3,8			2,9
A31	To create a safe situation for the older person	30,0	47,0	17,0	3,0		3,0
B31	Protect against mistreatment of the older person	51,0	26,7	13,0	4,0	0,6	4,7

TABLE 17: Cluster IX: possibilities for caring communion.

		Distribution function for Cluster IX (percent)					
		5	4	3	2	1	Missing
B11	Person-centred care	30,2	49,7	17,7			2,4
E41	The desire to listen to the older person	41,9	44,8	9,5			3,8
D11	Monitoring of older person's satisfaction about care	56,2	29,5	11,4	0,9		1,9
B41	True presences	44,8	42,9	9,5			2,9
C11	Flexibility	4,6	45,9	41,7	6,5		1,5
C41	Encourage participation	41	41,9	13,3	1		2,9
F/E11	Respect for the older person's own decisions	3,8	13,3	34,3	29,5	10,5	8,6

TABLE 18: Effects on distribution function when C11 "4" = 100%.

		5	4	3	2	1	Missing
B11	Person-centred care	5,57	−0,57	−3,48			−1,52
E41	Listen to the older person	2,21	−1,15	−1,25			4,01
D11	Monitoring of older person's satisfaction about care	14,17	−3,01	−10,58	−0,55		
B41	True presences	5,09	0,25	−5,82			1,47
C41	Encourage participation	−1,54	0,5	2,03	−0,05		−0,92
F/E11	Respect for the older person's own decisions	−3,55	−6,64	1,7	9,32	4,13	−4,97

regardless of the health and functional status, and feeling respected is important entity for the experience of dignity. Wadensten and Carlsson [31, 33, 34] showed in their studies of the previous phenomena, that the caregivers did not properly perceive and comprehend the older person. In order to guarantee ethical care for the elderly, it seems likely that the view of the elderly needs to be changed, and the elderly should be seen as an adult with her own life to live, regardless of health or illness. Wadensten and Carlsson [31, 33] state that caregivers have not observed the value shifts as Tornstam [29] explained in his study.

Earlier research and findings [8–10, 12, 20] from this study are consistent with each other. Opportunities for unethical manners and ethical challenges are in previous research described in a rather context dependent and descriptive way, and often without prospective and prognostic aspects. This study aims to include foresightedness and to highlight the probable effects on and prospects of ethical care. If we do not take these negative attitudes seriously, as we can see in the findings section, good ethical care will be at risk.

On the basis of the present study, we can only state that there are differences in caregivers attitudes. Some caregivers felt it was "almost" or "every time" possible to act in an ethical manner, while others did not feel they had sufficient possibilities to act ethically. The reasons for those possibilities being limited is not confirmed in the present study but appear in some previous research [13, 35, 36]. In addition to the views of the elderly and knowledge about the ageing process, we should further include observations about situations where the total resources are not in balance to meet the needs of the elderly [37, 38]. Different opinions within the care unit about the caregivers ability to provide care in accordance with the ideals, related to good ethical care, moral anxiety, and guilt, are further circumstances [36] to be considered beyond the scope of this study.

This stress is clearly related to the quality of care. The situation can become very serious. Earlier research reports about serious medical errors and even death, illness, indifference, and arrogance [35–37].

We cannot overlook leader's responsibilities, as leadership sets the norms and upholds a culture [39]. The leaders support and create conditions for caregivers to act in accordance with the collective agreements about ethical good care, but they also explicitly provide and disseminate the ethical care criteria for and within the organisation. Leaders also take questions about resource allocation seriously, by creating human and material conditions for caregivers to act in accordance with their ethical ideals [39].

This study is unique in its kind, both concerning the selected approach and methodological questions. BBNs have not been used significantly in nursing research, nor are there any studies that examine the ethical possibilities with focus on the probable effects upon changing conditions.

An important point to make is that results must be understood given the translation of symbolic data from numbers to logical concepts and statements. Ethical ideals and ethical manners are phenomena that indeed make no sense to be explained exclusively by numeric data. The data represented and presented in the study are seen as symbolic data and appear, for example, as clusters of ethical ideals and attitudes which obtain their special character of the entities (nodes) and forms the network within the cluster. The character of a given cluster depends on the explanation given the cluster. The nine clusters within the study are interpreted from caring science perspective [7, 24–26] and earlier research about ethical questions in the daily work with the older person. In view of this transformation from numeric to statements, we have thus moved along the path *from statistics to logic*.

4. Conclusion

The study has opened up new opportunities to prevent services from becoming increasingly impersonal and stereotypical, and instead becoming care-based concerning ethos with ethical manners.

The nodes that describe the cluster's character may in the future not only serve as a basis for ethical discussions and decision-making, but also be starting points for caregiver's individual development.

The structure of the cluster with the underlying entities, that the study generated, seems to be an interesting development of the ISAEC instrument. The clusters with underlying nodes could be used as a framework for the continued development of instruments to identify caregiver attitudes to ethical values and ethical approach.

In summary, we can state that the study has enriched the ethical discussion and opened up new "what-if" questions. That in turn creates awareness of barriers to ethical good care.

Ethical Approval

Ethical permission for the realization of the study was provided by the Community Board of Social Care (§180/2005) for the municipality in which this study took place. Good scientific praxis in accordance with the directives of the National Advisory Board on Ethics (2002) and the Helsinki declaration (2008) has been followed.

Disclosure

The paper has been planned, written, and evaluated in close cooperation with the other authors.

Conflict of Interests

The authors declare that no conflict of interests exists and that no financial relationship exists to any organization.

References

[1] I. Å. Bolmsjö, L. Sandman, and E. Andersson, "Everyday ethics in the care of elderly people," *Nursing Ethics*, vol. 13, no. 3, pp. 249–263, 2006.

[2] I. Berggren, I. Bégat, and E. Severinsson, "Australian clinical nurse supervisor's ethical decision-making style," *Nursing and Health Sciences*, vol. 4, no. 1-2, pp. 15–23, 2002.

[3] M. Mahlin, "Individual patient advocacy, collective responsibility and activism within professional nursing associations," *Nursing Ethics*, vol. 17, no. 2, pp. 247–254, 2010.

[4] J. Pearl, "Fusion, propagation, and structuring in belief networks," *Artificial Intelligence*, vol. 29, no. 3, pp. 241–288, 1986.

[5] S. L. Lauritzen and D. J. Spiegelhalter, "Local computations with probabilities on graphical structures and their application to expert systems," *Journal of the Royal Statistical Society: Series B*, vol. 50, pp. 157–194, 1988.

[6] M. Frilund, L. Fagerstrom, and K. Eriksson, "The caregivers' possibilities of providing ethically good care for older people— a study on caregivers' ethical approach," *Scandinavian Journal of Caring Science*, 2012.

[7] K. Eriksson, "Ethos," in *Gryning II. Klinisk Vårdvetenskap. Institutionen för Vårdvetenskap*, K. Eriksson and U. Å. Lindström, Eds., pp. 21–33, Åbo Akademi, Vaasa, Finland, 2003.

[8] A. Mamhidir, M. Kihlgren, and V. Sorlie, "Ethical challenges related to elder care. High level decision-makers' experiences," *BMC Medical Ethics*, vol. 8, article 3, 2007.

[9] E. V. Boisaubin, A. Chu, and J. M. Catalano, "Perceptions of long-term care, autonomy, and dignity, by residents, family and care-givers: the Houston experience," *Journal of Medicine and Philosophy*, vol. 32, no. 5, pp. 447–464, 2007.

[10] I. Randers and A. Mattiasson, "Autonomy and integrity: upholding older adult patients' dignity," *Journal of Advanced Nursing*, vol. 45, no. 1, pp. 63–71, 2004.

[11] B. McCormack, B. Karlsson, J. Dewing, and A. Lerdal, "Exploring person-centredness: a qualitative meta-synthesis of four studies," *Scandinavian Journal of Caring Sciences*, vol. 24, no. 3, pp. 620–634, 2010.

[12] M. E. Cameron, M. Schaffer, and H. Park, "Nursing students' experience of ethical problems and use of ethical decision-making models," *Nursing Ethics*, vol. 8, no. 5, pp. 432–447, 2001.

[13] L. Fagerström, Y. Gustafson, G. Jakobsson, S. Johansson, and P. Vartiainen, "Sense of security among people aged 65 and 75: external and inner sources of security," *Journal of Advanced Nursing*, vol. 67, no. 6, pp. 1305–1316, 2011.

[14] K. Eriksson, "The theory of caritative caring: a vision," *Nursing Science Quarterly*, vol. 20, no. 3, pp. 201–202, 2007.

[15] M. Edlund, *Människans Värdighet ett Grundbegrepp inom Vårdvetenskapen [Akademisk avhandling]*, Åbo Akademis, Vaasa, Finland, 2002.

[16] S. Davies, "Promoting autonomy and independence for older people within nursing practice: an observational study," *Journal of Clinical Nursing*, vol. 9, no. 1, pp. 127–136, 2000.

[17] P. Anderberg, M. Lepp, A. Berglund, and K. Segesten, "Preserving dignity in caring for older adults: a concept analysis," *Journal of Advanced Nursing*, vol. 59, no. 6, pp. 635–643, 2007.

[18] G. A. Brilowski and M. C. Wendler, "An evolutionary concept analysis of caring," *Journal of Advanced Nursing*, vol. 50, no. 6, pp. 641–650, 2005.

[19] B. Pauly, C. Varcoe, J. Storch, and L. Newton, "Registered nurses' perceptions of moral distress and ethical climate," *Nursing Ethics*, vol. 16, no. 5, pp. 561–573, 2009.

[20] R. Suhonen, M. Stolt, V. Launis, and H. Leino-Kilpi, "Research on ethics in nursing care for older people: a literature review," *Nursing Ethics*, vol. 17, no. 3, pp. 337–352, 2010.

[21] A. Clarke, E. J. Hanson, and H. Ross, "Seeing the person behind the patient: enhancing the care of older people using a biographical approach," *Journal of Clinical Nursing*, vol. 12, no. 5, pp. 697–706, 2003.

[22] L. Nygård, U. Grahn, A. Rudenhammar, and S. Hydling, "Reflecting on practice: are home visits prior to discharge worthwhile in geriatric inpatient care? Clients' and occupational therapists' perceptions," *Scandinavian Journal of Caring Sciences*, vol. 18, no. 2, pp. 193–203, 2004.

[23] K. Nydén, M. Petersson, and M. Nyström, "Unsatisfied basic needs of older patients in emergency care environments—obstacles to an active role in decision making," *Journal of Clinical Nursing*, vol. 12, no. 2, pp. 268–274, 2003.

[24] K. Eriksson, "Caring science in a new key," *Nursing Science Quarterly*, vol. 15, no. 1, pp. 61–65, 2002.

[25] K. Eriksson, "Becoming through suffering—the path to health and holiness," *International Journal of Human Caring*, vol. 11, no. 2, pp. 8–16, 2007.

[26] U. Å. Lindström, L. Lindholm, and J. E. Zetterlund, "Katie Eriksson: Theory of caritative caring," in *Nursing Theorists and Their Work*, A. M. Marriner Tomey and M. R. Alligood, Eds., pp. 191–223, Mosby, St. Louis, Mo, USA, 6th edition, 2006.

[27] I. Berggren, I. Bégat, and E. Severinsson, "Australian clinical nurse supervisor's ethical decision-making style," *Nursing and Health Sciences*, vol. 4, no. 1-2, pp. 15–23, 2002.

[28] I. Berggren, A. Barbosa da Silva, and E. Severinsson, "Core ethical issues of clinical nursing supervision," *Nursing and Health Sciences*, vol. 7, no. 1, pp. 21–28, 2005.

[29] L. Tornstam, "Gerotranscendence—a theoretical and empirical exploration," in *Aging and the Religious Dimension*, L. E. Thomas and S. A. Eisenhandler, Eds., Greenwood Publishing Group, Westport, Conn, USA, 1994.

[30] K. Hyse and L. Tornstam, *Recognizing Aspects of Onself in the Theory of Gerotranscendence*, Online publication from The Social Gerontology Group, Uppsala, Sweden, 2009.

[31] B. Wadensten and M. Carlsson, "Nursing theory views on how to support the process of ageing," *Journal of Advanced Nursing*, vol. 42, no. 2, pp. 118–124, 2003.

[32] L. Tornstam, *Gerotranscendence: A Developmental Theory of Positive Aging*, Springer, New York, NY, USA, 2005.

[33] B. Wadensten and M. Carlsson, "A qualitative study of nursing staff members' interpretations of signs of gerotranscendence," *Journal of Advanced Nursing*, vol. 36, no. 5, pp. 635–642, 2001.

[34] B. Wadensten and M. Carlsson, "Theory—driven guidelines for practical care of older people, based on the theory of gerotranscendence," *Journal of Advanced Nursing*, vol. 41, no. 5, pp. 462–470, 2003.

[35] A. Nordam, K. Torjuul, and V. Sørlie, "Ethical challenges in the care of older people and risk of being burned out among male nurses," *Journal of Clinical Nursing*, vol. 14, no. 10, pp. 1248–1256, 2005.

[36] A.L. Glasberg, *Samvetsstress bidragande orsak till utbrandhet i vården [Doktorsavhandling]*, Umeå University Medical Dissertations, 2007.

[37] K. Murphy, "A qualitative study explaining nurses' perceptions of quality care for older people in long-term care settings in Ireland," *Journal of Clinical Nursing*, vol. 16, no. 3, pp. 477–485, 2007.

[38] L. H. Aiken, Y. Xue, S. P. Clarke, and D. M. Sloane, "Supplemental nurse staffing in hospitals and quality of care," *Journal of Nursing Administration*, vol. 37, no. 7-8, pp. 335–342, 2007.

[39] L. Fagerström and S. Salmela, "Leading change: a challenge for leaders in Nordic health care," *Journal of Nursing Management*, vol. 18, no. 5, pp. 613–617, 2010.

15

Adolescents' Perceptions of Their Consent to Psychiatric Mental Health Treatment

Anthony James Roberson[1] and Diane K. Kjervik[2]

[1] Capstone College of Nursing, The University of AL, Tuscaloosa, Alabama 35487-0358, USA
[2] Health Care Environments Division, School of Nursing, University of North Carolina at Chapel Hill, 528 Carrington Hall, Chapel Hill, NC 27599-7460, USA

Correspondence should be addressed to Anthony James Roberson, ajroberson@ua.edu

Academic Editor: Patrick Callaghan

The purpose of this paper is to present the findings of a small-scale study in which the decision-making process of adolescents who consent to psychiatric mental health treatment was examined. Sixteen (16) adolescents were interviewed about their decisions related to initial and continued treatment, along with their understanding of minor consent laws. Interviews were audio-recorded, and transcripts were analyzed through concept analysis. Findings are presented in the context of the decision-making steps and research questions. Most adolescents did not recognize consequences related to psychiatric mental health treatment and did not assimilate and integrate information provided to them about treatment choices. Adolescents disagreed with current minor consent laws that allow minors to consent to certain healthcare treatments without the required consent of the parent. Further, adolescents reported that a collaborative approach in making decisions about the adolescent's psychiatric mental health treatment was most facilitative of achieving the goals of treatment.

1. Introduction

Adolescence is uniquely different from all other stages of human development, especially from physiological and cognitive perspectives, and it can be argued that it is the most challenging of all developmental periods [1]. The physical changes that occur during this developmental stage are perhaps more obvious than the cognitive changes. The adolescent experiences genital development, breast development, pubic and axillary hair development, skin changes, and at times rapid changes in height and weight [1]. The physiological changes of development will be realized eventually for each adolescent. Further, physiological changes generally occur earlier in girls than boys.

The cognitive changes of adolescents occur with great diversity. "Many adolescents are as egocentric in some respects as preschool children, while others reach the stage of abstract thinking that characterizes advanced cognition" [1, page 351]. Adolescence is the period of development that the individual is usually attempting to break parental bonds, establish themselves in certain social groups, and develop a sense of self [2].

In addition to establishing one's identity, the adolescent is also striving to become more independent. Adolescence is perhaps the phase of development in which the individual is making the most effort to seek independence and control over their lives, which includes the desire to start making more of their own decisions [3, 4]. Piaget defines the cognitive developmental stage of formal operational thinking as the phase in which adolescents aged 12 years and older can think about hypothetical concepts and are able to contemplate consequences related to decision choices [1]. Part of the cognitive development of adolescents aged 12 years and older includes the adolescent's increased ability to solve problems and "speculate about the possible as well as the real" more independent of others [1, page 56].

One area of decision-making research that has recently been examined more closely is that of adolescents making independent decisions about their healthcare treatment [5–7]. These researchers suggest that adolescents are capable of

TABLE 1: Gender and race frequency distribution by age group.

| Age group | Caucasian ($n = 6$) | | African-American ($n = 10$) | |
Total (n)	Female ($n = 1$)	Male ($n = 5$)	Female ($n = 8$)	Male ($n = 2$)
12 to 14 (9)	0	3	5	1
15 to 17 (7)	1	2	3	1

TABLE 2: Diagnosis and frequency by age group.

Diagnosis	12 to 14 years old ($n = 9$)	15 to 17 years old ($n = 7$)
ADHD	3	1
ODD		2
MDD		2
PTSD	1	
Social phobia	1	
ADHD/DBD	2	
ADHD/ODD	1	
ADHD/MDD		2
ADHD/PTSD/ODD	1	

Note: ADHD: attention deficit hyperactivity disorder; ODD: oppositional defiant disorder; MDD: major depressive disorder; PTSD: post traumatic stress disorder; DBD: disruptive behavior disorder.

making complex healthcare decisions. However, adolescents have shown that they are more interested in having their developmental needs, such as independence and autonomy, met and at times may forgo the recommended treatment in order to meet these needs [8].

Research studies support that parents and peers influence the decision-making of adolescents in hypothetical healthcare situations [9–11]. Parents are more influential than peers when the adolescent is making a decision that has a moral or value slant, such as deciding to report someone who has destroyed property or has engaged in stealing. Peers are more influential when the adolescent is deciding on non-life-threatening issues, such as whom to date and what to wear to an event. However, the influence that parents and peers have on the adolescent who is deciding to consent in a real life healthcare situation is not fully understood. Further, we do not understand the influences of parents, family, and peers on outcomes in psychiatric mental health situations.

The informed consent rights of minors have been expanded in recent years [12, 13]. English and Kenney [13] have provided a comprehensive monograph describing each state's minor consent laws related to healthcare treatments. Although these laws vary in the types of healthcare treatments, the adolescent may consent, most states allow minors to consent to certain medical procedures, such as mental health services, including outpatient and crisis intervention for mental health reasons, without the required consent of the parent or legal guardian [13].

The purpose of this paper is to provide the findings of a descriptive qualitative study in which the decision-making process of adolescents who consent to psychiatric mental health treatment in real life situations was examined.

Considering the minor consent laws that provide adolescents the right to consent to psychiatric mental health treatment without the consent of the parent, the following research questions were addressed in the study.

(1) How do 12-to-17-year-old adolescents who consent to psychiatric mental health treatment (medication intervention, psychotherapy, or a combination of both) perceive the process of deciding to accept treatment?

(2) How do 12-to-17-year-old adolescents who consent to psychiatric mental health treatment (medication intervention, psychotherapy, or a combination of both) perceive the goals of treatment?

2. Methods

2.1. Subjects. Sample size in qualitative research is determined by theoretical data saturation, rather than power analysis, which is associated with quantitative research [14]. The sample size for this study consisted of 16 adolescents. The age range of the adolescents was 12 to 17 years (nine 12 to 14 years old and seven 15 to 17 years old). These age groups represent the major adolescent developmental stages. The study included a relatively equal number of females (9) and males (7). The intent for this inclusion was to identify any differences between genders in problem-solving abilities. The study included 10 African American and 6 Caucasian adolescents.

An outline of the demographic information for the adolescent and parent participants is provided in Tables 1, 2, and 4.

Full approval for this research was obtained from the University of North Carolina at Chapel Hill Public Health and Nursing Institutional Review Board. Adolescents whose only language was English were recruited and included in this study. All adolescents who participated in this study were from lower socioeconomic families. The sample was purposeful in that adolescents recruited for the study had consented to treatment and were receiving out-patient psychiatric mental health treatment. Psychiatric mental health treatment is defined as a combination of medication and psychotherapy intervention.

Only adolescents who were receiving maintenance psychiatric mental health treatment were considered for this study. Maintenance treatment was defined by the American Psychiatric Association [15] criteria as a period of treatment when the patient is not experiencing recurrent signs and symptoms of the illness being treated. Although *maintenance phase* is not defined by the number of weeks or months, the criteria established for this study were as follows: over the

TABLE 3: Frequency of current management regimen by age group.

Age group Total (n)	Medication only ($n = 4$)	Therapy only ($n = 6$)	Combined ($n = 6$)
12 to 14 (9)	2	3	4
15 to 17 (7)	3	2	2

TABLE 4: Participant grade level progression frequency by age group.

Age group total (n)	On time grade	1-year behind grade	≥2-years behind grade
12 to 14 (9)	4	4	1
15 to 17 (7)	2	4	1

past four weeks, the adolescent's medications had not been changed or adjusted either in dosing or type, and new issues in therapy were not being addressed.

2.2. Setting. Data collection took place in a community-based out-patient psychiatric mental health practice located in a mid-sized city in the Southeast. Services provided by the facility include medication intervention, individual psychotherapy, group therapy, and case management services. Psychiatric Mental Health Nurse Practitioners provide medication management in addition to individual and family therapy for patients. Master's and doctoral level therapists provide individual and group therapy. Case management is provided by bachelor's prepared therapists.

2.3. Procedure. After the appropriate informed consents were obtained by this researcher, adolescents were interviewed using a semistructured interview script [16]. Although the intent was to consistently follow the interview script [16], participants were encouraged to discuss other matters not included in the interview questions that were related to the research topic. The final interview script was pilot-tested with three adolescents to ensure that the interview questions could be understood and comprehended. The adolescents who participated in the pilot test were not included in the final data analysis of this study.

Interviews with the adolescent were audio-recorded with the use of an Olympus digital recorder and took place in a private, sound-proof room at the study facility. Each interview lasted for approximately one hour. Specific consent for this author to read the medical records of the adolescents was obtained. The information extracted from the medical records included demographic data about the adolescent, such as year of birth, ethnicity, mental health diagnosis, medical diagnosis, and education level.

2.4. Data Management and Analysis. Data analysis was a continuous process throughout the study [17]. The researcher transcribed the data after each interview. All field notes were transcribed by the principal investigator (PI). Field notes contained a detailed description of the events that occurred during the interview, such as the location, date, and time of the interviews and any events that were observed during the interview. These notes also included what was learned by this author from one interview to the next. The field notes were organized chronologically in a loose-leaf binder [14].

Each participant was assigned a number that was only identifiable by this researcher. Each document that included data (transcripts from adolescent, demographic information, field notes) was assigned the participant number. No participant-identifying information was linked to the transcripts, audiotapes, field notes, or demographic information. All collected data were categorized according to date and time of interview, and the deidentifying number assigned to each participant.

The data analysis process was completed using several components. Verbatim transcripts were read iteratively [18]. A system of data reduction, through open, *in vivo*, and axial coding [19] techniques was used when appropriate. Members of the research team and psychiatric mental health therapists and nurse practitioners assisted in evaluating the coding schemes. The components and subcomponents of coded data were analyzed to develop themes, and then the themes were related to the research questions and synthesizing framework [18, 20, 21]. Collected field notes were used to enhance the insights provided by the transcripts [18].

Content analysis [22] of the data was completed for this study. This approach was helpful considering the limited knowledge on the topic of the decisions adolescents make in psychiatric mental health situations [22, 23]. Data were categorized, in this case according the interview questions [23]. The categories were further separated into indexes and are represented by exemplaries included as support for the findings. The units that were analyzed in this study were primarily phrases and sentences from the adolescent interviews.

Validation of data was crucial to ensure the accuracy of the data and reliability of the findings. To make certain, validity was optimized, accuracy of the transcripts was thoroughly scrutinized by this researcher. Creswell and Miller [24] state that validity in qualitative studies is defined by how accurately the account of the study participants' realities is presented in the data analysis. The researcher was most concerned with the inferences drawn from reported study results and whether the realities of the participants were provided. Therefore, validity of the findings was checked by asking the study participants themselves if the interpretations by the PI truly captured the essence of their experiences [18]. Another test of validity involved the PI sharing the descriptions and the steps of analysis with qualitative experts [14, 18].

3. Results

The following decision-making step model was used as the framework in formulating the interview questions and will serve as a guide to present the findings: (a) the adolescent's recognition that a treatment decision is required, (b) the adolescent's understanding of treatment goals, (c) the ability of the adolescent to determine the consequences of the treatment decisions, and (d) the adolescent's ability to understand that each consequence is likely to occur, which includes assimilating and integrating the information provided about treatment options [25–27]. In addition to the decision-making model, the study findings were also presented in terms of the research questions.

4. Research Question No. 1: Adolescents' Perceptions of Their Decision-Making Process about Treatment

4.1. Recognizing That a Treatment Decision Was Required. Adolescents were first asked about the decisions they made in initiating psychiatric mental health treatment with the following: "tell me about the initial decisions you made about getting treatment" and "how did you decide that you needed treatment?" The researcher was specifically interested in how the adolescents came to the decision that they were in need of treatment. Particular attention was given to those decisions that the adolescent made without the parent or legal guardian to initiate treatment. It was important to distinguish between those decisions that the adolescent made without others and those made with others in order to fully understand if the adolescent recognized that a decision about their mental health treatment was required.

"*I knew I needed to get some help, I had to.*" (John, 17-year-old male) All adolescents reported that during the initial meeting with the nurse practitioner or therapist, they realized that a decision about treatment choices would be needed. Most ($n = 12$) adolescents stated that the initial decision to seek treatment was completed in collaboration with their parent or legal guardian. Some adolescents ($n = 4$) reported that decisions made about initiating treatment were made without the parent. All adolescents felt their own input was taken seriously by their parent and nurse practitioner, whether in making independent decisions or decisions in conjunction with their parent or legal guardian.

There was strong evidence to support the adolescent's ability to identify that a decision about treatment was needed or ultimately required. For example, a common response among adolescents was that they knew when the initial appointment was made at the treating facility; there would ultimately be a decision made about accepting or rejecting treatment. All adolescents identified that the general purpose of the initial visit to the facility was to receive psychiatric mental health treatment and that a decision about their treatment would be required. Although all adolescents engaged in discussions about their initial decisions to seek treatment, the older adolescents (15 to 17 years old) provided more detailed and focused descriptions regarding their perceptions of need for treatment.

The interview questions included asking adolescents about the initial treatment-related decisions. Each adolescent was asked about the purpose of seeking treatment and more specifically about starting treatment. The purpose of posing questions in this manner was to determine exactly what decisions the adolescents made about their treatment. It is evident that all adolescents could recognize that a decision to seek mental healthcare was needed, based on their negative experiences behind and ahead of them:

> *I was on drugs real bad and I started, when I, I felt real bad one day. I was like crying all of the sudden, I donot know. I had this feeling that something werenot right so I went to [private hospital]. I told my mom that I wasnot feeling great, so she took me to the hospital and I was the one who wanted to go but she kind of helped me out with that. Then I wanted to come here because [private hospital] didnot think I needed to be in the hospital. So, I knew I needed to get some help, I had to.* (John, 17-year-old male)

Understanding the Goals of Treatment. Adolescents were asked specific questions related to their goals of treatment to understand whether the adolescent could identify personal treatment goals, rather than those established by others (i.e., nurse practitioner, therapist, parents). Each adolescent voiced specific goals for treatment, including those independently formulated and those that seemed influenced by others.

"*I just wanted to feel better.*" Most adolescents based their goals of treatment on the struggles experienced in living with their mental illness. One 17-year-old male diagnosed with a major depressive disorder, severe type, communicated that his goal in treatment was to "feel better and to not be so depressed...I was not doing well in school because of the depression and I needed to get my grades better...but I had to get over the depression first." Other examples of goals were

> *I wanted to, uh, stop stressing all the time and stop fighting and stuff and fighting to [sic] my little sister.* (Lauren, 15-year-old female)

> *I wanted to be able to control myself better and bring my grades up...I was feeling real bad and I just wanted to feel better.* (John, 17-year-old male)

"*To not end up like my mother.*" It was evident in some responses ($n = 3$) that some adolescents may have formulated an answer about their goals in treatment based on what they had been told by others. For example, a 12-year-old male who had been sexually molested by his mother for many years reported his goal in treatment was "to not end up like my mother because she molested us [siblings] when we were little and I do not want to molest my kids when I get older." The concept that certain behaviors, such as molestation, are somehow "passed down" is at a higher level of logic and abstraction that would normally be expected of an older adolescent, but not of a 12-year-old's thought pattern. This response suggests that an adult discussed this particular goal with him. Regardless of his age, this adolescent was capable of stating a treatment goal and he had learned from prior experiences.

"*To feel better now.*" Initially, questions about their short-term goals and responses were highly detailed. However, when questioned about any long-term goals that were established in the initial stages of treatment, adolescents would consistently refer back to the short-term goals of feeling better now, improving grades, or to stop being angry. The adolescents were unsuccessful in identifying long-term goals established at the onset of their treatment. But, they were successful in discussing immediate goals such as to feel better now.

Determining the Consequences of Treatment Decisions. To understand whether adolescents could determine the consequences and risks associated with taking medication or engaging in individual or group psychotherapy, the participants were asked to identify the reasons for taking the medications or receiving psychotherapy.

"*The medication helps me calm down.*" Identifying the reasons for any treatment is an important step to being able to identify the consequences. All adolescents spoke easily about their reasons for taking medication. Each rationale was linked with past behavioral experiences that were perceived as negative with positive medication effects. Each related to a context important to the adolescent school performance, emotions, and relationships. The extent of knowledge about the specific reasons for the medications and the elaboration provided by the participants varied, but not by a specific age group. The following are examples of responses when the adolescents were asked to identify the reasons for taking the medications:

> I take Metadate so, it help keep me calmed down a little bit and help me in school...I do better in school, my grades are better...it were given to me because I were hyper a lot, and were gettin' in trouble at school a lot. (James, 12-year-old male)

> I know the medicine, it [Concerta] helps me concentrate more. (Sue, 14 year-old female)

"*Wellbutrin influences dopamine levels.*" One 16-year-old adolescent provided a more technical response as to the reason and purpose of the medications he was prescribed. His response differed from other adolescents because he made no mention of how the medication helped him feel better or for what purpose the medication was intended. Even with the use of probes, the adolescent did not seem to make the connection between the goal to feel better and taking an antidepressant. Discussion by the adolescent about the intended purpose and reason for the medication remained at a medical terminology level:

> Um, Wellbutrin, um, influences your dopamine levels, while Lexparo is an SSRI,which focuses more on serotonin, but it does, I think, influence overall levels...like all three brain chemicals. (Tim, 16-year-old male)

This adolescent's father is a healthcare professional and frequently discusses with his son the reasons for the medications, perhaps on a more technical level than an emotional one.

"*Therapy can relax you.*" Adolescents were also capable of identifying reasons for receiving therapy:

> He's [therapist] teaching me like, um, stuff like tell me do not do bad stuff and what not do and what is good to do. Like he told me I got, um gotta start talking and stuff about stuff that could help me. (Lauren, 15-year-old female)

"*Antidepressants increase risk for suicide.*" In terms of adolescents identifying consequences and risks associated with medication or psychotherapy intervention, the responses varied according to age. Each adolescent understood the meaning of *risk* as they were asked to provide a definition of the word and an example of "taking a risk". For example, one adolescent (13-year-old male) defined "taking a risk" as "taking a chance". He further provided an example by describing, "if you drink and drive, that's a risk of getting a ticket for driving drunk, or it's a risk of hitting someone while you're drunk...having a car accident." Out of the 11 adolescents taking medications, only one (16-year-old male) provided a clear understanding of the risks involved with taking the medications he was prescribed. This was also the adolescent (*Tim, 16-year-old male*) who discussed the goals of the medication in more technical terms:

> Um, Lexapro, like it has a side effect of, like, like tiredness, which at the beginning I felt a lot, like collapsing in the middle of class until we the times I given [sic] it were switched. I know that Wellbutrin can, is like, has a real risk for seizures...so you always have to be careful about your dose. I know that all antidepressants, especially for adolescents, can increase, like, risk of suicide, well for all ages, but particularly focusing on adolescents because you suddenly have that energy to do things, while it's (antidepressant) not necessarily treating your behavior yet. (Tim, 16-year-old male)

"*There are no risks.*" Tim's identification of risks associated with taking medications was not typical. In fact, a common theme among the adolescent participants was their inability to identify risks associated with taking the medications they were prescribed. Out of the remaining ten adolescents taking medications, eight stated the medication(s) they were taking had no risks. Two adolescents responded with "I did not know" when asked if the medication(s) they were taking had any risks. The examples reflect that the notion of no risks may be related to the adolescent's perception that they had not experienced any side effects or adverse events, thus there must not be any risks involved in taking the medication:

> *No, there ain't no risks. . .it [Concerta] hadn't done anything wrong to me for the past two years that I been taking it.* (James, 12-year-old male)

> *Nothing really. . .I do not remember what the risks was if there was any. . .cause I guess they really weren't that bad even if there was em [risks]. I do not know of any [risks].* (Angela, 15-year-old-female)

One 15-year-old female adolescent identified a side effect of taking Zoloft by stating, "I think I've got to eat with it [Zoloft] so I won't get sick." One adolescent provided the following response to the risk associated with her medication. Similar responses were shared by others (n = 6), but this was the only response this particular adolescent provided in explaining the risks associated with taking Zoloft:

> *If I take, if I take a lot of them I know it can do, make an overdose.* (Sue, 14-year-old female)

"*If therapy is helping, how could it hurt?*" No adolescent receiving psychotherapy was able to provide a description of any risks involved in this form of treatment. Each adolescent was asked why they did not think there were any risks associated with receiving therapy. The overwhelming response was similar to "if therapy is helping, how could it hurt?"

In summary, most adolescents did not identify risks associated with taking certain psychotropic medications or receiving psychotherapy. No adolescent identified risks associated with receiving therapy. However, in the adolescent's eyes, the positive effects of improving sadness, providing increased ability to focus, and improving energy levels, satisfied their goals without any thought or consideration to risks or consequences.

Understanding That Each Consequence Is Likely to Occur. This step of the decision-making process involves the adolescent assimilating all of the treatment options presented and deciding on the desirability of each consequence. Each adolescent involved in this study was receiving medication, psychotherapy, or a combination of both. To obtain information about the process of assimilation, adolescents were asked questions about their initial treatment decisions in addition to those decisions made about continued treatment. The information gleaned from this interview approach provided an understanding of the process the adolescent went through to incorporate the psychiatric mental health treatment information presented.

5. Initial Treatment Decisions

"*We made them together.*" Most (n = 12) adolescents perceived that they made the initial decisions about treatment with their parents. Adolescents spoke of the collaboration with their parents in the initial phase of treatment. This collaboration consisted of discussions about whether or not to start medication or psychotherapy intervention:

> *We decided that I was going to get treatment and that I would take the medicine that I'm taking.* (Joe, 13-year-old male)

> *She [grandmother] wanted me to take the medication and I wanted to take it too, so we decided that together.* (Mack, 15-year-old male)

"*I made the choice.*" Other (n = 4) adolescents perceived that they were the ones who decided upon initial treatment, including what kinds of interventions they would consider:

> *I'm the one that told them [parents] that I wanted to go [to treatment] andEverything.* (Jim, 17-year-old male)

> *I made the choice about me getting into group therapy.* (Jill, 13-year-old female)

6. Research Question No. 2: Adolescents' Perceptions of the Goals of Treatment

6.1. Continued Treatment Decisions. "*We made those together too.*" The perception among all adolescents was that most decisions made related to continued treatment (those made after the initial treatment decisions) were made with their parents. Examples of continued treatment decisions included goals related to making changes in medications, either in type, dosing levels or timing, or discontinuing therapy:

> *Um, I was asked if I wanted to be switched to a different dose and me and my parents talked about that to see if I needed.* (Tim, 16-year-old male)

> *My mother asked me if I wanted to stay here [treatment facility], because she would have take me somewhere else if I really wanted to, because I wanted to go to therapy.* (Jill, 13-year-old female)

"*I decided on the mentor I wanted.*" Some (n = 6) adolescents reported making some decisions about continued treatment without their parents. These decisions included those made about staying on medications, choosing a mentor, or getting to the appointments at the facility:

> *I think the biggest choice I made [about treatment] was not making a big deal out of it, I just kind of went along, but the fact that I just stayed on it [medication], that was not really influenced by my parents.* (Tim, 16-year-old male)

> *I decided if I'm feeling something, to just tell my therapist and not hold back like I usually do.* (Barbara, 14-year-old female)

7. Adequacy of Adolescent Treatment Decisions

Given the significant decisions made about their treatment, it was important to understand the adolescents' perceptions about the best decisions that were made in treatment. Adolescents were asked "which decisions about your continued treatment do you consider the best; those made without your parent, by your parents without you, or with you and your parents?" "Best" was defined as those decisions that have most led to the adolescent's current psychiatric stability.

7.1. The Best Treatment Decisions. The overwhelming theme was that the adolescents (*n* = 16) perceived that the best decisions made about their continued treatment were the ones made in collaboration with their parents. When asked about why they perceived that the best decisions about treatment have been made with their parents, a common response was that collaboration with parents provided them with the opportunity to reflect on the information about treatment more effectively and that some of the treatment decisions could not have been made without their parent. The time spent to mull over the information with their parents prior to deciding was described as important. The discussions with parents about treatment were viewed as helpful in the process and supportive for decision making.

"The decision me and my grandmom have made" (Sue, 14-year-old female). Among those (*n* = 11) taking medications, most (*n* = 8) relayed that they would not have been able to make a decision about what type of medication to agree to if this decision would have been made independent of their parent(s)/legal guardian. Although some adolescents (*n* = 2) taking medications relayed that initial decisions related to their treatment were made primarily by their parents, these adolescents perceived that their parents played an integral role in the decisions made about the adolescent's continued treatment.

8. Parental Influence from the Adolescent Perspective

When adolescents were asked if parent(s)/guardians were influential in their remaining on the prescribed medication(s) and remaining in therapy, the adolescents' comments indicated the important roles of parents in facilitating treatment through a variety of mechanisms. The adolescents' description of these roles is represented by the following labels: *encourager*, *transporter*, *administrator*, and *purchaser*.

"She [mother] just helps me." (Jill, 13-year-old female) Fifteen adolescents viewed the most influential role of the parent as that of *encourager*. The adolescents contributed their continued commitment and followup to treatment to the consistent encouragement that their parents provided them throughout treatment. Adolescents voiced a strong need for parental encouragement during treatment and discussed this particular role of the parent as essential to their continued stability:

"She makes sure I get there [mental health facility]." Several adolescents (*n* = 7) described that one manner in which

their parents/guardians were influential in contributing to their stability was the role the parent played as a *transporter*. Although this role did not receive the emphasis of the *encourager* role, adolescents from both age groups identified this role as an essential component to their overall continuation in treatment.

"She [mother] makes sure I take it [medication] everyday." (Angela, 15-year-old female) Adolescents also identified their parent as the *administrator* of their medications. Of the eleven adolescents currently receiving medication intervention, six discussed this particular role of their parent/guardian in terms of the significant influence on their continued stability. Further probes provided information on how the adolescent perceived this particular role. Among those taking medications, four viewed this role in a positive light, stating that the reminders from parents to take their medication(s) were helpful, while the remaining two viewed the parent's reminders as annoying.

"She buys it for me." (John, 17-year-old male) Another influential parental role described by adolescents (*n* = 3) was that of a *purchaser*. The adolescents considered the task of their parents purchasing the medications as a positive influence on them remaining stable and continuing in treatment:

> She calls over here [mental health facility] and gets the prescription and then she buys it for me. If she did not do that I wouldn't have 'em…that would not be a good thing for me, so, that's important for me to stay stable. (John, 17-year-old male)

"I encouraged myself." Seven adolescents (four 12 to 14 years old and three 15 to 17 years old) stated that in addition to their parents, their own influence led them to remain in treatment:

> I just wanted to stay in therapy because I think it helps me…so I guess you could say that I encourage myself because I see what good it does for me. (Angela, 15-year-old female)

9. Others Who Influence

Two 12 to 14 years old and one 15 to 17 years old identified the nurse practitioner as influential in their remaining on medication(s) and two 12-to-14-year-old participants identified their therapist as influential in them remaining in therapy. Mentors were identified as influential in the adolescent remaining in treatment by three 12 to 14 years old, and two 15 to 17 year-olds identified a relative who was influential on them remaining in treatment.

10. Definition of "Consent to Treatment"

Minor consent laws afford adolescents the right to seek and receive psychiatric mental health treatment without the permission of their parents. Given these adolescents have consented to medication therapy, psychotherapy, or both, exploring their understanding of consent to treatment is integral to understanding the decision-making process of adolescent consenting. Eleven participants (six 12 to 14 years old and five 15 to 17 years old) provided examples to explain their understanding of the minor consent laws.

"*You say you want to come to treatment.*" Of the eleven adolescents who provided a definition of "consent to treatment", five provided examples that paralleled the technical definition of "consent to treatment":

> *It's like you allow…you say that you want to go to treatment and you're willing to go.* (John, 17-year-old male)

> *That you say you want to come to treatment…that you say that you want to get help.* (Jill, 13-year-old female)

> *It's like you get, you say "okay", I will do it [receive treatment]…that it means I will do something or do it and I agree to it.* (Dave, 13-year-old male)

Two adolescents provided a definition of "consent to treatment" that was partly correct. Based on the current North Carolina minor consent law, the sections identified by italic bold are not accurate:

> *Well, it means that you have to be willing to have treatment, and no one can force you into doing anything…* **you have to have a parent or a guardian with you to sign the papers and everything**. (Barbara, 14-year-old female)

> *Consent to treatment, is, um, like not only, um, not only affirmative, but just kind of like an agreement to, um, carry out all the, all of the components, like, well, the ask, well the assent of* **the, um, minor is just kind of agreeing with the consent** [of the parent]. (Tim, 16-year-old male)

"*Somebody can make you take it.*" The responses of the remaining four participants who provided a definition of "consent to treatment" spoke of this concept in terms of what was required or expected of them related to continued treatment, or what services they might receive at the facility:

> *It means that like the doctor give you some medication and you have to take it…that you just do what they [doctor] tell you to do.* (Mack, 15-year-old male)

> *Consent mean [sic] that somebody can make you take it [medication]. But parent consent means parent permission.* (Elaine, 17-year-old female)

> *It means that I will get a mentor and sign up for anger management.* (Jill, 13-year-old female)

> *Consent to me means that I will accept it [medication and/or therapy], that I will take whatever they [treatment facility] give me without any problem, that I won't make a big deal about it or*

fight about it…that I will come and whatever they suggest, I will agree to, like if they think it's best to have you put on medication, I'll take it. (Lauren, 15-year-old female)

"*I do not know.*" When asked "what does *consent to treatment* mean to you?" five of the adolescent participants answered "I do not know." Further probes included "what does it mean to you when you agree to treatment?", or "what is involved in your agreeing to treatment?" These five respondents (three 12 to 14 years old and two 15 to17 years old) held to their original answer, "I do not know." It was clear from this response that these participants either did not understand the question, or the adolescent was not aware that there was some level of required agreement on their part in consenting to treatment.

As indicated by these examples, younger and older adolescents were equally represented among those who understood and those who did not understand the concept of "consent to treatment."

11. Evaluation of Minor Consent Laws

Adolescents were asked to describe their thoughts about a law that provides minors the right to consent to psychiatric mental health treatment without their parent's permission.

"*Kids should not be making those type of decisions.*" An overwhelming number of adolescent participants (*n* = 13) did not agree with a law that allows someone their age to consent to treatment without their parent's permission. The most common theme among these respondents (*n* = 11) was they did not possess the *confidence* in making healthcare decisions without their parent's input. In addition to lack of confidence, some adolescents (*n* = 5) discussed their opposition to the minor consent law solely on the *age* of the adolescent. For example, "older than 16 or 17" was a representative response among those who referred to age as a strict determinant of when a minor should be allowed to consent without their parent's required permission:

> *Some kids should not be making those type of decisions without their parent…they just donot know what to ask about and they may end up not asking about something or telling the doctor something that's important.* (Vivian, 16-year-old female)

> *Well, I think deciding about something like that should be a family thing…that's how we did it, so we decided as a family to do the treatment, to come here, so that's why I did it because it was a family thing.* (James, 12-year-old male)

> *I donot think anyone younger than fifteen could decide on that stuff without their parent, not no 12 year or 13 year-old, for sure. I donot even know about a fifteen year-old, if they could do it [decide on treatment without parent]. Cause they still donot know what's good for them at that age*

[fifteen], and then maybe there's some 12 year-olds who think they know a lot but they be having babies and stuff... they donot know nothing, but I think maybe 16 year-olds could, maybe, it just depends on what they have to decide, maybe therapy, but I sure donot know about medicine. (Elaine, 17-year-old female)

Our parents should let us pick what we want to be in, like group and stuff, but they (parents) should be, should know about my health, because they have to know about what's going on with me and my health, because if something goes bad and they do not know what's goin' on, then I could be in trouble. (Barbara, 14-year-old female)

Only one adolescent (17-year-old male) emphatically believed that adolescents should be allowed to consent to psychiatric mental health treatment without the required permission of parents, regardless of age, mental health diagnosis, or treatment involved. Two adolescents considered the *type of treatment* involved when expressing their perception of whether it was acceptable for an adolescent to consent to treatment without their parent's permission:

I think it's okay with some things, like therapy maybe, it's okay with if they decide on their own, but they may not be in the position to do it on their own, like when medicines involved, then they cannot, I cannot see how they decide on that, that's something more serious, taking medicine, and they then the parent should decide, that's what I think. (Elaine, 17-year-old female)

Like medicine obviously, I think the parent should be there when deciding on that. If it were up to me I would have never taken the medicine, and I'd probably still be failing every class, or I'd probably be dead if it were up to me to not do the treatment. (Lauren, 15-year-old female)

11.1. Voice in Treatment Decisions. Eleven adolescents (six 12 to 14 years old and five 15 to 17 years old) discussed that they should be allowed a voice in treatment decisions, but the inclusion of parents in the decision-making process was important to them:

I think that would be good [a law that allows her to decide on her own healthcare without her parent], that's kind of good, because I get to make my own decisions, but I think asking my mom would help out a lot...asking her about the treatment first before I do it, that would be helpful. (Jill, 13-year-old female)

You know, we should be able to make our own decisions about our healthcare, but we do need our parents...they can help us out with that kind of stuff. (Dave, 13-year-old male)

It would be okay to have something like that [a law that allows her to decide on her own healthcare without her parent] cause I like to make my own decisions, but I donot think I could make those decisions without my mom, like treatment stuff. (Jean, 12-year-old female)

Yeah, I like that idea [a law that allows her to decide on her own healthcare without her parents], yeah the child should have some rights, but the child ain't so smart she know everything that the parent know...the parent, they look into things a little bit more then their child do. (Vivian, 16-year-old female)

I think maybe the kid should have opinions in the situation, like, if the child really thinks that he doesnot need whatever, then they should consider that. But, if they really need it, therapy and stuff, if they think they do not need therapy and they have scars going all up and down their arm and they're threatening suicide, then obviously they need some help, so I think the parent should definitely be involved when it comes to that type of stuff, especially with the medicine stuff. (Lauren, 15-year-old female)

Further probing about inclusion of parents provided more detailed information about this aspect of consenting. One adolescent (17-year-old male) viewed requiring permission from the parent as unnecessary when it came to deciding on his psychiatric mental health treatment and that the input from his parents would most likely not make a difference in the decisions he made about treatment. One adolescent (12-year-old male) stated "I think it [treatment decisions] should be talked over with the kid and they decide about things with the parent." Three adolescents (two 12 to 14 years old and one 15 to 17 years old) argued that the reason the current minor consent law should not exist is that the parent should be the one who decides on healthcare treatment and that the minor is not capable of making such decisions. When the term "capable" or similar terms were used by the adolescent, they were further asked to explain their meaning of "capable". The adolescents described *capable* in terms of their inability to make decisions about issues that they had limited knowledge about, specifically related to choosing between different medications.

12. Discussion

The findings of this study suggest that younger and older adolescents are successful in completing the first two steps of the decision-making process (recognizing that a decision is required and understanding the goals). Adolescents in this study readily recognized that a decision from them about initial treatment and goals was necessary. However, it was typical for adolescents to complete the first two steps of the decision-making process in collaboration with their parents.

One consistent finding related to the first two steps of the decision-making process was that adolescents discussed the decisions they made and the desired goals of treatment in specific terms of their psychiatric mental health symptomatology, such as the desire to feel or act better now. For example, adolescents spoke of deciding on treatment and establishing short-term goals based on their desire to decrease sadness and tearfulness and increase their ability to focus and concentrate in school. Although, adolescents consistently made strong connections between what they were feeling or experiencing and the initial decisions made about treatment, the goals never moved beyond those of the short-term goals to feel better and act better. From a developmental perspective, this would be expected given that adolescents generally focus on the here and now when it comes to making decisions [4].

In relation to the first two steps of the decision-making process, the findings of this study are in contrast to what is observed in clinical settings [28]. In outpatient psychiatric mental health settings, younger adolescents seem to be less aware than older adolescents that a decision about treatment is needed. However, based on the findings of this study, younger and older adolescents equally recognize that decisions about their treatment are needed. One explanation for younger adolescents appearing to be less likely to recognize the requirement of a decision may be as simple as the clinician not consulting with the younger adolescent about this step, but with the parent instead. With older adolescents, clinicians may discuss initiation of treatment directly. However, when it comes to addressing the initial treatment decisions of the younger adolescent, the clinician may direct the discussion to the parents only, thus taking the younger adolescent out of the communication forum. This study provides greater insight into the ability of younger and older adolescents to recognize that treatment decisions are required, stating treatment goals, and verbalizing the details of these two decision-making steps in their own words.

Although younger and older adolescents readily identified the benefits of taking the medications and receiving psychotherapy, their ability to identify the risks and consequences related to these interventions was limited. The findings from this study are similar to researchers [7, 29] who examined risks identification of adolescents in healthcare situations. Adolescents in these studies did not readily identify risks of healthcare interventions, especially if the adolescent had not experienced previous side effects or adverse reactions to the intervention. From a cognitive developmental perspective, the expectation would be that younger adolescents would not think at a level other than immediate [4, 23]. Therefore, the findings of this study are in line with what others have reported in that younger adolescents experience difficulty in identifying the risks and consequences of treatment choices.

Identifying future consequences requires the adolescent to think in abstract terms, which is a defining characteristic of the formal operational stage of development [23]. Bloom [30] identifies six levels of learning. Within these levels, consideration is given to the concept of critical-thinking. It is important for the adolescent to develop critical-thinking skills in order to make decisions [23]. The development of critical thinking skills is dependent on the adolescent's ability to analyze, synthesize, and evaluate information [30]. For example, in the current study, in order to understand the future consequences of psychiatric mental health treatment choices and assimilate and integrate information about treatment options, the adolescent had to be able to analyze and synthesize the information presented. Based on the participants' ages (12 to 17 years old), it was expected that the older adolescents (15 to 17 year-olds) would respond more than younger adolescents (12 to 14 years old) to interview questions from a formal operational stage of development perspective, which includes the ability of the adolescents to synthesize and evaluate the initial treatment information presented to them [28].

Adolescents in this study did not recognize the future consequences of their treatment decisions. Most importantly, adolescents did not assimilate and integrate the information presented to them about their treatment options. These findings are similar to those of Lewis [29] and Urberg and Rosen [31] who reported that younger and older adolescents in their study were not capable of integrating information about the treatment interventions represented in their studies. The findings of this study are similar to the findings of others in that adolescents do not independently inquire about future implications of the treatment options. Further, adolescents in this study did not assimilate and integrate information unless this process was completed in collaboration with their parents. There was no evidence that adolescents in this study were functioning in the formal operational stage of development, nor were they using critical thinking skills (synthesis and evaluation) when it came to consenting to psychiatric mental health treatment.

13. Conclusions

In summary, findings of this study suggest that, unless completed in collaboration with their parents or legal guardians, 12-to-17-year-old adolescents do not identify consequences (step 3) and assimilate and integrate information (step 4) when it comes to deciding about psychiatric mental health treatments. These findings support the argument of those who oppose the expansion of the minor consent laws. However, the extraordinary experiences of adolescents gleaned from the current study provide support for those arguing in favor of minor consent laws. For example, the description of one particular adolescent's experiences reverberates. James is the 12-year-old male participant who was sexually molested by his mother and friends of his mother, for several years. James had a supportive and caring grandmother to disclose the details about the sexual abuse inflicted upon him. However, the possibility of James living with this abuse without a confidante is easily contemplated. Proponents of the current minor consent law would argue that James represents those for whom minor consent laws were intended. Specifically, proponents of minor consent laws would posit that adolescents like James benefit from these laws because they allow the adolescent to consent to psychiatric mental health treatment when it is the parent who is instigating the problem or substantially contributing to the adolescent's mental health issues. In the case of parental abuse, it is unlikely that the parent would agree to the adolescent receiving psychiatric mental health treatment. Current minor consent laws would allow the adolescent to seek treatment without the parent knowing, which is perhaps the only way that some adolescents would seek refuge when it is the behaviors of the parents that are contributing to their mental illness. The overall findings of this study support those who oppose the current minor consent laws. However, based on the experience of James, which is representative of many adolescents, the negative implications of changing this law cannot be overlooked.

Finally, the findings of this study indicate that knowledge and understanding of the minor consent laws by adolescents is significantly limited. Most adolescents in this study were not aware of an existing law that allows minors to consent to psychiatric mental health treatment without their parent's permission. Considering the findings of this study, there is a need for increased dialogue among adolescents, parents, healthcare professionals, and legislators related to this law. This dialogue should focus on three main topics. First, for clinical and legal reasons, societal awareness of minor consent laws should be increased. If increased awareness leads to more adolescents seeking treatment without their parents, then further research is warranted in order to thoroughly evaluate the outcomes of the law. Second, if further research supports the findings of this study, that adolescents make their best decisions in psychiatric mental health settings when collaborating with parents, then minor consent laws should be considered for amendment to better reflect the decision-making process and cognitive development of adolescents. Third, consideration should be given to the voice of the parents. Perhaps a change in the law would not only reflect any concerns expressed by parents, but also provide clear legal and clinical guidelines related to adolescents consenting to psychiatric mental health treatment.

References

[1] K. S. Berger, *The Developing Person Through the Life Span*, Worth, New York, NY, USA, 8th edition, 2012.

[2] L. M. Langer and G. J. Warheit, "The Pre-Adult Health Decision-Making Model: linking decision-making directedness/orientation to adolescent health-related attitudes and behaviors," *Adolescence*, vol. 27, no. 108, pp. 919–948, 1992.

[3] D. F. Bjorklund, "Piaget and the neo-piagetians," in *Children's Thinking: Cognitive Development and Individual Differences*, Thomson Wadsworth, 2005.

[4] J. W. Santrock, *Physical and Cognitive Development in Adolescence*, McGraw-Hill, Boston, Mass, USA, 13th edition, 2010.

[5] B. Ambuel and J. Rappaport, "Developmental trends in adolescents' psychological and legal competence to consent to abortion," *Law and Human Behavior*, vol. 16, no. 2, pp. 129–154, 1992.

[6] R. T. Bastien and H. S. Adelman, "Noncompulsory versus legally mandated placement, perceived choice, and response to treatment among adolescents," *Journal of Consulting and Clinical Psychology*, vol. 52, no. 2, pp. 171–179, 1984.

[7] N. Kaser-Boyd, H. S. Adelman, L. Taylor, and P. Nelson, "Children's understanding of risks and benefits of psychotherapy,"

Journal of Clinical Child Psychology, vol. 15, no. 2, pp. 165–171, 1986.

[8] A. M. La Greca, "Issues in adherence with pediatric regimens," *Journal of Pediatric Psychology*, vol. 15, no. 4, pp. 423–436, 1990.

[9] H. J. Emmerich, "The influence of parents and peers on choices made by adolescents," *Journal of Youth and Adolescence*, vol. 7, no. 2, pp. 175–180, 1978.

[10] C. G. Ortiz, *Teenage pregnancy: factors affecting the decision to carry or terminate pregnancy among Puerto Rican teenagers*, Doctoral dissertation, University of Massachusetts Amherst, Dissertation Abstracts International, 43, 2559, 1983.

[11] M. Poole, G. H. Cooney, and A. C. S. Cheong, "Adolescent perceptions of family cohesiveness, autonomy and independence in Australia and Singapore," *Journal of Comparative Family Studies*, vol. 17, no. 3, pp. 311–332, 1986.

[12] C. A. Ford and A. English, "Limiting confidentiality of adolescent health services: what are the risks?" *JAMA*, vol. 288, no. 6, pp. 752–753, 2002.

[13] A. English and K. E. Kenney, *State Minor Consent Laws: A Summary*, Center for Adolescent Health and the Law, Chapel Hill, NC, USA, 2nd edition, 2003.

[14] P. L. Munhall, "Ethical considerations and qualitative," in *Nursing Research: A Qualitative Perspective*, pp. 501–511, Jones and Bartlett, Boston, Mass, USA, 4th edition, 2007.

[15] American Psychiatric Association, "Domains of the clinical evaluation," in *Practice Guides for the Treatment of Psychiatric Disorders*, American Psychiatric, Arlington, Va, USA, 2006.

[16] J. M. Morse, "The semistructured questionnaire," in *Qualitative Health Research*, pp. 361–362, Sage, Thousand Oaks, Calif, USA, 1991.

[17] P. R. Ulin, E. T. Robinson, and E. E. Tolley, *Qualitative Methods in Public Health: A Field Guide for Applied Research*, Jossey-Bass, San Francisco, Calif, USA, 2005.

[18] R. R. Parse, "The qualitative descriptive method," in *Qualitative Inquiry: The Path of Sciencing*, Jones and Bartlett, Boston, Mass, USA, 2001.

[19] A. L. Strauss and J. M. Corbin, *Basics of Qualitative Research: Techniques and Procedures for Developing Grounded Theory*, Sage, Thousand Oaks, Calif, USA, 1998.

[20] N. K. Denzin and Y. S. Lincoln, *Handbook of Qualitative Research*, Sage, Thousand Oaks, Calif, USA, 2000.

[21] K. Krippendorff, *Content Analysis: An Introduction to Its Methodology*, Sage, Thousand Oaks, Calif, USA, 2004.

[22] M. Sandelowski, "Focus on research methods: whatever happened to qualitative description?" *Research in Nursing and Health*, vol. 23, no. 4, pp. 334–340, 2000.

[23] L. Rew, "Adolescent health and health-risk behaviors," in *Adolescent Health: A Multidisciplinary Approach to Theory, Research, and Intervention*, pp. 1–22, Sage, Thousand Oaks, Calif, USA, 2005.

[24] J. W. Creswell and D. L. Miller, "Determining validity in qualitative inquiry," *Theory into Practice*, vol. 39, no. 3, pp. 124–130, 2000.

[25] B. Fischhoff, N. A. Crowell, and M. Kipke, Eds., *Decision-Making. Board on Children, Youth, and Families Commission on Behavioral Social Science and Education National Research Council*, Institute of Medicine, National Academy Press, Washington, DC, USA, 1999.

[26] I. L. Janis and L. Mann, *Decision-Making: A Pscyhological Analysis of Conflict. Choice, and Commitment*, The Free Press, New York, NY, USA, 1977.

[27] L. Mann, R. Harmoni, and C. Power, "Adolescent decision-making: the development of competence," *Journal of Adolescence*, vol. 12, no. 3, pp. 265–278, 1989.

[28] E. D. Sturman, "The capacity to consent to treatment and research: a review of standardized assessment tools," *Clinical Psychology Review*, vol. 25, no. 7, pp. 954–974, 2005.

[29] C. C. Lewis, "How adolescents approach decisions: changes over grades seven to twelve and policy implications," *Child Development*, vol. 52, pp. 538–544, 1981.

[30] R. Bloom, *A Taxonomy of Educational Objectives: Handbook 1 Cognitive Domain*, David McKay, New York, NY, USA.

[31] K. A. Urberg and R. A. Rosen, "Age differences in adolescent decision-making: pregnancy resolution," *Journal of Adolescent Research*, vol. 2, no. 4, pp. 447–454, 1987.

16

Dealing with a Latent Danger: Parents Communicating with Their Children about Smoking

Sandra P. Small,[1] Kaysi Eastlick Kushner,[2] and Anne Neufeld[2]

[1] *School of Nursing, Memorial University of Newfoundland, St. John's, NL, Canada A1B 3V6*
[2] *Faculty of Nursing, University of Alberta, 11405 87 Avenue, Edmonton, AB, Canada T6G 1C9*

Correspondence should be addressed to Sandra P. Small, ssmall@mun.ca

Academic Editor: Sheila Payne

The purpose of this study was to understand parental approach to the topic of smoking with school-age preadolescent children. In-depth interviews were conducted with 38 parents and yielded a grounded theory that explains how parents communicated with their children about smoking. Parents perceived smoking to be a latent danger for their children. To deter smoking from occurring they verbally interacted with their children on the topic and took action by having a no-smoking rule. There were three interaction approaches, which differed by style and method of interaction. Most parents interacted by discussing smoking with their children. They intentionally took advantage of opportunities. Some interacted by telling their children about the health effects of smoking and their opposition to it. They responded on the spur-of-the-moment if their attention was drawn to the issue by external cues. A few interacted by acknowledging to their children the negative effects of smoking. They responded only when their children brought it up. The parents' intent for the no-smoking rule, which pertained mainly to their homes and vehicles, was to protect their children from second-hand smoke and limit exposure to smoking. The theory can be used by nurses to guide interventions with parents about youth smoking prevention.

1. Introduction

Tobacco use continues to be the leading cause of preventable morbidity and mortality in many countries and has been described as a global epidemic [1]. Smoking is most commonly tried and established in adolescence [2]. Tobacco dependence typically occurs in the early years of use, even at low levels of smoking [3, 4] and is considered a childhood condition [1]. Early age of smoking initiation is associated with heavy smoking over time [2]. Further, smoking during youth is associated with subsequent alcohol and illicit drug use during youth and for that reason it has been referred to as the gateway drug. The developing brain may be particularly susceptible to addiction, which makes primary prevention of smoking in youth all the more important [2, 5].

Despite a decline in some countries in recent years, youth smoking remains a major public health concern in many countries world-wide [6]. Within Canada cigarette smoking among adolescents aged 15 to 19 is at 14% [7]. Among younger children, ages 11 to 14 years, 22% have at least tried a cigarette [8]. Typically, smoking rates are based on cigarette use. Unfortunately, that tells only part of the story as many youths world-wide smoke other forms of tobacco, for example, little cigars and pipes [6, 8, 9].

Research efforts in the area of youth smoking primarily have focused on adolescents with the main emphasis being on identifying factors that influence them to smoke. Numerous studies have been carried out and a large number of correlates and predictors of the behavior have been identified, which may be broadly classified as social, psychological, personality, developmental, and genetic factors. One type of social influence that has been studied extensively is parental influence. Many parental characteristics and behaviors have been examined including smoking status, sociodemographic factors (e.g., education, income, and marital status), beliefs about smoking, attitude toward smoking, disciplinary measures for the child, rules restricting child exposure to smoking, and discussion with the child concerning smoking.

However, an area that needs more research attention concerns parental communication with their children about the topic of smoking. In studies that have been carried out, generally the focus was narrow (e.g., whether discussion occurred or there were antismoking rules, or a particular aspect of communication such as frequency of discussion) and a comprehensive examination to gain an in-depth understanding was not taken. The studies largely were about communicating with adolescent or late preadolescent children and many were from the children's, not the parents', perspectives. Inconsistencies in findings make it difficult to draw conclusions about particulars of parental smoking-specific communication. No studies were found about parental smoking-specific communication with young school-age children. As well, a theory was not found that addresses parental communication with children about smoking.

Increasingly, it has been acknowledged that interventions to curb smoking should be broad, taking into account the varied influences [1, 10]. Yet, little has been done to engage parents in prevention efforts; for the most part, programs are not available to parents that would promote youth smoking prevention and media campaigns tend to be directed to youth themselves rather than to parents. Because adolescence is the key period for smoking initiation, to have an impact on prevention parents would need to take measures before the adolescent years. An important first step is to determine the approach parents typically take with their children before they become adolescents. The purpose of this study, therefore, was to understand from parents' perspectives their approach to the topic of smoking with their school-age preadolescent children.

2. Method

We chose grounded theory method as it is suited to studying an area for which little is known or findings are unclear and gaining an in-depth understanding of a phenomenon through theory development [11, 12].

2.1. Sample. The study was approved by affiliated university ethics boards and written informed consent was obtained from the participants. The study took place in a city in eastern Canada. The participants were recruited through three means: (a) study information brochures sent home to parents through elementary schools; (b) study brochures and posters displayed in community centers, and (c) the snowball technique, whereby study participants identified other potential participants. Prospective participants were told that the purpose of the study was to learn about the approaches that parents take with their children about the topic of smoking. The purposive sample was comprised of 28 mothers and 10 fathers, including 6 mother-father pairs. The parents had at least one child 5 to 12 years of age (i.e., kindergarten to grade 6), with the majority (60%) having 2 or 3 children in that age range. There was about an equal number of boys and girls in the referent children. See Table 1 for a description of the sample characteristics.

TABLE 1: Parent characteristics.

Characteristics		n^a
Marital status	Single	10
	Spouse or partner	28
Household income^b (Canadian dollars)	Low (< $29,000)	12
	Middle ($30,000–$89,000)	13
	High (> $90,000)	12
Education	Less than high school	5
	High school graduate	3
	Some university or college	13
	University or college graduate	17
Occupation	Professional	12
	Services, sales	5
	Skilled trades	6
	Stay-at-home mother	10
	Unemployed, disabled, student	5
Smoking status	Current smoker	9
	Mother	5
	Father	4
	Former smoker	17
	Mother	11
	Father	6
	Never smoker	12
	Mother	12
	Father	0

Note. $^a N = 38$.
^{b} Missing data for one parent.

2.2. Data Collection and Analysis. Consistent with grounded theory method, data collection and beginning analysis occurred concurrently. Interviews were carried out with the parents to encourage them to discuss their thoughts and feelings about youth smoking and smoking prevention and how they approach the topic with their children. Broad open-ended questions were employed such as "Would you tell me about your thoughts on children smoking?" "What are your thoughts on factors that influence children to smoke? "How has the topic of smoking come up?" "Can you think of a specific time when your child mentioned smoking or asked questions about it? Would you describe the situation for me?" "What do you find helpful to you (hinders you) in addressing the topic of smoking with your children?" "What are your thoughts on barriers to preventing smoking among children?" Parents' responses were probed for details. The interviews ranged in length from 30 to 60 minutes. Four parents who were interviewed early in the study were interviewed a second time to expand upon points in the first interviews. The interviews were held in private, and when both parents in a family participated in the study, they were interviewed separately. All interviews were conducted by the first author. They were digitally-recorded and then transcribed verbatim to form the text for analysis. After each interview, the interviewer recorded journal notes about her impressions of the interview and any questions that needed to be raised in future interviews, particular observations of the participant, thoughts about the data, and feelings the interview provoked personally. Those insights were used to guide subsequent data collection and inform analysis.

The analysis was carried out primarily by the first author with team meetings to discuss findings and finalize the analysis. The procedure for constructing theory from the parent data was based on the approach of Strauss and Corbin [12] and involved coding and theoretical sampling. Coding consisted of three integrated steps. In the first step, open coding was used to identify concepts in the data and their properties and dimensions. Incidents were compared through constant comparison analysis for similarities and differences both within and across interviews. Incidents that were conceptually similar were grouped and labeled using *in vivo* codes, as possible, or substantively derived codes. In the second step, axial coding and the coding paradigm were used to link category with category and category with subcategory. This coding yielded the different types of interaction and the action the parents took with their children concerning smoking, the conditions that influenced their action and interaction, and the outcomes for them as a consequence of their action and interaction. In the third step, selective coding was used to integrate and refine categories and abstract a central category to form an explanatory whole. Throughout the coding process, memos were written to facilitate data analysis. Diagrams were created to help sort out relationships among the categories and culminated in Figure 1, the theoretical model.

Theoretical sampling was used during data collection and analysis to achieve theoretical saturation. As concepts and relationships were identified in the data, those analytic leads were followed up with subsequent study participants. Previous interviews also were reviewed to consider whether there was any fit of new categories with previously identified categories. Theoretical sampling was conducted and data were collected until there was replication, no new information was arising during coding, and variation was accounted for.

3. Results

The results represent a substantive theory that explains how parents communicated with their children about smoking. The central category *dealing with a latent danger: parents communicating with their children about smoking* represents the problem for the parents and their response to it (see Figure 1). The problem was that although their children were not smoking at that point in time, the possibility was there for them to begin in the future. As one parent said "you're dealing with a threat that's not immediate" (OA) (participants are identified by fictitious acronyms for multiword quotations). Although some parents thought of it as a more remote possibility because of their children's negative reaction to smoking, they had misgivings and a lingering uncertainty.

I would be surprised. That would be my initial reaction to it because right now she has a real

aversion to smoke.... I don't think that at this point... she would definitely not do [it]. Now like when she's a teenager it's going to be a different... you just don't know. (AM)

Other parents thought that the possibility of their children beginning to smoke was more likely.

Yes, I would be hurt but I wouldn't be surprised knowing that children are children and they're going to try different things.... You can't be like an ostrich and put your head in the sand.... You'll just be fooling yourself because then you're going to find out they're smoking, right, or found cigarettes in their pocket...[You] know because you did it yourself. (FU)

This story illustrates the source of a mother's doubt.

When she was about 6 or 7 she said, "When I get older I'm going to smoke" and I looked at her and said, "[Daughter], it's not good. It can do a lot of damage to your lungs." I said, "It can give you cancer." I said, "It's not a good habit to have." "But," she said, "daddy does smoking." I said, "Yea, but daddy tells you everyday how he feels towards smoking. It's just a nasty habit." And, he tells them that he don't like smoking, right. But, it's just a habit that.... And I said to her, "Why would you [say that]?" "I don't know," she said, "mom." She said, "Just wondering what it would be like if I smoked when I got older." I'm like, "It's not a good habit."... Now that she's 8, she says it is yucky. But, I mean, there's always a doubt in my mind. Is she going to smoke when she gets older? (CR)

Hence, the meaning that parents applied to youth smoking relative to their children is that it is a latent danger. That meaning was shaped by their knowledge of the serious health effects of smoking and by their knowledge of youth smoking. Their response was to deter the behavior from materializing by communicating with their children, which involved verbally interacting with them on the subject and taking action in the form of having a no-smoking rule. Their verbal interaction and action produced outcomes for them in the form of feelings and thoughts.

3.1. Parental Verbal Interaction. Parents verbally interacted with their children about smoking through using one of three approaches: (a) discussing smoking with their children by intentionally taking advantage of opportunities, (b) telling their children about the health effects of smoking and their opposition to it by responding on the spur-of-the-moment if their attention was drawn to the issue by external cues, or (c) acknowledging to their children the negative effects of smoking by responding only when their children brought it up (see Figure 1). Each approach is composed of interaction style, which refers to the manner in which the parents interacted with their children, and interaction method, which refers to what the parents did to interact with their children. The styles and associated methods reflect differences in the quality and extent of the parents' interaction. Each approach also is marked by underlying properties that reflect the purpose, timing, and intensity of the interaction and the character of the message conveyed. These reveal differences and similarities among approaches and within-category variation within approach. It is difficult to tell whether smoking status or any specific sociodemographic factor, including the sex of the referent children, was associated with a particular verbal interaction approach. However, there seemed to be a pattern of relatively fewer smoking parents, and more mothers, more parents who had a spouse or partner, and more parents with any of higher household income, education, and occupational status located in the category *discussing smoking with their children by intentionally taking advantage of opportunities* than in the other two categories.

3.1.1. Discussing Smoking with Their Children: Intentionally Taking Advantage of Opportunities. The majority of parents (22 of 38) interacted verbally with their children about smoking by discussing smoking with them, which reflects an open communication style. They encouraged their children to talk about smoking, engaged them in discussion, and participated with them in a two-way exchange of ideas. Their method was to take advantage of everyday ordinary opportunities. "It's utilizing whatever comes up at the time.... Every now and then something triggers it and we talk about it." (AM) The discussions occurred "naturally" but were deliberate and "purposeful" nonetheless. "I look for a kind of teachable moment. I don't just say, okay, we're going to talk about smoking today and go from there." (JV) Those parents had thought about it beforehand and had conscious intent to talk with their children about smoking.

Purpose. The purpose of the parents' interaction was to clarify or validate their children's understanding of smoking, give information about smoking, and reinforce the antismoking message.

Timing. Opportunities to discuss smoking occurred either from the parents noticing something themselves while with their children, such as seeing someone smoking, or from their children noticing something and making comments or asking questions about smoking.

> We just look for the opportunities. If there's an ad on TV, we'll pick up on that or if we're driving in the car, if there is an ad on the radio about not smoking then we'll, I'll pick up on that and just chat about it a bit. (EQ)

In families where a parent smoked the topic came up often mainly because the child noticed and asked questions as to why the parent smoked or made negative comments about it. A mother, who smoked and whose husband also smoked, talked about her children's reaction, which gave her no choice but to discuss it. They would say things such as

> "You don't need to be smoking anyway. That stuff will kill you."... and then they're talking about, "[I] can smell it off you, Mom. Go brush your teeth."... The kids, they don't like it at all. They hate the fact that we smoke and they really get down on us.... Where I smoke I feel like I have to let the kids know what is going on with me. It is part of my life and it's part of their life so we have no other choice but to discuss it. (YK)

Intensity. Parents started talking with their children before school-age. They believed that when children are old enough to grasp messages about health and "start asking questions about [smoking] then they're old enough to probably understand a little bit about it." (JV) Some parents were sure to "take advantage of every opportunity" (IU) to convey an antismoking message. Other parents raised the topic more periodically, "not all the time but enough that it stays in their [children's] mind." (AM) However, parents acknowledged that they needed to be careful to not "force" the issue or "harp" on it. It is important not to make the topic so common that it loses its effect, to have the "right balance" between raising it enough but not too much.

Message. The parents' emphasis in discussing smoking was on health effects including effects that were directly relevant to their children's personal situation such as effect on asthma and sports activity. They also tended to discuss other issues such as environmental tobacco smoke (ETS), the unacceptability of "pretend" smoking, and factors that influence people to smoke including, for current and some former smokers, their own addiction. Those parents thought that sharing their experience was a good teaching strategy. Other former smokers had not told their children they had smoked and were unsure whether they would for fear of it being a negative influence.

Although the parents gave an "honest" health message based on facts, some who formerly smoked or never smoked stressed the importance of using an "age-appropriate," "progressive" approach. They took into account developmental level and tried to give a message that they thought the child would understand at his or her age. They used general messages about health and avoided talking specifically about cancer and death and giving graphic messages.

> I wouldn't introduce pictures or anything like you see sometimes on the back of cigarette packages.... Sometimes you'll see a picture of someone's mouth. It's been eaten away by cancer, or a set of lungs from a smoker or something.... I wouldn't want to shock them with horrible pictures. (JY)

They thought that detailed and explicit messages about health consequences were more appropriate for children who were nearing or at adolescence; that is, once they are better able to understand disease, risk, probability, and long-term outcomes. Those parents were particularly mindful of what they said to their children if the other parent or a close relative such as a grandparent smoked as they didn't want to cause the children to become scared or worried. As the mother of young school-age children said

> I'm not going to talk to my children about that, especially with their father smoking. You don't really want to let them know that he might die from this.... They'd still get the message... it smells bad and it doesn't look very nice and it'll make you sick, even though their father is a smoker, being exposed to seeing him smoke. I still think they need that negative message... so I still give them everything negative that they can understand at their age about smoking. (IX)

Other parents, regardless of smoking status, were less cautious in their approach. They always gave a strong, frank message to their children, even preschool children. They thought that children need and should not be protected from the blatant facts about smoking and that young children can understand about serious consequences. Where possible, those parents used real-life situations to show the serious health effects of smoking, for example, the illness or death of a grandparent. A mother conveyed that her father had died of lung cancer when her son was five years old and that she told him at the time why her father had died.

> We have been very up front in having discussions with him to let him know that poppy smoked for a long period of time.... and what smoking does and that smoking causes lung cancer and that the result of lung cancer is that in all likelihood you will die. And we have not kept that from him.... I want him to know that smoking does a lot of damage to your body, that ultimately it could kill you and I think that's the important message because I think that's the truth of it, and it's important for him and kids generally to know the truth about smoking. (EQ)

Parents who had relatives who smoked and the parents who smoked themselves recognized that such messages can cause children to worry. However, they thought that, regardless of any emotional impact, it still was important for their children to know about the serious health effects. As one mother who smoked said "we discussed that smoking is not good for you and this [serious effects] is what happens. I've showed him the pictures on the cigarette packages and the nasty teeth and explained stuff to him." (TI) For children who indicated that they might be troubled by the facts, parents tried to reassure them by explaining that while smoking is always harmful not every person who smokes ends up with serious disease or dies because of it and serious effects happen later in life. The parents who smoked tried to further comfort their children by indicating that they were fine and wanted to quit and would continue trying. A mother explained how she dealt with the situation when her son saw a television commercial of a smoker who had a tracheotomy and asked her

> "Like mommy, could that happen to you?" I couldn't say, no. When they ask you questions like that, what do you say cause you can't say no and I just said to him, "No, please God, mommy won't

> be smoking by then. Please God that won't happen to mommy." Cause what can you say to them.... I just said, "No, hopefully mommy will never have to go through that."(TI)

3.1.2. Telling Their Children about the Health Effects of Smoking and Their Opposition to It: Responding on the Spur-of-the-Moment If Their Attention Was Drawn to the Issue by External Cues. Some parents (9 of 38) interacted verbally with their children about smoking by telling them their thoughts about it, which reflects a directive style of communication. They did not engage their children in conversation about smoking as such. Their method was to comment about smoking if their "attention" was drawn to it by some smoking-specific external cue. For instance, a father said "if a commercial comes on TV about smoking and if they're [the children] doing something, I get their attention, "Look at that, look at that, pay attention", right." (AP) Their comments tended to be random and in the moment. "We don't have one specific time, one specific moment. It's just at that particular time and moment when it pops up." (TH) Although parents' comments were goal-driven, that is, meant to deter smoking, their overall approach was not deliberately planned. It was spur-of-moment and is likened to a hit-or-miss approach.

Purpose. The purpose of the parents' interaction was to inform their children of the health effects of smoking and ensure they knew that the parents were opposed to it in an effort to persuade them not to smoke, "to make sure they do not get involved with it." (NC)

Timing. The parents remarked about smoking when prompted by such cues as a question or comment about smoking from their children, exposure to smoking, and smoking-attributable illness in the family. As one father revealed, he had not said anything about smoking to his children before their grandfather had become ill with lung cancer and died because of it.

Intensity. The topic of smoking had first come up with their children before the children were school-age. Most parents had commented about smoking only occasionally over time and those parents tended to be moderate in their approach. Others varied in the frequency with which they "reiterated" their message about smoking, from occasionally to often, but they tended to be hardline in their approach. As one father said "I'm not going to sit there every day and tell them don't you smoke today.... But if the topic does come up, well I give [them] more than a mouthful." (AP)

Message. The parents who had a moderate approach kept information about the health effects simple such as "it can make you sick." (GV) Those parents thought that their children, who ranged from early to middle school-age, were too young to understand the serious health consequences and they would give a stronger message about the health effects when their children were older. Parents who were hardline in their approach told their children about the serious health consequences of smoking. They did not differentiate their message based on the child's age but believed that children should receive the strongest message regardless of age so "they'll listen and they'll remember." (AP) They wanted their children to know the "real reality of it" (AP) and believed that fear was good for them. They used examples of family members, where possible.

> *I had an aunt that died with lung cancer and I told them it had to do with smoking and I had an uncle that had to have his throat sliced on both sides and opened because of throat cancer and I told them that it all had to do with smoking.... And like your arteries are blocking and like that's what I explain to my 9 year old and she understands it. (NC)*

To send a strong message, those parents made firm, unequivocal statements such as "smoking kills." A father said that he wanted his children to have the "message" that

> *It'll kill them.... Not it'll make you sick, not it'll make you unpopular... just it'll kill you. You will die from this soon. I don't like the idea that you can say that someday this'll probably make you sick.... It [cancer] will kill you if you get it. This will give it to you. No sense of correlation. An absolute sense of causation. (OA)*

Parents who had smoked or who were currently smoking also had commented on their own smoking in an effort to reinforce the health message.

Regardless of the strength of their health message, parents voiced their opposition to smoking by making sure their children knew that they were against the behavior or that they expected them not to smoke. The smoking parents realized they were not being good role models and wanted their children to get the message "do not do as I do, do as I say." (GV)

> *Well, basically, like he knows it's wrong. I know it's wrong.... Just because daddy does it, doesn't make it right. Just because daddy does it all the time, everyday whatever, you know, it's not right.... It's just the way I guess that they were raised. Since day one, it was put in their head that smoking is wrong even though I do it. Just because I do it doesn't make it right. It's wrong. (DS)*

Hard-line parents gave their children warnings that smoking would not be tolerated or told them of the punitive consequences they would get if ever caught smoking.

> *I tell them, "You better not go smoking anyway cause I'll come get you. I'll find you." So, if they goes having a smoke they're looking around the corner to see if I'm there cause I got that put in their head.... I just put it there and keep it there in a good way, you know, there's no harm, right. I tell them they'll get everything out of their room, all of their toys, the TVs, everything, gone.... And we always check their clothes. (AP)*

3.1.3. Acknowledging to Their Children the Negative Effects of Smoking: Responding Only When Their Children Brought It Up. For a small group of parents (6 of 38), their verbal interaction with their children about smoking consisted of acknowledging to them the negative effects of the behavior. These parents had a nonassertive style of interacting with their children in that they did not raise the topic or enter into a conversation with them. As one mother of an 11-year-old daughter said "I just have not really had a conversation about that yet." (HW) Rather, the parents simply confirmed the children's understanding of smoking. Their method was to comment only when their children brought it to their attention. For instance, one mother said that the topic had come up with her daughter only since grade 6 and it was the daughter who had raised it. Although these parents believed that in order to prevent smoking it is important for children to be informed, they did not take on an active role themselves. Their responses were routine rather than considered.

Purpose. Up to that point in their children's development, the parents had not given much consideration to smoking as an issue that needed their attention. However, they did not want their children to smoke, so their responses to them were to convey the message that smoking is not good for you or that it is harmful to health and that "no one should smoke." (KZ)

Timing. The parents' interaction with their children about smoking was dependent on the children bringing it up. They simply responded to questions or comments the children made when they were provoked by such things as having done something in school about smoking or having seen antismoking signage or someone smoking. As one mother who was referring to her five year old said "I've never approached it.... He's had a few questions about what it is and so I've responded to his questions. I've never actually said anything just outright about it." (LA)

Intensity. The parents had not initiated discussion with their children about smoking so there was no intensity on their part. However, some children had noticed and had asked about smoking before they were school-age, whereas others had not commented until they were older. Similarly, some of the children had raised the topic only occasionally; others had raised it often.

Message. The parents let their children know that they were correct about the negative attributes of smoking, but they did not offer extra detail or explanation about the behavior or explicit information about the health effects.

> *I assure him that he's right, like, "Hey, you're right, you're not allowed smoking around here."... Most of the times, after he points out that there's a no smoking sign, he'll say, "Smoking is bad for you" and I'm like, "You're right, smoking is very bad for you."(KZ)*

The parents who smoked invariably had been confronted by their children about it in such ways as pointing out the discrepancy between what the parents were saying and doing and urging them to quit. "I try to tell them, when it comes up, that it's not good. It will make you sick. Of course they shoot back and say, "Well why do you smoke?"... and give me grief for smoking." (WI) A mother said that her son had told her "that I should quit and he doesn't want me to smoke and it's bad for me and he wants me to be around to take care of him." (QF) The parents tried to appease their children by indicating that they knew they should not smoke or suggesting that they would like to or intended to quit. "I put them off and say, "Daddy's going to quit soon. One of these days Daddy's going to throw them down.".... My famous escape is "soon.".... It's easy to brush it off and carry on to the next conversation." (WI)

3.1.4. Conditions for Parental Verbal Interaction. Whether because of direct personal experience as a smoker or former smoker, knowledge as a result of having relatives or friends who smoked, or knowledge acquired more generally, parents knew that smoking causes serious illnesses and is a serious addiction and knew about youth smoking (see Figure 1). Many of the parents had family members or friends who had smoking-related illness or who had died as a consequence of such illnesses. Parents who formerly or currently smoked had experienced or were experiencing respiratory symptoms and had firsthand knowledge of addiction.

> *I know what smoking does to you and how hard it is to quit. Like I'm after trying umpteen times.... I just cannot quit. I'm after trying the patch and the gum... but I just become so irritable that I actually find it hard to be a good mom when I don't smoke. But when I get out and have that cigarette, I come in and I can clean up my house. I can play with my children, read stories.... Once you get that craving it's just the worst thing in the world.... I just can't help myself. I just get the shakes and I just start crying and I just get really emotional and just got to have a cigarette. (YK)*

They especially knew how easy it is to start smoking and how quickly one becomes addicted. The parents' knowledge of the health consequences of smoking was the main reason for their verbal interaction. Because of the health effects the parents did not want their children to smoke.

The parents had good knowledge of the nature of youth smoking and factors that influence children to smoke, which heightened their awareness of the vulnerability of children to smoking and gave them increased reason for their interaction. Although they thought that youth smoking was less common than when they were growing up, they believed that many youths still take up the behavior as they regularly saw them smoking. They knew that it more commonly occurs in adolescence but younger children also might try or even start smoking. Commenting about how young he was when he started smoking, a father said "I think I got caught smoking Camel cigarettes when I was 9 years old." (AP) Some parents had seen smoking among preadolescents, even

currently. Parents believed that children may begin to smoke for reasons such as exposure to other youths who smoke, role models who smoke (e.g., parents, siblings, and popular idols), and prosmoking messages in society (visibility of smoking and tobacco products) and relatively easy access to tobacco products. However, smoking by peers and family members generally was recognized as the most important. Many of the parents could relate personally to peer pressure because they had experienced it themselves when they were growing up. "It put you in a higher bracket like as in being cool around the school." (XJ) Similarly, many of the parents who formerly or currently smoked could relate personally to the negative influence of family members, especially their own parents, who smoked. Some thought that their parents' smoking had been the "root" cause of their own smoking. Smoking parents acknowledged that their smoking was a negative influence for their own children.

> *Growing up for me, I saw my parents smoke, figured it was okay, so I tried. Then I got hooked, been smoking ever since basically. But definitely parents play a humungous role in how their kids react and what their kids do. If they see their parents... smoking... obviously they're going to think it's okay and they're going to try it. If mom and dad can do it, why can't I, basically. (DS)*

Whereas their knowledge influenced the parents to verbally interact with their children about the topic of smoking, the saliency of the issue for them and their belief concerning communicating with children about smoking influenced the particular verbal interaction approach they took (see Figure 1). For some parents, their knowledge about the serious health consequences of smoking caused them strong emotions, such as deep concern or worry, sadness, and guilt, which kept smoking foremost in their minds or as one father said "top of mind." (JY) Because smoking was so present in their consciousness or salient for them, when opportunities arose, and in an effort to deter the behavior, they intentionally took advantage and discussed the behavior with their children to ensure that they were well informed. The parents' emotions were evoked for any of several personal experiences: (a) being exposed to the health risks as a smoker or former smoker, regardless of whether there was any evidence of ill effects; (b) having a close family member who smoked and was at risk for illness, had serious illness, or had died from such illness; (c) having a child who had asthma, which could be worsened by smoking; and (d) having negative parental role modeling in the family because they or the other parent smoked.

> *I think it makes me more desperate... to try to get that message across than it would if I wasn't a smoker cause I'd probably just tell them stuff. And it'd be like ... that's nasty, blah, blah, blah. I think as a smoker, it's almost like I know if they grow up and they smoke I'm going to feel like I failed and I'm going to have guilt. So, I think like that's a big thing, is trying to avoid that whole thing by making sure they don't smoke. (TI)*

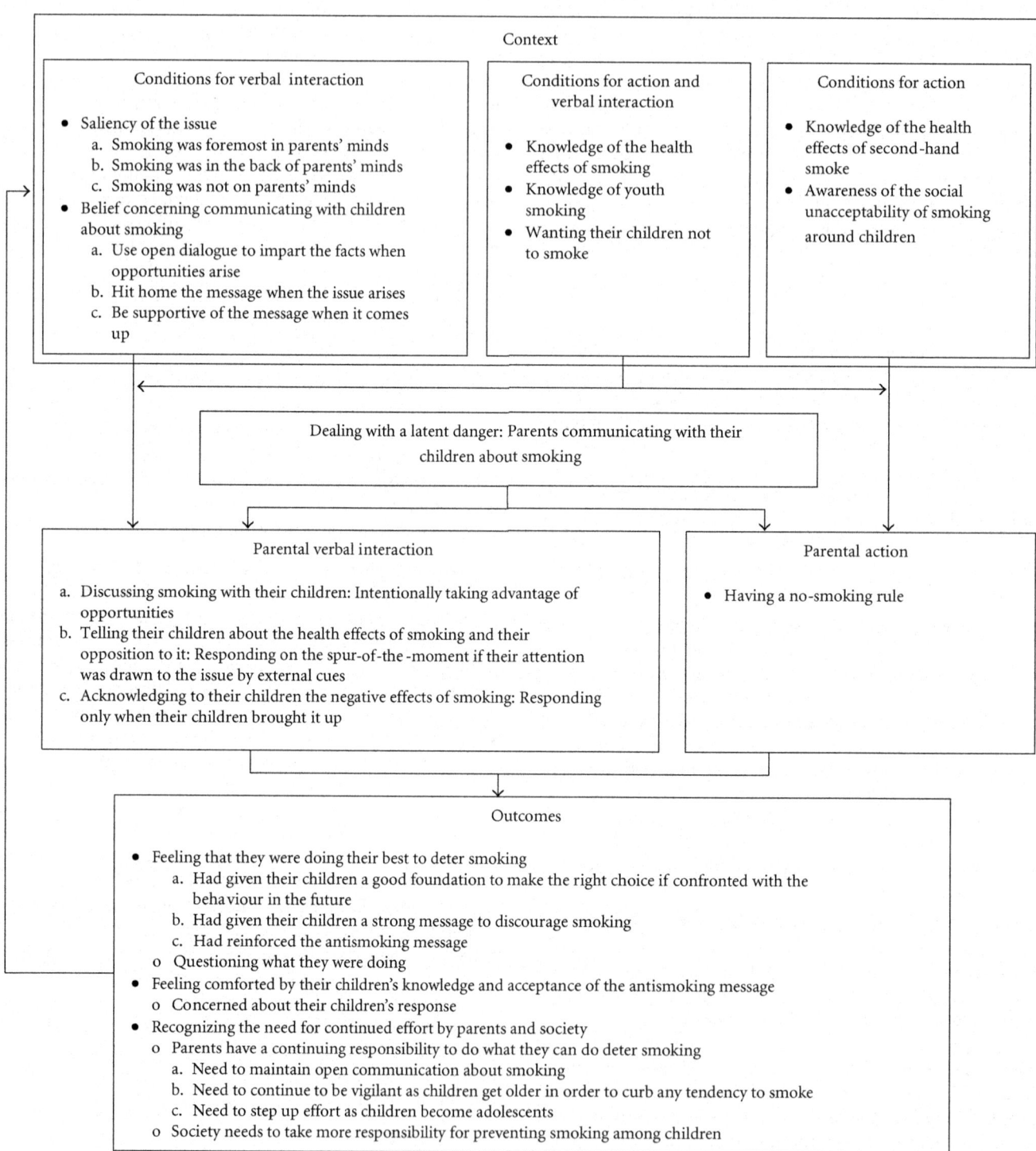

FIGURE 1: A theoretical model of the process that parents used in communicating with their children about smoking. Verbal interaction and action were influenced by conditions and resulted in outcomes for the parents. The outcomes fed back and contributed to the context for the parents' continuing action and interaction to deal with the latent danger. Note. The letters for conditions and outcomes correspond with the respective letters for the verbal interaction approaches and indicate variation according to the particular interaction approach.

For other parents smoking was in the back of their minds rather than being foremost. Their response was not emotional but was matter-of-fact, a gut reaction that smoking is "horrible," "disgusting," and "atrocious by far ... [so just] don't do it." (DS) Those parents told their children about the health effects of smoking and their opposition to it if their attention was drawn to the issue by external cues. There also were parents for whom smoking was not on their minds. Although they did not condone smoking, they also did not respond emotionally to it. Their response was more neutral as reflected in the view that "I think everybody knows the cons of it, the health [effects]." (WI) Their approach was to acknowledge the negative effects of smoking by responding only when their children brought it up.

A similar pattern of variation in verbal interaction was noted for parental belief regarding communicating with children about smoking. Some parents believed it is important to use "open dialogue" to impart the facts when "opportunities" arise. Those parents discussed smoking with their children by intentionally taking advantage of opportunities. Their thoughts were that parents should be "honest... objective, non-punitive, and non-judgmental when discussing smoking." (LX) Talking to children about smoking is about "equipping [them] to deal with things [rather than simply telling them] don't smoke. [It should not be] the Ten Commandments." (RG) Open dialogue is the foundation for a positive relationship between children and their parents, increasing the chances that children will talk to their parents and accept the antismoking message in the long run. Parents believed that taking advantage of ordinary opportunities is a good strategy for initiating discussion with children about smoking and allows smoking education to be carried out in an ongoing manner throughout childhood.

Other parents believed it is important to "hit home" the message that smoking is "harmful" and "unacceptable" when the issue arises. They believed that smoking is an issue to which parents need to pay attention and address from time to time as well as on an as needed basis, that is, when the risk increases, such as with adolescence, or smoking actually materializes. Those parents told their children about the health effects of smoking and their opposition to it by responding on the spur-of-the-moment if their attention was drawn to the issue by external cues.

Yet, other parents believed there was no need for them to do anything more at the time except be supportive of the antismoking message when it came up because their children already had received information about smoking through social sources, especially school. The approach of those parents was to acknowledge to their children the negative effects of smoking by responding only when their children brought it up. Parents of young school-age children thought that young children need only simple messages and their children had received those. They thought that detailed and explicit messaging is more appropriate for older children. Parents of older school-age children thought their children were very well informed about smoking. "It's already being talked about. What more do you do if it's after being talked about." (HW)

3.2. Parental Action. The main intent of the parents' no-smoking rule (see Figure 1) was to protect their children from ETS but they also wanted to limit exposure of their children to smoking behavior. The rule was consistent with and lent support to the message they conveyed through their verbal interaction that smoking is unhealthy. Although the strictness of the rule varied among parents from stringent to less stringent, there did not appear to be a pattern in stringency according to smoking status, sociodemographic characteristics, or particular verbal interaction approach. The parents who had a stringent rule held strong views against exposure to ETS and smoking. They were strongly opposed to smoking in public places that were visible and accessible to children, had a total ban on smoking in their homes and vehicles, and made a point of not exposing their children to ETS and smoking in places outside their homes, including the homes of relatives.

> We won't even go to like activities that the family has if people are going to be smoking and everybody knows that.... [Grandparents] go outside now, like, on account of the kids cause they know that I'm totally against it and I wouldn't bring them [the children] if I knew they were smoking in the house. I'm that against it. (BQ)

They believed that a strict no-smoking rule demonstrates that it is not an "acceptable" behavior. The smoking parents always smoked outside and tried to do so inconspicuously so as to not draw their children's attention to it.

> First and foremost it's not allowed in my home. If I want to have one, like I said, snow, rain, whatever, I will go on outside and do my business.... I do go out by the door but I mean I don't announce and say, I'm going out to have a cigarette now. I kind of sneak out and do my thing and kind of sneak back in. I try to not let her even see me do it if I can. Like she knows that I do [smoke].... If somebody asked her if I did she wouldn't say no but can she say [I] see her do it all the time? She'd definitely have to say no there. (GV)

The parents who had a less stringent rule tended not to require total avoidance of tobacco smoke and smoking. For instance, some had only partial restrictions on smoking in that they prohibited smoking in their homes and vehicles when their children were present but otherwise allowed it. Although parents who smoked did so outside when their children were home, they did not take extra precautions to conceal from their children what they were doing. They tended not to make an issue of environmental exposure beyond the societal measures that already were in place and tended not to be rigid about exposure in relatives' homes. Former and never-smokers in that group had a less stringent rule to accommodate a spouse or other relatives who smoked.

3.2.1. Conditions for Parental Action. Parents, to one extent or another, knew that ETS can affect health. That knowledge was the main impetus for their no-smoking rule. In commenting on his rationale for smoking outside, a father said "it's bad enough that I'm polluting my lungs. Why would I want to pollute my child's." (DS) Parents also knew that smoking in the presence of children had become "socially unacceptable" and not smoking around children was the societal expectation. Although more directly related to their verbal interaction, their knowledge of the health effects of smoking, their knowledge of youth smoking, and wanting their children not to smoke influenced them to have a no-smoking rule to limit exposure of their children to the behavior, hence, reducing what they thought was a risk factor for youth smoking (see Figure 1).

3.3. Outcomes. Although there was variation that corresponded with the verbal interaction approach they had taken, parents felt that they were doing their "best" to deter smoking (see Figure 1). However, despite that feeling, a few parents, regardless of the approach they had taken with their children and their smoking status, questioned in their own minds what they were doing; if it was the most appropriate. They wondered about such things as whether their antismoking message was too strong or not strong enough, they talked about smoking too much or not enough, and they gave enough detail or not enough detail for the child's age.

> *They are well versed in what I have chosen to give them.... But whether it's the right thing, I don't know. What is the appropriate thing to tell any child about smoking... I'm a parent, I'm doing the best I can and I have no idea if it's right or wrong. (OA)*

Similar to the other parents in this study, those parents had not sought or used any particular smoking prevention resources in their efforts to deter their children from smoking. Like the other parents, they were guided by their knowledge about smoking and belief concerning communicating with children about the behavior. However, they acknowledged that they could benefit from having more information on youth smoking, prevention strategies, and communication with children about smoking and thought that a resource they could use with their children would be helpful.

In addition to feeling they were doing their best, parents also were feeling comforted by their belief that their children had knowledge of and accepted the antismoking message (see Figure 1). At the very least, the children knew that smoking is unhealthy and can make people sick and some knew about the serious illnesses and that smoking can cause death. The children demonstrated acceptance of the antismoking message through various reactions. However, some held stronger antismoking views than did others. Those children not only were "receptive" to the message but had "internalized" it. They were quite knowledgeable about smoking and could "make a very strong case for not smoking" (ZL) based on the health facts, were ardently opposed to it, made negative comments when they saw someone smoking, went out of their way to avoid tobacco smoke, expressed concern about relatives who smoked and wanted to encourage them to quit or actually tried by telling them about the dangers of smoking, and demonstrated

antismoking assertiveness with family members. They were tuned in to the issue perhaps even more so than were their parents.

> *He tells all of us... stuff like, "You'll get cancer. You're going to get cancer."... He'd read the cigarette packages and he'd read the labeling on it and he'd say... "Cigarettes cause lung cancer. Why are you smoking if it causes lung cancer? Why would you do that?" And he knew stuff. He'll say that to us, you know. "This is what's going to happen to your teeth. This is what's going to happen to your lungs." So, I'm hoping that he remembers that when he gets a teenager and someone passes him a cigarette. (TI)*

Some of the parents of those children, although pleased that their children were antismoking, had concern about their children's response. All were parents whose approach was to discuss smoking with their children by intentionally taking advantage of opportunities. Their children were inclined to inappropriately tell others, even strangers, that they should not smoke or to think negatively of people who smoked such as they are "bad." As a consequence the parents felt they had to be careful about the message they conveyed in order to temper their children's reaction and had to correct any unintended misperception about smokers.

> *My little boy will get so worked up that I have to stop him from marching up to other people and telling them not to smoke.... That's one of the reasons why I don't want to come on as strong as I do because I don't want him to get up on a soapbox and start. (RG)*

Although feeling they were doing their best and feeling comforted by their children's knowledge and acceptance of the message, parents recognized the need for continued effort. They knew that because of the nature of youth smoking and influencing factors, especially at adolescence, smoking was possible for their children and at some level wondered whether they would stay smoke-free when they were older. "And generally I'm wondering if they just toe the line. "Yes, mommy I'll never smoke" and they might." (PB) Hence, they thought that because of the continuing threat that might become more pronounced at adolescence, parents have an important continuing "responsibility" to do what they can to deter smoking. However, what they thought they would need to do varied with their overall approach (see Figure 1).

> *Say from 10 years old to say 18, 19 years old, if you can save them [in] that period of time like when the peer pressure is there all that, [if] you can save them from that, I think you're pretty well in the clear then. I do, right. And that's your responsibility because from the age of 10 to 18 they're your responsibility anyway. So do what you can, I guess. (AP)*

Parents also thought that because they can do only so much society needs to take more responsibility for preventing smoking among children (see Figure 1) and that children might be more inclined to accept a message that is received through different sources. Although generally pleased with societal efforts in recent years to curb smoking, parents thought that regulations should be further strengthened to reduce access by children to tobacco and to reduce public exposure of children to the behavior. However, the area parents thought would produce the greatest impact is with respect to smoking prevention education. When they were growing up there was little emphasis on smoking prevention in society generally. For many, aside from perhaps being told or warned not to smoke, their own parents had not raised the subject or talked with them about it. Parents believed that a lack of education about the health consequences was a main cause of the high rate of smoking in the past. They thought that "education is the best tool" (ET) for prevention. They recognized that there had been more smoking prevention education in recent years, but many thought that it was not enough. Although some parents thought that schools had good smoking prevention education, many thought that little was being carried out, especially in the early grades. They thought that smoking should be covered early and often in the school curriculum.

> I think that school is really important. They need to hear the message in school as well and they need to hear it not just once a year. It needs to come up on a fairly regular basis as part of the health program or whatever and I think it needs to start in kindergarten and repeat the message regularly and loudly every year. (BN)

Some wanted more done at the community level and identified children and parents as key targets. They thought there was little in the way of smoking prevention advertisements and that television advertisements against smoking were a particularly good way to get the message across to children. They suggested that antismoking messages be produced for young children, even preschool children, and conveyed through children's television programming. Although comfortable with what they were doing themselves, consistent with the parents who had questioned their own approach, some parents were of the view that there needs to be an ongoing prevention initiative to increase parent awareness of youth smoking, inform them about the important role they can play in smoking prevention, and guide their approach. They thought there are parents who do not address smoking with their children and suggested that smoking prevention education materials be readily available to parents through such venues as schools and health clinics.

3.4. The Context for Parental Continuing Verbal Interaction and Action. The parents' feelings and thoughts as a consequence of their verbal interaction and action were not endpoints but dynamic internal processes. Although some parents were uncertain about the appropriateness of the verbal interaction approach they had taken with their children and some were concerned about their children's strong reaction to the antismoking message, in general, parents felt they were doing their best to deter smoking and felt comforted by their children's knowledge and acceptance of the message. However, they recognized the need for continued effort and thought that parents have an ongoing responsibility to deter the behavior. Those feelings and thoughts gave them reason to continue their effort and as such contributed to the ongoing context for their continuing interaction and action to deal with the latent danger (see Figure 1).

3.5. A Negative Case. There was one parent in this study whose approach did not fit with the theory. He was a former smoker who had quit smoking before becoming a parent and his daughter was a late preadolescent. Similar to other parents in the study, this father had knowledge of smoking and factors that contribute to youth smoking and did not want his daughter to smoke. However, he had never raised the topic or discussed smoking with her or said anything at all about it to her as he thought there was no need to do so. He thought that his daughter had learned about smoking in school and had good knowledge of the health effects of smoking. Further, she demonstrated a negative attitude toward the behavior. Therefore, he believed she would never smoke; hence, not a latent danger, and he did not interact with her about it. For those reasons, the approach of that parent is considered a negative case. "I don't talk to her about it. She knows the dangers and that, right. I don't think she'll ever smoke.... Not the way she acts now like [about] people smoking and that.... I can't imagine her smoking." (BC)

4. Discussion

Although they differed in what they had done, parents in this study had communicated in some manner with their children about smoking. No studies were found in the literature concerning younger children, but similar to the parents in this study, there is evidence that many parents at least raised the topic of smoking with their late preadolescent or adolescent children (e.g., [13–16]). It is difficult to tell from most studies how much parents talked with their children and the type and extent of content. However, similar to some of the parents in this study, it was noted in other studies that parents did not talk often about smoking with their adolescent children [17, 18]. Like many of the parents in this study, it seems that the main focus of any communication about smoking was on health effects, although expectations or warnings not to smoke, financial cost, and peer pressure were addressed in some cases [19–22].

The majority of parents interacted with their children by discussing smoking with them, which reflected an open style and they believed that communication with children should be an open dialogue. Their style fits with what has been characterized as good quality communication and which has such attributes as attentive, responsive, acceptant, open (back-and-forth), meaningful, honest, nonjudgmental, nonpunitive, and relaxed. That type of communication is effective for positive child outcomes. Communication that is characterized by such attributes as one-sidedness, superficial, strained, conflictual, controlling, judgmental, or punitive does not facilitate positive child outcomes [23–25]. The overall approach of the parents who discussed smoking with their children also closely matches recommendations by authorities in the field of smoking prevention [26–28]. This includes their open style, method of taking advantage of opportunities, deliberateness, early initiation of discussion, and comprehensive message addressing health and influencing factors.

Two areas in which parents who discussed smoking with their children varied in their approach are with respect to age-appropriate messaging and discussion of their former smoking. Some parents took into account their children's developmental level and tried to give age-appropriate messages, whereas others gave a strong message about serious health effects irrespective of their children's age. It is recommended in the literature that parents take a developmental approach to discussing smoking with their children [27, 28]. However, there does not appear to be any hard-and-fast rule about what to discuss with children at particular ages. It is suggested that since children mature at different rates and since parents know their children best, they may have a better sense of what is appropriate at different ages for their own children. Similarly, some formerly smoking parents had talked with their children about their past addiction; whereas, others were uncertain as to whether they would. There does not appear to be a specific recommendation in the literature about whether parents who formerly smoked should raise and discuss with their children their past experience with smoking. However, it is argued that parents who smoke should talk with their children about their experience [27], which is consistent with what the smoking parents in this study had done.

In addition to verbal interaction with their children, parents in this study had a no-smoking rule albeit, for some parents, their rule was not strict. It is well accepted that ETS is harmful to health [29] and that exposure to smoking is a risk factor for youth smoking because of modeling and because it engenders a perception of acceptability [30–32]. Consequently, and consistent with the measures of the parents in this study who had a stringent rule, it is recommended that homes and vehicles should be completely smoke-free and parents who smoke should not do so in the presence of their children [26, 27, 33]. Whereas in the past it commonly was the case that parents did not have any restrictions on smoking in their homes [34–36], consistent with the findings in this study, many parents now at least have partial restrictions with the majority having a total ban [8, 13, 33, 37, 38].

5. Implications for Practice, Theory, and Research

It is generally accepted that parents are a potentially powerful influence on children's decisions to smoke and have an important role to play in smoking prevention [27, 39].

Consistent with that view, parents in this study recognized the need for parental intervention to deter children from smoking. Although different in style and method of interaction, many parents had taken it upon themselves to address smoking with their children and all had a no-smoking rule. Parents across the three verbal interaction approaches thought that they had a continuing responsibility to do what they could to deter smoking as their children get older. The parents had knowledge about the health effects of smoking, the nature of youth smoking, and factors that influence youth to smoke that is consistent with what is known about smoking. However, although parents felt they were doing their best to discourage smoking, some wondered whether what they were doing was the most appropriate and they thought that they could benefit from having more information on the matter. Similarly, although parents were feeling comforted by their children's knowledge and acceptance of the antismoking message, some were concerned about their children's strong reaction.

Nurses are encouraged to work with parents through an empowerment model whereby parents' strengths and efforts are acknowledged and fostered and they are supported to participate in smoking prevention social policy [40, 41]. Those whose approach is consistent with recommendations in the literature need to be encouraged to continue their interventions with their children and offered reassurance about their approach. Parents need to know that children might react strongly to messages about smoking and be offered guidance on how to address it. Those whose approach differs from recommendations should be offered guidance on how to address the topic with their children to build on and enhance their efforts. Appropriate educational resources to assist parents need to be made available to them. There is evidence to support such interventions. Parents have suggested that interventions for parents about alcohol, tobacco, and other drugs should focus on practical information concerning how to successfully talk with children, how to raise the topic, and what to talk about, rather than on factual information about specific drugs [42]. Interventions with parents that promoted their involvement in prevention efforts concerning smoking resulted in more discussion with their children [43–46]. As suggested by the parents in this study and endorsed by smoking prevention advocates in the field, youth smoking prevention requires a multifaceted approach which involves the efforts of parents, schools, and society at large [1, 10, 26, 47]. Some parents thought there needs to be more smoking prevention education for children both in school and at the larger community level. Parents also thought that regulations concerning access to tobacco and exposure to the behavior need to be strengthened. Nurses are encouraged to partner with parents to enable their active engagement in smoking prevention advocacy. Because they *want their children not to smoke*, parents could be a strong force for supportive public policy.

The theory generated from this study is about parental communication with children who are younger than adolescence. Because adolescence is a high risk period for initiation of smoking, parents might have a different approach with their adolescent children than with younger children. Indeed, some parents in this study indicated that they would give more detail or a stronger message to older children or would need to change their approach (i.e., step up their effort as their children become adolescents). Hence, research needs to be carried out with parents of adolescent children to determine whether and how approaches to the topic of smoking change with adolescent children. That knowledge may then be used to extend the theory derived in this study or generate another substantive theory to explain the phenomenon for that age group. Smoking is one of a number of risk behaviors in which adolescents engage. Others include drinking alcohol, using illicit drugs, and having unsafe sex [9, 48]. There is a need for a formal theory that explains how parents address with their children risk behaviors in general in an effort to prevent them.

There was one parent in this study whose approach did not fit the substantive theory. Although not invalidating the theory, that case draws attention to another approach parents might take with their children about smoking, *not addressing the topic of smoking at all*. All the parents in this study were self-selected for participation. Hence, it is conceivable that there are other parents whose approach aligns with that case. It also is conceivable that there are other parental approaches to the topic of smoking that were not identified by this study. For instance, there might be parents whose behaviour indicates approval of smoking. There is evidence in the literature that some parents engaged in prompting behaviors, such as asking their children to bring them cigarettes, which actually could facilitate their children towards smoking [49, 50]. In future studies on parental communication with children about smoking it is important to explore for other parental approaches that might exist. Such findings could be used to further develop this substantive theory. However, little is known about the effectiveness of parental communication for smoking prevention. Research to establish the effectiveness of parental approaches to the topic of smoking could further inform health promotion practice.

This study was about parental approaches to the topic of smoking from the perspective of parents. In studies of adolescent children, there is evidence they have different perceptions of their parents' communication than do their parents [14, 51–53]. Further, there is evidence of differences between mothers and fathers and adolescent girls and boys in perceptions of parent-child communication [54]. In future studies it would be important to examine children's perspectives about their parents' approaches to the topic of smoking and their receptivity to parental messages. Parenting children about smoking happens within the context of the family with interactions occurring among parents and children. Research using a family approach, involving parents and children, could lead to further understanding of the complexity involved. Observation as a source of data would provide important information about parent-child communication and would be useful to validating findings of this study. There was diversity among the parents in this study in terms of socio-demographic factors and smoking status, and there were boys and girls in the referent group of children. However, it was not possible to determine whether any such parent or child characteristics influenced parental approaches. Many of the parents had a high educational level and there were few fathers relative to mothers and few smoking parents relative to nonsmoking parents. There is a paucity of information in the literature on parent and child characteristics that influence parental smoking-specific communication. Research needs to be carried out to further examine those characteristics and to explore for other potential influences such as parenting styles. Findings could be used to elaborate the conditions component of the theory.

6. Conclusion

This theory contributes new knowledge about parents' communication with their children concerning smoking. Notwithstanding the need for more research in this area, the understanding gained from the theory can be used by nurses in their interventions with parents about youth smoking.

Conflicts of Interest

The authors declare no conflicts of interest with respect to this study or paper.

Acknowledgments

The authors acknowledge receipt of funding for this study from the Canadian Respiratory Health Professionals through the Canadian Lung Association and the Association of Registered Nurses of Newfoundland and Labrador.

References

[1] World Health Organization, *WHO Report on the Global Tobacco Epidemic 2011: Warning about the Dangers of Tobacco*, Geneva, Switzerland, 2011.

[2] U. S. Department of Health and Human Services, How TobaccoSmoke Causes Disease: The Biology and Behavioral Basis for Smoking-Attributable Disease—A Report of the Surgeon General, Atlanta, Ga, USA, 2010, http://www. surgeongeneral.gov/library/tobaccosmoke/reports/full_report.pdf.

[3] J. R. DiFranza, J. A. Savageau, N. A. Rigotti et al., "Development of symptoms of tobacco dependence in youths: 30 month follow up data from the DANDY study," *Tobacco Control*, vol. 11, no. 3, pp. 228–235, 2002.

[4] J. R. DiFranza, J. A. Savageau, K. Fletcher et al., "Symptoms of tobacco dependence after brief intermittent use: the development and assessment of nicotine dependence in youth-2 study," *Archives of Pediatrics and Adolescent Medicine*, vol. 161, no. 7, pp. 704–710, 2007.

[5] The National Center on Addiction and Substance Abuse (CASA) at Columbia University, Tobacco: The Smoking Gun, New York, NY, USA, 2007, http://www.casacolumbia.org/absolutenm/templates/PressReleases.aspx?articleid=508&zoneid=65.

[6] C. W. Warren, S. Asma, J. Lee, V. Lea, and J. Mackay, Global Tobacco Surveillance System: The GTSS Atlas, CDC Foundation, Atlanta, Ga, USA, 2009, http://www.cdc.gov/tobacco/global/gtss/tobacco_atlas/pdfs/tobacco_atlas.pdf.

[7] Health Canada, Health Concerns: CTUMS 2010 Wave 1 Survey Results, 2011, http://www.hc-sc.gc.ca/hc-ps/tobac-tabac/research-recherche/stat/_ctums-esutc_2010/w-p-1_sum-som-eng.php.

[8] Health Canada, Health Concerns: Summary of Results of the 2008-09 Youth Smoking Survey, 2010, http://www.hc-sc.gc.ca/hc-ps/tobac-tabac/research-recherche/stat/_survey-sondage_2008-2009/result-eng.php.

[9] Health Canada, Health Concerns: Canadian Tobacco Use Monitoring Survey (CTUMS) 2009—Summary of Annual Results for 2009, 2010, http://www.hc-sc.gc.ca/hc-ps/tobac-tabac/research-recherche/stat/_ctums-esutc_2009/ann_summary-sommaire-eng.php.

[10] Centers for Disease Control and Prevention, *Best Practices for Comprehensive Tobacco Control Programs—2007*, U.S. Department of Health and Human Services, Centers for Disease Control and Prevention, National Center for Chronic Disease Prevention and Health Promotion, Office on Smoking and Health, Atlanta, Ga, USA, 2007.

[11] J. Corbin and A. Strauss, *Basics of Qualitative Research 3e: Techniques and Procedures for Developing Grounded Theory*, Sage, Los Angeles, Calif, USA, 2008.

[12] A. Strauss and J. Corbin, *Basics of Qualitative Research: Techniques and Procedures for Developing Grounded Theory*, Sage, Thousand Oaks, Calif, USA, 2nd edition, 1998.

[13] J. L. Muilenburg and J. S. Legge, "Investigating adolescents' sources of information concerning tobacco and the resulting impact on attitudes toward public policy," *Journal of Cancer Education*, vol. 24, no. 2, pp. 148–153, 2009.

[14] L. A. Baxter, C. L. Bylund, R. Imes, and T. Routsong, "Parent-child perceptions of parental behavioural control through rule-setting for risky health choices during adolescence," *Journal of Family Communication*, vol. 9, pp. 251–271, 2009.

[15] T. Bush, S. J. Curry, J. Hollis et al., "Preteen attitudes about smoking and parental factors associated with favorable attitudes," *American Journal of Health Promotion*, vol. 19, no. 6, pp. 410–417, 2005.

[16] J. Wyman, J. H. Price, T. R. Jordan, J. A. Dake, and S. K. Telljohann, "Parents' perceptions of the role of schools in tobacco use prevention and cessation for youth," *Journal of Community Health*, vol. 31, no. 3, pp. 225–248, 2006.

[17] R. N. H. de Leeuw, R. H. J. Scholte, Z. Harakeh, J. F. J. van Leeuwe, and R. C. M. E. Engels, "Parental smoking-specific communication, adolescents' smoking behavior and friendship selection," *Journal of Youth and Adolescence*, vol. 37, no. 10, pp. 1229–1241, 2008.

[18] S. K. Riesch, L. Bush, C. J. Nelson et al., "Topics of conflict between parents and young adolescents," *Journal of the Society of Pediatric Nurses*, vol. 5, no. 1, pp. 27–40, 2000.

[19] S. T. Ennett, K. E. Bauman, V. A. Foshee, M. Pemberton, and K. A. Hicks, "Parent-child communication about adolescent tobacco and alcohol use: what do parents say and does it affect youth behavior?" *Journal of Marriage and Family*, vol. 63, no. 1, pp. 48–62, 2001.

[20] M. A. Miller-Day, "Parent-adolescent communication about alcohol, tobacco, and other drug use," *Journal of Adolescent Research*, vol. 17, no. 6, pp. 604–616, 2002.

[21] L. Throckmorton-Belzer, V. L. Tyc, L. A. Robinson, J. L. Klosky, S. Lensing, and A. K. Booth, "Anti-smoking communication to preadolescents with and without a cancer

[22] M. von Bothmer and B. Fridlund, "Promoting a tobacco-free generation: who is responsible for what?" *Journal of Clinical Nursing*, vol. 10, no. 6, pp. 784–792, 2001.

[23] M. D. Dixon, "Models and perspectives of parent-child communication," in *Parents, Children & Communication: Frontiers of Theory and Research*, T. J. Socha and G. Stamp, Eds., pp. 43–61, Lawrence Erlbaum, Hillsdale, NJ, USA, 1995.

[24] S. Jackson, J. Bijstra, L. Oostra, and H. Bosma, "Adolescents' perceptions of communication with parents relative to specific aspects of relationships with parents and personal development," *Journal of Adolescence*, vol. 21, no. 3, pp. 305–322, 1998.

[25] A. L. Robin, "Communication between parent and adolescent," in *Comprehensive Adolescent Health Care*, S. B. Friedman, M. Fisher, and S. K. Schonberg, Eds., pp. 643–648, Quality Medical Publishing, St. Louis, Mo, USA, 1992.

[26] American Academy of Pediatrics, "Policy statement-tobacco use: a pediatric disease," *Pediatrics*, vol. 124, pp. 1474–1487, 2009.

[27] Health Canada, "Help your child stay smoke-free: a guide to protecting your child against tobacco use," Catalogue no. H128-1/07-498E, Minister of Health, Ottawa, Canada, 2008.

[28] U.S. Department of Health and Human Services, For Parents: What Parents Can Do, 2009, http://www.womenshealth.gov/quit-smoking/parents/.

[29] U. S. Department of Health and Human Services, *The Health Consequences of Involuntary Exposure to Tobacco Smoke: A Report of the Surgeon General*, U.S. Department of Health and Human Services, Centers for Disease Control and Prevention, National Center for Chronic Disease Prevention and Health Promotion, Office on Smoking and Health, Atlanta, Ga, USA, 2006.

[30] N. L. Alesci, J. L. Forster, and T. Blaine, "Smoking visibility, perceived acceptability, and frequency in various locations among youth and adults," *Preventive Medicine*, vol. 36, no. 3, pp. 272–281, 2003.

[31] K. K. Corbett, "Susceptibility of youth to tobacco: a social ecological framework for prevention," *Respiration Physiology*, vol. 128, no. 1, pp. 103–118, 2001.

[32] L. Turner, R. Mermelstein, and B. Flay, "Individual and contextual influences on adolescent smoking," *Annals of the New York Academy of Sciences*, vol. 1021, pp. 175–197, 2004.

[33] S. U. Rainio and A. H. Rimpelä, "Home smoking bans in Finland and the association with child smoking," *European Journal of Public Health*, vol. 18, no. 3, pp. 306–311, 2008.

[34] L. Biener, D. Cullen, Z. X. Di, and S. K. Hammond, "Household smoking restrictions and adolescents' exposure to environmental tobacco smoke," *Preventive Medicine*, vol. 26, no. 3, pp. 358–363, 1997.

[35] P. I. Clark, A. Scarisbrick-Hauser, S. P. Gautam, and S. J. Wirk, "Anti-tobacco socialization in homes of African-American and white parents, and smoking and nonsmoking parents," *Journal of Adolescent Health*, vol. 24, no. 5, pp. 329–339, 1999.

[36] Health Canada, Health Concerns: Canadian Tobacco Use Monitoring Survey (CTUMS) 2000, 2007, http://www.hc-sc.gc.ca/hc-ps/tobac-tabac/research-recherche/stat/_ctums-esutc_2000/yanosc-vesfcc-eng.php.

[37] H. J. Binns, J. O'Neil, I. Benuck, and A. J. Ariza, "Influences on parents' decisions for home and automobile smoking bans in households with smokers," *Patient*

Education and Counseling, vol. 74, no. 2, pp. 272–276, 2009.

[38] M. C. Kegler, C. Escoffery, A. Groff, S. Butler, and A. Foreman, "A qualitative study of how families decide to adopt household smoking restrictions," *Family and Community Health*, vol. 30, no. 4, pp. 328–341, 2007.

[39] Centers for Disease Control and Prevention, Parents— Help Keep Your Kids Tobacco-Free, 2010, http://www.cdc.gov/tobacco/youth/information_sheet/index.htm.

[40] C. H. Gibson, "The process of empowerment in mothers of chronically ill children," *Journal of advanced nursing*, vol. 21, no. 6, pp. 1201–1210, 1995.

[41] D. D. Perkins and M. A. Zimmerman, "Empowerment theory, research, and application," *American Journal of Community Psychology*, vol. 23, no. 5, pp. 569–579, 1995.

[42] S. E. Beatty and D. S. Cross, "Investigating parental preferences regarding the development and implementation of a parent-directed drug-related educational intervention: an exploratory study," *Drug and Alcohol Review*, vol. 25, no. 4, pp. 333–342, 2006.

[43] S. E. Beatty, D. S. Cross, and T. M. Shaw, "The impact of a parent-directed intervention on parent-child communication about tobacco and alcohol," *Drug and Alcohol Review*, vol. 27, no. 6, pp. 591–601, 2008.

[44] C. Jackson and D. Dickinson, "Can parents who smoke socialise their children against smoking? Results from the Smoke-free Kids intervention trial," *Tobacco Control*, vol. 12, no. 1, pp. 52–59, 2003.

[45] E. M. Mahabee-Gittens, B. Huang, G. B. Slap, and J. S. Gordon, "An emergency department intervention to increase parent-child tobacco communication: a pilot study," *Journal of Child and Adolescent Substance Abuse*, vol. 17, no. 2, pp. 71–83, 2008.

[46] E. C. Tilson, C. M. McBride, and R. N. Brouwer, "Formative development of an intervention to stop family tobacco use: the parents and children talking (PACT) intervention," *Journal of Health Communication*, vol. 10, no. 6, pp. 491–508, 2005.

[47] Centers for Disease Control and Prevention, "Reducing tobacco use: a report of the surgeon general," *Morbidity and Mortality Weekly Report*, vol. 49, no. 16, pp. 1–27, 2000.

[48] M. Rotermann, "Trends in teen sexual behaviour and condom use," *Health Reports*, vol. 19, no. 3, pp. 53–57, 2008.

[49] C. Jackson, "Initial and experimental stages of tobacco and alcohol use during late childhood: relation to peer, parent, and personal risk factors," *Addictive Behaviors*, vol. 22, no. 5, pp. 685–698, 1997.

[50] R. Laniado-Laborín, J. I. Candelaria, A. Villaseñor, S. I. Woodruff, and J. F. Sallis, "Concordance between parental and children's reports of parental smoking prompts," *Chest*, vol. 125, no. 2, pp. 429–434, 2004.

[51] H. L. Barnes and D. H. Olson, "Parent-adolescent communication and the circumplex model," *Child Development*, vol. 56, pp. 438–447, 1985.

[52] Z. Harakeh, R. H. J. Scholte, H. de Vries, and R. C. M. E. Engels, "Parental rules and communication: their association with adolescent smoking," *Addiction*, vol. 100, no. 6, pp. 862–870, 2005.

[53] D. F. Herbert and K. M. Schiaffino, "Adolescents' smoking behavior and attitudes: the influence of mothers' smoking communication, behavior and attitudes," *Journal of Applied Developmental Psychology*, vol. 28, no. 2, pp. 103–114, 2007.

[54] R. Rosnati, R. Iafrate, and E. Scabini, "Parent-adolescent communication in foster, inter-country adoptive, and biological Italian families: gender and generational differences," *International Journal of Psychology*, vol. 42, no. 1, pp. 36–45, 2007.

17

Pregnancy-Related Lumbopelvic Pain: Listening to Australian Women

Heather Pierce,[1] Caroline S. E. Homer,[2] Hannah G. Dahlen,[3] and Jenny King[4]

[1] Faculty of Nursing, Midwifery and Health, University of Technology, Sydney, P.O. Box 123, Broadway, NSW 2007, Australia
[2] Centre for Midwifery, Child and Family Health, Faculty of Nursing, Midwifery and Health, University of Technology, Sydney, P.O. Box 123, Broadway, NSW 2007, Australia
[3] Family and Community Health Research Group, School of Nursing and Midwifery, University of Western Sydney, Locked Bag 1797 Penrith, NSW 2751, Australia
[4] Pelvic Floor Unit, Department of Women's and Children's Health, Westmead Hospital, P.O. Box 533, Wentworthville, NSW 2145, Australia

Correspondence should be addressed to Heather Pierce, aqwhaphysio@optusnet.com.au

Academic Editor: Ciara Hughes

Objective. To investigate the prevalence and nature of lumbo-pelvic pain (LPP), that is experienced by women in the lumbar and/or sacro-iliac area and/or symphysis pubis during pregnancy. *Design.* Cross-sectional, descriptive study. *Setting.* An Australian public hospital antenatal clinic. Sample population: Women in their third trimester of pregnancy. *Method.* Women were recruited to the study as they presented for their antenatal appointment. A survey collected demographic data and was used to self report LPP. A pain diagram differentiated low back, pelvic girdle or combined pain. Closed and open ended questions explored the experiences of the women. *Main Outcome Measures.* The Visual Analogue Scale and the Oswestry Disability Index (Version 2.1a). *Results.* There was a high prevalence of self reported LPP during the pregnancy (71%). An association was found between the reporting of LPP, multiparity, and a previous history of LPP. The mean intensity score for usual pain was 6/10 and four out of five women reported disability associated with the condition. Most women (71%) had reported their symptoms to their maternity carer however only a small proportion of these women received intervention. *Conclusion.* LPP is a potentially significant health issue during pregnancy.

1. Introduction

During pregnancy there are many discomforts experienced by women. The effects of these discomforts on the lifestyles of women are usually minor and self-limiting. Musculoskeletal complaints such as lumbopelvic pain (LPP) are described as "minor discomforts" [1, 2] or "unpleasant symptoms" [3]; however women may suffer considerable levels of pain and disability, with social and economic consequences [4]. Analgesic medications and mobility aids can be required, and life threatening conditions such as venous thrombosis have been reported as a complication of immobility [5]. LPP can impact sick leave, influence psychological health, and become a chronic pain condition [4, 6]. An increasing number of women are requesting an early induction of labour or an elective caesarean in order to achieve relief from their pain [7].

There are limited obstetric guidelines for the diagnosis and management of LPP during pregnancy. The Antenatal Care Guidelines from the National Collaborating Centre for Women's and Children's Health [8] refer to the conditions of "backache" and "symphysis pubis dysfunction" during pregnancy and recommend that more research is needed on the safety and efficacy of management strategies [9]. Over the last decade, systematic reviews [7, 10–12] have sought to bring clarification to the understanding of the conditions, and the publication of European guidelines [13] has added further to this knowledge [13]. These guidelines recommend that pelvic girdle pain (PGP) during pregnancy is a specific form of low back pain (LBP), with risk factors of a previous history of LBP and previous trauma to the pelvis. PGP can be diagnosed by pain provocation tests [14], and the recommended treatment includes adequate information, reassurance [15], and individualised exercises [16, 17].

Limited guidelines for pregnancy-related LPP may be attributable to the belief that the condition is not a serious health risk to the mother or fetus. It could also be argued that acknowledgement of pregnancy-related LPP as a pain condition creates pathology of a process that is "normal" in pregnancy, perhaps reinforcing pain catastrophising behaviour and fear avoidance beliefs [18, 19]. Guidelines for the management of nonspecific LBP in the general population emphasize that acute and chronic LBP should be viewed not just as pathoanatomical conditions, with mechanical or injury-based causes, but as conditions with psychosocial influences and consequences [20, 21]. The attitudes and beliefs of both the woman and health care practitioner shape the significance attributed to pain, clinical decision making, and recovery outcomes [22]. Whatever belief is held, pregnancy-related LPP is a condition that deserves further exploration, with translation of knowledge across countries, cultures, and health disciplines. Listening to women will add to existing knowledge and promote further understanding as to the degree of seriousness of this common complaint.

Almost half of all pregnant women and one-quarter of postpartum women are reported to experience LPP [10]. The point prevalence of pelvic girdle pain (PGP) during pregnancy is thought to be 20% [13]. The prevalence of "back pain" related to pregnancy in an Australian population has been described from population-based surveys as 35.5% and 80% [23, 24]; however the prevalence of LPP as differentiated as low back pain (LBP) and/or pelvic girdle pain (PGP) and the associated degree of pain and disability suffered by Australian women is currently unknown.

2. Research Aims

The aim of this research was to determine the prevalence of LPP in a sample of pregnant women attending an Australian public hospital antenatal clinic. The secondary aim was to explore the experiences of women reporting LPP, through assessment of pain and disability, differentiating low back pain (LBP) and pelvic girdle pain (PGP).

3. Method

A cross-sectional descriptive study was undertaken. A survey was self-administered to a cross-sectional cohort of 105 primiparous or multiparous women in their third trimester (from 28 weeks gestation) with a singleton pregnancy. Women with insufficient knowledge of the English language were excluded from the study as lack of funding did not allow for the use of interpreters and translation of the survey into other languages. Women were approached for recruitment to the study as they presented for their antenatal appointment with either a midwife or doctor. The study sample included women from medical clinics with conditions such as hypertension and diabetes. Women with inflammatory arthritis, a recent fracture or surgery to the back, hip, or pelvic area (in the previous 12 months) and/or any other serious pathology were excluded due to

the possible influence on the reporting of pain. Sample size was not calculated for statistical power but selected as one manageable for the time constraints of the project.

Data were collected in the Women's Health Clinic, Westmead Hospital between 17th and 23th March, 2010. Westmead Hospital is a tertiary level hospital in Western Sydney, New South Wales, with around 4,500 births per year. The initial survey gathered data on the woman's demographics, exercise habits and lifestyle using dichotomous variable. Women who reported symptoms of LPP (LBP and/or PGP) completed a second survey including a pain diagram, Visual Analogue Scale, and the Oswestry Disability Index (version 2.1a). Closed and open-ended questions further explored the experiences of the women, for example, whether they had reported their pain to their maternity care, whether they had treatment, and whether the treatment helped. The study received the approval of Sydney West Area Health Service (Westmead Campus) Human Research Ethics Committee.

4. Measurement of Pain

The pain diagram was used to self-report LPP (Figure 1). Areas marked above the level of the 5th lumbar vertebra (L5) were classified as LBP, areas marked below the level of L5 and the iliac crests (anterior, posterior, and/or lateral view) were classified as PGP, and those marked both above and below were classified as combined LBP and PGP. The Visual Analogue Scale (VAS) was used to measure pain intensity, consisting of a horizontal line, 100 mm in length, anchored by word descriptors at each end: no pain and pain as bad as it could possibly be [25, 26]. Women were asked to select the point on the scale that best represents the perceived level of pain. Pain intensity was measured for usual pain during the pregnancy and pain on the day of the survey.

5. Measurement of Function

At the time of data collection there were only a few tools reported for the measurement of function specifically during pregnancy [27, 28], none with proven validity [13]. The Oswestry Disability Index (ODI) (Version 2.1a) is a condition-specific tool in the management of spinal disorders that attempts to quantify the level of pain interference with physical activities by providing an estimate of disability expressed as a percentage score [29]. The index is a questionnaire with ten sections covering the assessment of pain intensity, personal care, lifting, walking, sitting, standing, sleeping, sex life, social life and travelling. The scores are calculated as a percentage; a higher percentage score indicates a greater disability. The ODI (vs2.1a) was chosen because of its use in previous studies of pregnancy-related LPP [30] and because it measures disability not just as mobility dysfunction but as a social and environmental construct. An instrument for the assessment of symptoms and activity limitation for people with PGP has recently been published [31]. This instrument is reported to have high reliability and validity both during pregnancy and postpartum and would be useful in future studies of PGP.

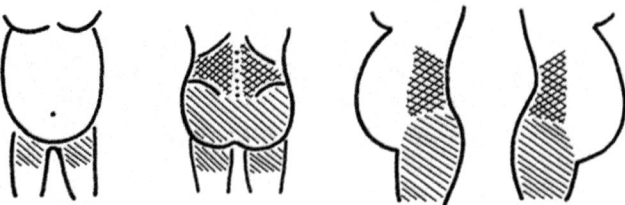

FIGURE 1: The pain diagram for self-report of LBP and/or PGP.

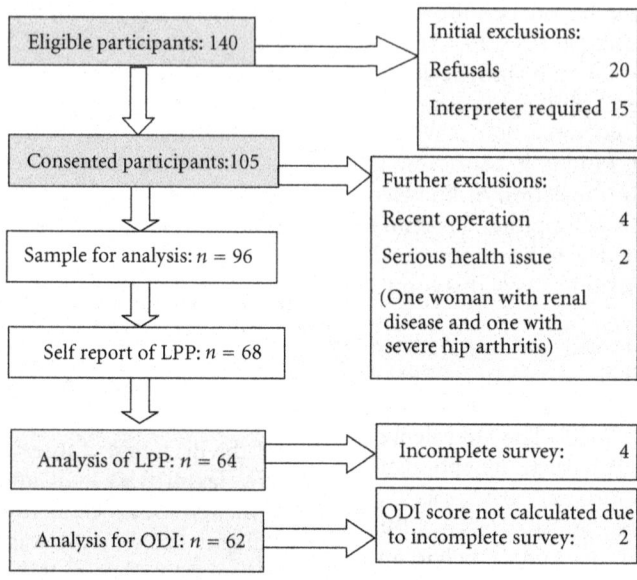

FIGURE 2: Flow chart of participants.

6. Analysis

The period prevalence of self-reported LPP (a retrospective recollection of pain throughout the pregnancy) and point prevalence (pain on the day of data collection) were calculated from the sample. The relationship between LPP, LBP and/or PGP and study sample characteristics was investigated. Data were analysed descriptively using PASW statistics 18, with calculation of means and standard deviations for parametric data. Pearson's Chi-Square (X^2) or Fisher's Exact Test was used to test the difference between groups for categorical, nonparametric data. The significance level was set at $P \leq 0.05$. Segmentation of the VAS by verbal descriptors within the scale was used in subgrouping of pain level for data analysis [25]. The guidance for subgrouping of the ODI was taken from a previous study of pregnancy related LBP and PGP [30]. The Kruskal-Wallis Test tested the differences between groups for nonparametric data. Statistical methods to control for confounding variables were not employed due to the limited sample size. A thematic analysis was conducted on the open-ended question: "Is there anything else you would like to tell us about your experience of pain?" Responses were categorised according to the identification of themes and key words as written by the women.

7. Results

One hundred and forty women were approached at their antenatal appointment. One hundred and five women consented and completed the initial survey. Nine women were initially excluded due to incomplete survey (3), recent surgery (4), renal disease (1), and severe hip arthritis (1), leaving a final study sample of 96 women (Figure 2).

8. Study Participants

Of the 96 women in the analysis, 46 (48%) were attending a midwives' clinic and 49 (51%) a medical clinic (1 missing clinic data). Analysis of variables within the sample demonstrated no significant differences between the clinic groups in terms of age, parity, country of birth, gestation, and booking-in body mass index (BMI). The mean gestation of the sample was 34.8 weeks (range: 28–41 weeks). One-third of women were born in Australia (38.5%); 36 (37%) Asia (including 18 (20%) from India/Sri Lanka); 23 (24%) women were grouped as "other"; the largest subgroup of 6 (6%) was Middle Eastern. These data revealed a broad and reasonably representative sample of Western Sydney when compared to local demographics from the Australian Bureau of Statistics,

TABLE 1: Participant characteristics.

Participant characteristic (n = 96)	Percentage of total sample	Percentage in NSW (2008) Total births = 94,864
Age		
<35	85.4	76.4
≥35	14.6	23.6
Parity		
Primiparous	54.2	41.6
Multiparous	45.8	55.3
BMI*		
<25	57.3	Not reported
≥25	41.7	
Country of Birth**		
Australia	38.5	69.3
Asia	37.4	12.9
Other	24	14.2

* BMI from "booking in" visit; unable to calculate BMI for one woman due to missing height/weight. **3.6% not stated in NSW report.

[32] which show a high culturally and linguistically diverse population. Population characteristics as comparable to the wider geographic region of New South Wales tabled in the report: NSW Mothers and Babies, 2008 [33], are found in Table 1.

9. Prevalence of LPP, LBP, and/or PGP

The period prevalence of self-reported LPP during the current pregnancy was 68 (71%) and the point prevalence was 33 (34%). Of the women who reported LPP (n = 64) when differentiated by the pain diagram, 11 (17%) women reported LBP only, 21 (33%) reported PGP only, and 32 (50%) reported both LBP and PGP (4 excluded due to incomplete survey/pain diagram).

10. Risk Factors

Multiparous women were more likely to report LPP than primiparous women ($P = 0.05$). If the woman reported a past history of LPP unrelated to pregnancy, she was more likely to report LPP on the day of data collection ($P = 0.005$). Women were also more likely to report LBP ($n = 8$) or PGP ($n = 18$) if they used stairs regularly ($P = 0.04$). There was an association between regular bending and LPP reported on the day of the survey ($P = 0.002$). There was no association found between LPP and age, ethnicity, booking-in body mass index, exercise (regular, abdominal, or pelvic floor), regular lifting, or the presence of support in the home (Tables 2, 3, and 4).

11. Pain and Disability

The mean pain score for LPP reported by women for usual pain was 6.5 (range 1–9) and on the day of data collection

was 3.8 (range 0–10). The VAS scores were subgrouped into four categories: no pain (<1), mild pain (1 to 3.9), moderate pain (4 to 6.9) and severe pain (7–10) (Figure 3). There were significant differences in pain intensity levels across the three groups: "LBP", "PGP", and "both LBP and PGP", for usual pain ($P = 0.002$) and for pain today ($P = 0.02$).

The mean Oswestry Disability Index (ODI) score for women with LPP ($n = 62$) was 29% (range: 0–74%). The ODI scores were sub-grouped into three categories: "minimal disability": score ≤ 10%; "mild disability": score 11 to 39%; and "moderate disability": score ≥ 40%. Most women ($n = 40$, 65%) were classified as having a mild disability. Seven women (11%) were classified as having "minimal disability"; 14 women (23%) had a moderate disability; four of these women scored 60% or higher (Figure 4). There was a significant difference in the ODI scores across the distribution ($P = 0.03$). Women with both LBP and PGP scored a higher mean score (33.5%), therefore higher disability level than women with PGP (26%) or LBP alone (18%) (Table 5).

12. Listening to Women

Even though 45 (71%) of the women in the LPP sample had reported their pain to their maternity carer, only 16 women (25%) had received any form of treatment. Twelve of the women who received treatment reported benefit from the intervention. When asked why they had not received treatment, some women responded: "I was told during the last pregnancy that there was nothing that there could be done to help"; "I asked the doctor but they said it is normal in pregnancy"; "No one cared or suggested any treatment." Other women stated: "I do not think it's necessary"; "I did not think I needed treatment"; "The pain [is] manageable". A majority of women (70%) agreed that "LPP was to be expected because of the pregnancy."

Eighteen women (29%) provided a response to the question: "Is there anything else you would like to say about your experience of pain?" Responses were categorised according to key words and four themes emerged from this process: pain described as a physical symptom, the impact of pain on lifestyle, the impact of pain on psychological health, and what helped the pain including coping strategies (Figure 5). Further details of the qualitative results of this study will be provided in another paper.

13. Discussion

The results of this study support a high prevalence of lumbopelvic pain (LPP) for pregnant women, both during the pregnancy (71% period prevalence) and on the day of the survey (34% point prevalence). This period prevalence is comparable to other studies which use similar definitions and a cross-sectional survey design. For example, a survey of 891 women in Sweden within 24 hours of birth reported the prevalence of LPP during pregnancy as 72% [34]; a period prevalence of 72% is calculated from a study of 213 Japanese women who were greater than 36 weeks' gestation [35]. The

TABLE 2: LPP and participant characteristics.

Participant response to survey Q ($n = 96$)	LPP during pregnancy yes (n)	LPP during pregnancy no (n)	P	LPP on day of survey yes (n)	LPP on day of survey no (n)	P
Age						
<35	56	26	0.2	28	54	1.0
≥35	12	2		5	9	
Parity						
Primiparous	32	20	0.05*	17	35	0.8
Multiparous	36	8		16	28	
Ethnicity						
Australia	28	9		17	20	
Asia	27	9	0.2	10	26	0.2
Other	13	10		6	17	
BMI						
<25	37	18	0.5	18	37	0.8
≥25	30	10		14	26	
LPP in the past (unrelated to pregnancy)						
Yes	20	8	1.0	16	12	0.005**
No	48	20		17	51	

*X^2 ($n = 96$) = 4.7, $P = 0.05$, phi = −0.2; **X^2 ($n = 96$) = 9.08, $P = 0.005$, phi = 0.3.

TABLE 3: LPP, exercise habits, and lifestyle.

Participant response to survey Q ($n = 93$) (3 surveys not completed)	LPP during pregnancy yes (n)	LPP during pregnancy no (n)	P	LPP on day of survey yes (n)	LPP on day of survey no (n)	P
Regular exercise*						
Yes	39	21	0.2	18	42	0.2
No	26	7		14	19	
PF exercise*						
Yes	16	7	1.0	7	16	0.8
No	49	21		25	45	
Abdominal exercise*						
Yes	9	6	0.4	5	10	1.0
No	57	22		28	51	
Regular bending						
Yes	42	13	0.1	26	29	0.002**
No	23	15		6	32	
Regular lifting						
Yes	30	8	0.2	16	22	0.3
No	35	20		17	38	
Regular stairs						
Yes	44	19	0.8	21	42	0.6
No	22	8		12	18	
Support at home						
Yes ($n = 91$)	46	17	0.3	24	39	0.5
No	19	11		9	21	

*≥ once per week; **X^2 ($n = 93$) = 9.9, $P = 0.002$, phi = 0.3.

TABLE 4: LBP, PGP, or combined pain, exercise habits, and lifestyle.

Initial survey: Exercise and lifestyle	$n = 61^{**}$ (%)	LBP	PGP	Both LBP and PGP (%)	P
Regular exercise					
≥once per week	36 (59)	7 (70)	12 (57)	17 (57)	0.7
No regular exercise	25 (41)	3 (30)	9 (43)	13 (43)	
Regular bending					
Yes	39 (64)	7 (70)	14 (67)	18 (60)	0.8
No	22 (36)	3 (30)	7 (33)	12 (40)	
Regular lifting					
Yes	28 (45)	3 (30)	13 (62)	11 (40)	0.1
No	34 (55)	7 (70)	8 (38)	19 (62)	
Regular stairs					
Yes	43 (69)	8 (80)	18 (86)	17 (55)	**0.04***
No	19 (31)	2 (20)	3 (14)	14 (45)	

*X^2 ($n = 62$), $P = 0.04$, phi = 0.3; **3 surveys not completed.

TABLE 5: The VAS and ODI scores for self report of LPP.

Self-report of LPP	$n = 64$ (%)	ODI % ($n = 62$)* Mean (SD)	VAS: usual pain Mean (SD)	VAS: pain today Mean (SD)
LBP only	11 (17)	18 (10.8)	4.3 (2)	2.5 (2.6)
PGP only	21 (33)	26 (15.6)	6.5 (2.2)	3.0 (2.4)
Both LBP/PGP	32 (50)	33.5 (17.4)	7.1 (1.7)	4.7 (2.7)

*Two ODI scores unable to be calculated due to incomplete survey.

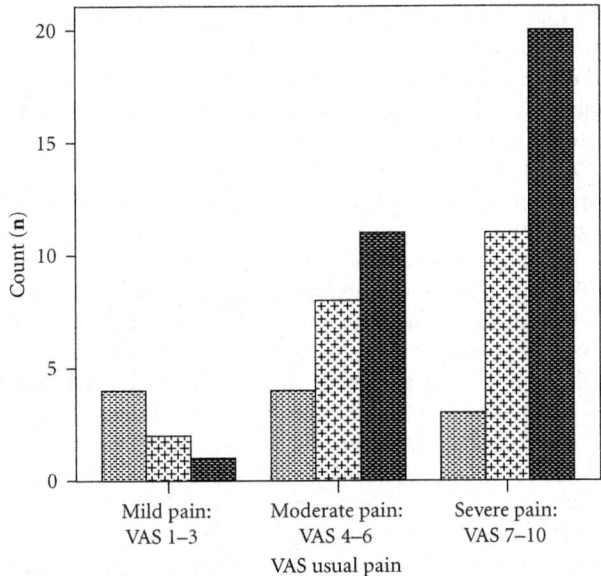

FIGURE 3: Distribution of categorised VAS scores for "usual pain" across the 3 categories: LBP, PGP, and both LBP and PGP.

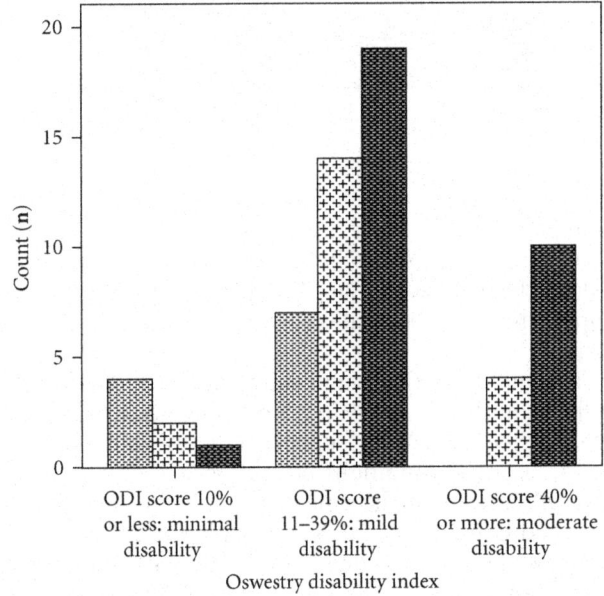

FIGURE 4: Distribution of categorised ODI scores across the 3 categories: LBP, PGP, and both LBP and PGP.

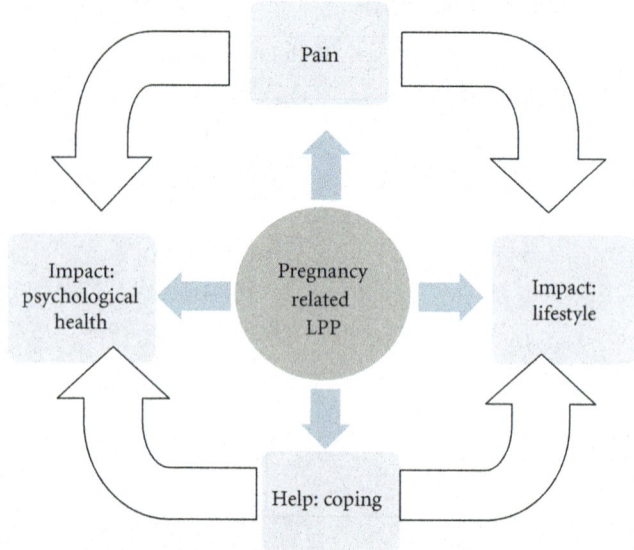

FIGURE 5: The relationship between pregnancy-related LPP and the four themes.

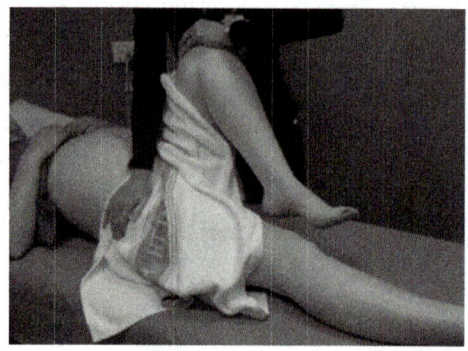

FIGURE 6: The posterior pelvic pain provocation test.

mean pain intensity score reported by women for this study (6.5) and the mean disability score (29%) are also similar to several other studies [34, 36, 37]. These comparable findings support this study population as a reasonably representative sample.

The importance of investigating pregnancy-related pelvic girdle pain (PGP) as distinct from low back pain (LBP) within reported LPP is supported in the literature [10, 13, 14, 30]. The conditions of LBP and PGP may coexist; however different management strategies are required for each condition [13, 38–40]. Sub-grouping of LPP also assists in identifying those women most at risk of long-term dysfunction [38, 41]. The prevalence rate of reported LBP only for this study was 17%, which is similar to that described by Gutke [30], and lower than the prevalence of PGP (33%) or combined LBP and PGP (50%) [30, 42]. When a review is made of the pain and disability levels for each of the subgroups, women with PGP only or both PGP and LBP reported higher median pain scores of 7 out of 10 for usual pain when compared to the LBP only median score of 4. These results support other research findings that LBP is less

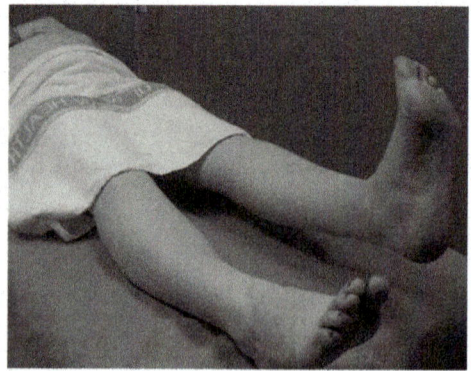

FIGURE 7: The active straight leg raise.

intense and less disabling during pregnancy when compared to PGP or combined pain groups [14, 30].

Many clinicians consider LPP as a normal discomfort of pregnancy. Women's comments, however, focused on a lack of acknowledgement of LPP by their maternity carer and the negative impact of pain on their lifestyle. It is apparent that for some women the pain was minimal and could be considered a discomfort, but for others, the pain was perceived as considerable. The Oswestry Disability Index attempts to measure pain interference with common daily activities. Forty women (65%) scored a mild disability (11–39%) and 14 women (23%) a moderate disability (≥40%). At least four out of five pregnant women with LPP encountered negative lifestyle consequences due to pain and disability, with one in five women experiencing a moderate level of pain-related disability. From the thematic analysis it can be hypothesized that the impact of LPP on a woman's lifestyle and psychological health is a balance between perceived pain, disability, and her capacity to elicit help and employ coping strategies (Figure 5).

Whilst most women recover from pregnancy-related LPP, some do not. Ten percent of women with pelvic pain during pregnancy still have moderate to severe pain and disability at 18 months postpartum [41]. High pain intensity scores (≥ 6 on VAS) are predictive ongoing pain and disability after birth [39, 43], and women with combined LBP and PGP recover to a lesser degree than those with PGP or LBP alone [40]. The challenge of assisting women who suffer long-term problems has been narrated in distressing case studies, including stories of surgical intervention and dramatic alterations in the lifestyles of women [44]. The complexity of chronic pain disorders drives the need for early recognition and effective management during pregnancy [40, 45].

The identification and treatment of women at risk of chronic pain disorders could reduce the number of women with pregnancy-related LPP and impact future pregnancies [14, 35, 46]. This study supports previous findings for the identifiable risk factors for the reporting of LPP of more than one pregnancy and a previous history of LPP; however sample size lacks statistical power to make definitive conclusions. Knowledge of risk factors and aggravating activities can assist maternity carers in advising women about their condition. Objective physical assessments such as the posterior pelvic pain provocation test (see the appendix and Figure 6) have a high sensitivity and specificity [47] and can be used with pain mapping (pain diagram) to assist in diagnosing women with PGP [35, 46, 48]. The active straight leg raise (see the appendix and Figure 7) is a test of load transfer for the pelvic girdle and is predictive of pain and disability at 3 months postpartum [46].

The main limitation of this study was the sample size: as this restricted the statistical tests available for use and conclusions are therefore conservative. The authors acknowledge the possibility of bias in the study sample as women with LPP may have been more likely to agree to participate in the study. Another drawback was the need to exclude 11% of women from participating due to lack of competency in English. As previously discussed, the ODI is not a scale for pregnancy, and this limits the interpretation of the scale and the results of the study.

14. Conclusion

This is the first known Australian study to report both the period and point prevalence of pelvic girdle pain as well as low back pain during pregnancy from a prospective cross sectional cohort. These results are similar to research conducted in other countries using similar methodology, however further investigation with a larger sample size is needed to provide more support to these findings.

It is recommended that low back and/or pelvic girdle pain should not be universally accepted as normal during pregnancy. In this study, the mean pain intensity score for usual pain was 6/10, and four out of five women reported disability scores with negative lifestyle consequences. Women with combined LBP and PGP, or PGP alone, experienced higher levels of pain and disability when compared to women with LBP alone. Only one-quarter of women surveyed received treatment, despite levels of pain and disability.

Future research in this area should investigate the benefit of early identification and the initiation of interventions for women with pregnancy-related LPP who are at risk of long-term problems. This may limit the development of comorbidities and chronic pain conditions. In conclusion, it would seem wise for maternity carers to listen to the concerns of women regarding pregnancy-related LPP, in order to optimise the health and lifestyle of the women in their care.

Appendix

Physical Tests Used for PGP [13]

Tests during pregnancy should be conducted with minimal time spent in the supine position. A wedge can be provided for left lateral tilt if the woman reports supine hypotension.

Posterior Pelvic Pain Provocation Test [14] and (Figure 6)

Woman: Supine with the hips and knees flexed.

Examiner: Standing at the woman's side.

Palpate: Flex the ipsilateral hip and knee to 90°. Gently stabilise the contralateral anterior superior iliac spine with one hand.

Test: Apply a posterior force gently through the axis of the femur to the ilium thus posteriorly shearing the sacroiliac joint. Test is considered positive if pain is reproduced in sacroiliac joint or symphysis.

The Active Straight Leg Raise [49] and (Figure 7)

Woman: Supine lying, legs extended.

Examiner: Monitor the anterior superior iliac spines bilaterally.

Test: Instruct the woman to raise their leg with an extended knee (20 cm above couch). Note the ease with which they are able to do so, the provocation of any symptoms, as well as any compensatory motions of the trunk during the test. When the active (neuromuscular) system is dysfunctional, the pelvic girdle will tend to rotate towards the leg which is being raised.

Conflict of Interests

The authors declare that they have no conflict of interests.

Authors' Contribution

H. Pierce was the principle author of the concept for research and research design; she conducted the collection and analysis of data and writing of paper. C. Homer was the principal supervisor and provided guidance with research concept and design, assistance with data analysis, and editing of all manuscripts. H. Dahlen was the assistant supervisor and provided guidance with research design, data analysis, and editing of paper. J. King was the onsite (Westmead Hospital) principal investigator of study and provided guidance with research design, assistance with ethics approval, and editing of paper.

Ethical Approval

Ethical approval was gained from Sydney West Area Health Service (Westmead Campus) Human Research Ethics Committee.

Acknowledgments

The authors wish to acknowledge the assistance of Westmead Hospitals' statistician Karen Byth in the early analysis of data. The encouragement and support of staff at Westmead Hospital in the Women's Health Clinic, the Birth Unit, the Maternity Ward, and the Physiotherapy Department is also acknowledged.

References

[1] C Grigg, "Working with women in pregnancy," in *Midwifery: Preparation for Practice*, S. Pairman, J. Pincombe, C. Thorogood, and S. Tracey, Eds., Elsevier Churchill Livingstone, Sydney, Australia, 2006.

[2] M. Yerby, "Minor disorders of pregnancy," in *Physiology in the Childbearing Year: with Anatomy and Related Biosciences*, D. Stables and J. Rankin, Eds., Elsevier, Edinburgh, UK, 2005.

[3] M. Enkin, M. Keirse, J. Neilson et al., *A Guide to Effective Care in Pregnancy and Childbirth*, Oxford University Press, 2000.

[4] I. M. Mogren, "Perceived health, sick leave, psychosocial situation, and sexual life in women with low-back pain and pelvic pain during pregnancy," *Acta Obstetricia et Gynecologica Scandinavica*, vol. 85, pp. 647–656, 2006.

[5] I. A. Babarinsa, I. F. Adewole, A. O. Fatade, and A. B. Ajayi, "Obstetric pubic symphysis arthropathy: a study of nine cases," *Journal of Obstetrics and Gynaecology*, vol. 19, no. 6, pp. 620–622, 1999.

[6] C. Olsson and L. Nilsson-Wikmar, "Health related quality of life and physical ability among pregnant women with and without back pain in late pregnancy," *Acta Obstetricia et Gynecologica Scandinavica*, vol. 83, pp. 351–357, 2004.

[7] E. Vermani, R. Mittal, and A. Weeks, "Pelvic girdle pain and low back pain in pregnancy: a review," *Pain Practice*, vol. 10, no. 1, pp. 60–71, 2010.

[8] Collaborating Centre for Women's and Children's Health National, *Antenatal Care: Routine Care for the Healthy Pregnant Woman*, RCOG Press, London, UK, 2008.

[9] V. E. Pennick and G. Young, "Interventions for preventing and treating pelvic and back pain in pregnancy," *Cochrane Database of Systematic Reviews*, no. 2, Article ID CD001139, 2007.

[10] W. H. Wu, O. G. Meijer, K. Uegaki et al., "Pregnancy-related pelvic girdle pain (PPP), I: terminology, clinical presentation, and prevalence," *European Spine Journal*, vol. 13, no. 7, pp. 575–589, 2004.

[11] R. E. Leadbetter, D. Mawer, and S. W. Lindow, "Symphysis pubis dysfunction: a review of the literature," *Journal of Maternal-fetal and Neonatal Medicine*, vol. 16, no. 6, pp. 349–354, 2004.

[12] J. M. A. Mens, A. Pool-Goudzwaard, and H. J. Stam, "Mobility of the pelvic joints in pregnancy-related lumbopelvic pain: a systematic review," *Obstetrical and Gynecological Survey*, vol. 64, no. 3, pp. 200–208, 2009.

[13] A. Vleeming, H. B. Albert, H. C. Östgaard, B. Sturesson, and B. Stuge, "European guidelines for the diagnosis and treatment of pelvic girdle pain," *European Spine Journal*, vol. 17, no. 6, pp. 794–819, 2008.

[14] H. C. Ostgaard, "Assessment and treatment of low back pain in working pregnant women," *Seminars in Perinatology*, vol. 20, no. 1, pp. 61–69, 1996.

[15] C. H. G. Bastiaenen, R. A. de Bie, J. W. S. Vlaeyen et al., "Long-term effectiveness and costs of a brief self-management intervention in women with pregnancy-related low back pain after delivery," *BMC Pregnancy and Childbirth*, vol. 8, article no. 19, 2008.

[16] J. Kluge, D. Hall, Q. Louw et al., "Specific exercises to treat pregnancy-related low back pain in a South African population," *International Journal of Gynecology & Obstetrics*, vol. 113, pp. 187–191, 2011.

[17] B. Stuge, I. Holm, and N. Vøllestad, "To treat or not to treat postpartum pelvic girdle pain with stabilizing exercises?" *Manual Therapy*, vol. 11, no. 4, pp. 337–343, 2006.

[18] A. T. Hirsh, S. Z. George, J. E. Bialosky, and M. E. Robinson, "Fear of pain, pain catastrophizing, and acute pain perception: relative prediction and timing of assessment," *Journal of Pain*, vol. 9, no. 9, pp. 806–812, 2008.

[19] D. A. Walsh and J. C. Radcliffe, "Pain beliefs and perceived physical disability of patients with chronic low back pain," *Pain*, vol. 97, no. 1-2, pp. 23–31, 2002.

[20] SBU-The Swedish Council on Technology Assessment in Health Care, "Back pain, neck pain: an evidence base review (Summary and conclusions)," Stockholm, Sweden, 2000, http://www.sbu.se/en/Published/Yellow/Back-and-neck-pain/.

[21] National Collaborating Centre for Primary Care, "Low back pain: early management of persistent non-specific low back pain," NICE, London, UK, 2009, http://www.nhmrc.gov.au/guidelines/publications/cp94-cp95.

[22] C. J. Main, N. Foster, and R. Buchbinder, "How important are back pain beliefs and expectations for satisfactory recovery from back pain?" *Best Practice and Research: Clinical Rheumatology*, vol. 24, no. 2, pp. 205–217, 2010.

[23] M. D. Smith, A. Russell, and P. W. Hodges, "Is there a relationship between parity, pregnancy, back pain and incontinence?" *International Urogynecology Journal and Pelvic Floor Dysfunction*, vol. 19, no. 2, pp. 205–211, 2008.

[24] D. B. Stapleton, A. H. MacLennan, and P. Kristiansson, "The prevalence of recalled low back pain during and after pregnancy: a South Australian population survey," *Australian and New Zealand Journal of Obstetrics and Gynaecology*, vol. 42, no. 5, pp. 482–485, 2002.

[25] H. Breivik, P. C. Borchgrevink, S. M. Allen et al., "Assessment of pain," *British Journal of Anaesthesia*, vol. 101, no. 1, pp. 17–24, 2008.

[26] A. M. Boonstra, H. R. Schiphorst Preuper, M. F. Reneman, J. B. Posthumus, and R. E. Stewart, "Reliability and validity of the visual analogue scale for disability in patients with chronic musculoskeletal pain," *International Journal of Rehabilitation Research*, vol. 31, no. 2, pp. 165–169, 2008.

[27] G. van de Pol, J. R. J. de Leeuw, H. J. van Brummen et al., "The pregnancy mobility index: a mobility scale during and after pregnancy," *Acta Obstetricia et Gynecologica Scandinavica*, vol. 85, pp. 786–791, 2006.

[28] R. E. Leadbetter, D. Mawer, and S. W. Lindow, "The development of a scoring system for symphysis pubis dysfunction," *Journal of Obstetrics and Gynaecology*, vol. 26, no. 1, pp. 20–23, 2006.

[29] M. Davidson, "Rasch analysis of three versions of the oswestry disability questionnaire," *Manual Therapy*, vol. 13, no. 3, pp. 222–231, 2008.

[30] A. Gutke, H. C. Ostgaard, and B. Oberg, "Pelvic girdle pain and lumbar pain in pregnancy: a cohort study of the consequences in terms of health and functioning," *Spine*, vol. 31, pp. E149–E155, 2006.

[31] B. Stuge, A. Garratt, H. K. Jenssen, and M. Grotle, "The pelvic girdle questionaire: a condition specific instrument for measuring activity limitations and symptoms in people with pelvic girdle pain," *Physical Therapy*, vol. 91, pp. 1096–1108, 2011.

[32] "Australian Bureau of Statistics: 4102.0 Australian Social Trends," ABS, 2007.

[33] NSW Department of Health, "NSW Mothers and Babies 2008," Centre for Epidemiology and Research Population Health Division, Better Health Centre, North Sydney, Australia, 2010.

[34] I. M. Mogren and A. I. Pohjanen, "Low back pain and pelvic pain during pregnancy: prevalence and risk factors," *Spine*, vol. 30, no. 8, pp. 983–991, 2005.

[35] F. Ando and K. Ohashi, "Using the posterior pelvic pain provocation test in pregnant japanese women," *Nursing and Health Sciences*, vol. 11, no. 1, pp. 3–9, 2009.

[36] M. A. Mohseni-Bandpei, M. Fakhri, M. Ahmad-Shirvani et al., "Low back pain in 1,100 iranian pregnant women: prevalence and risk factors," *Spine Journal*, vol. 9, no. 10, pp. 795–801, 2009.

[37] S. J. Mousavi, M. Parnianpour, and A. Vleeming, "Pregnancy related pelvic girdle pain and low back pain in an iranian population," *Spine*, vol. 32, no. 3, pp. E100–E104, 2007.

[38] I. Ronchetti, A. Vleeming, and J. P. Van Wingerden, "Physical characteristics of women with severe pelvic girdle pain after pregnancy: a descriptive cohort study," *Spine*, vol. 33, no. 5, pp. E145–E151, 2008.

[39] H. B. Albert, M. Godskesen, and J. Westergaard, "Prognosis in four syndromes of pregnancy-related pelvic pain," *Acta Obstetricia et Gynecologica Scandinavica*, vol. 80, pp. 505–510, 2001.

[40] A. Gutke, H. C. Östgaard, and B. Öberg, "Predicting persistent pregnancy-related low back pain," *Spine*, vol. 33, no. 12, pp. E386–E393, 2008.

[41] C. C. M. Rost, J. Jacqueline, A. Kaiser, A. P. Verhagen, and B. W. Koes, "Prognosis of women with pelvic pain during pregnancy: a long-term follow-up study," *Acta Obstetricia et Gynecologica Scandinavica*, vol. 85, pp. 771–777, 2006.

[42] H. S. Robinson, A. M. Mengshoel, E. K. Bjelland, and N. K. Vøllestad, "Pelvic girdle pain, clinical tests and disability in late pregnancy," *Manual Therapy*, vol. 15, no. 3, pp. 280–285, 2010.

[43] H. C. Ostgaard, G. Zetherstrom, E. Roos-Hansson, and B. Svanberg, "Reduction of back and posterior pelvic pain in pregnancy," *Spine*, vol. 19, no. 8, pp. 894–900, 1994.

[44] P. B. O'Sullivan and D. J. Beales, "Diagnosis and classification of pelvic girdle pain disorders-part 1: a mechanism based approach within a biopsychosocial framework," *Manual Therapy*, vol. 12, no. 2, pp. 86–97, 2007.

[45] H. B. Albert, M. Godskesen, L. Korsholm et al., "Risk factors in developing pregnancy-related pelvic girdle pain," *Acta Obstetricia et Gynecologica Scandinavica*, vol. 85, pp. 539–544, 2006.

[46] H. S. Robinson, A. M. Mengshoel, M. B. Veierød, and N. Vøllestad, "Pelvic girdle pain: potential risk factors in pregnancy in relation to disability and pain intensity three months postpartum," *Manual Therapy*, vol. 15, no. 6, pp. 522–528, 2010.

[47] H. C. Ostgaard, E. Roos-Hansson, and G. Zetherstrom, "Regression of back and posterior pelvic pain after delivery," *Spine*, vol. 21, pp. 2777–2780, 1996.

[48] H. S. Robinson, M. B. Veierød, A. M. Mengshoel, and N. K. Vollestad, "Pelvic girdle pain—associations with risk factors in early pregnancy and disability or pain intensity in late pregnancy: a prospective cohort study," *BMC Musculoskeletal Disorders*, vol. 11, article 91, 2010.

[49] J. M. A. Mens, A. Vleeming, C. J. Snijders, B. W. Koes, and H. J. Stam, "Reliability and validity of the active straight leg raise test in posterior pelvic pain since pregnancy," *Spine*, vol. 26, no. 10, pp. 1167–1171, 2001.

18

The Impact of Nursing Characteristics and the Work Environment on Perceptions of Communication

Dana Tschannen[1] and Eunjoo Lee[2]

[1] Division of Nursing Business and Health Systems, School of Nursing, University of Michigan,
  400 N Ingalls, Room 4152, Ann Arbor, MI 48109-5482, USA
[2] College of Nursing, Kyungpook National University, Daegu 702-701, Republic of Korea

Correspondence should be addressed to Dana Tschannen, djvs@umich.edu

Academic Editor: John Daly

Failure to communicate openly and accurately to members of the healthcare team can result in medical error. The purpose of this study was to explore the impact of nursing characteristics and environmental values on communication in the acute care setting. Nurses ($n = 135$) on four medical-surgical units in two hospitals completed a survey asking nurses' perceptions of communication, work environment, and nursing demographics. LPNs perceived significantly higher levels of open communication with nurses than did RNs ($P = .042$). RNs noted higher levels of accuracy of communication among nurses than did LPNs ($P < .001$). Higher experience levels resulted in greater perceptions of open communication. Only environmental values (e.g., trust, respect) were a significant predictor of both openness and accuracy of communication. These findings suggest understanding the environment (e.g., presence or absence of trust, respect, status equity, and time availability) is a foundational step that must occur before implementing any strategies aimed at improving communication.

1. Introduction

A significant cause of medical error in health care is poor communication [1, 2]. For the past three years, miscommunication has been identified as one of the most frequently identified root causes of sentinel events reported to The Joint Commission, with 82% of the sentinel events in 2010 identifying communication as the primary root cause [3]. According to Rucker and colleagues, up to 75% of clinical decisions are made without all pertinent clinical information [4]. Differences in status and discipline may be part of the confounding factors associated with poor communication. This includes various job categories (supervisor/supervisee), expertise level (novice/expert), and discipline (doctor/nurse) [2].

Although variations in status and discipline are abundant in the healthcare environment, it is critical for all members of the healthcare team to communicate effectively with one another, despite these differences. In an effort to understand how status and discipline differences may impact perceptions

of communication, the purpose of this study was to explore the impact of nursing characteristics (e.g., job category, education, experience, and expertise) on perceptions of communication in the acute care setting, while also considering the impact of the work environment.

2. Literature Review

The act of communication between nurses and physicians is a central activity in healthcare, and a failure to communicate has been linked with poor quality and patient errors [5]. Effective communication and collaboration among nurses and physicians has been shown to result in improved quality of care [6, 7], increased patient and professional satisfaction [6, 8], and greater intent to stay [8, 9]. Specifically, the presence of poor communication among nurses and physicians may result in an almost doubled risk for mortality and length of stay among intensive care unit (ICU) patients [8, 10, 11]. Manojlovich and colleagues, while surveying nurses in 25

ICUs, found timeliness of communication to be inversely correlated with pressure ulcer development ($r = -.38$, $P = .06$) [12]. In addition, higher variability of understanding—which can occur with a variety of education and experience levels—was significantly correlated with ventilator associated pneumonia ($r = .43$, $P = .03$).

Current research evaluating the impact of nursing characteristics on communication has resulted in mixed findings. Miller and colleagues, while examining the presence of individual characteristics and perceptions of nurse-physician interactions, found nurses with greater than six years of experience rated openness of communication and problem solving higher than less experienced nurses ($P = .04$) [13]. Foley and colleagues found a significant relationship between nurse-physician relationships and nursing expertise and the number of professional certifications ($P = .05$) [14]. In contrast, Mark and colleagues evaluated the relationship between nurse staffing, professional practice, and several patient outcomes and found no significant relationship between nurse staffing variables (education, experience, and skill mix) and professional practice [15].

Although nursing characteristics such as education and expertise level may determine levels of communication and collaboration (i.e., physicians may respect nurses who are more educated), values supported in the environment in which care is delivered may also impact communication patterns. When the values of the organization include trust, respect, and teamwork, collaborative relationships are more likely to ensue. According to Schmalenberg and colleagues, who conducted interviews with physicians and nurses, environmental values play a role in fostering the development of effective communication/collaboration [16]. One interviewee described collaboration as "a prevailing unit and organizational norm based on mutual trust, respect, teamwork, and open communication." Findings from focus groups of nurses and physicians conducted by Simpson and colleagues identified an agreement among participants that many interactions and experiences with one another over time were the basis for trust and confidence in one another [17].

In summary, communication among the healthcare team is critical for optimal patient outcome. The current literature has failed to identify specific communication strategies that have consistently impacted quality of care and patient safety [18]. This may be due to the failure to consider individual characteristics, such as education, experience, and expertise levels, as well as the values present in the environment. In addition, little work has been done beyond the critical care areas—ICUs, emergency rooms, and operating rooms. For this reason, the purpose of this study was to identify the relationship between individual nursing characteristics (education, experience, expertise, and job type), environmental values, and perceptions of communication with the healthcare team in the acute care setting.

3. Methods

3.1. Design. This study used a cross-sectional, descriptive design with a convenience sample of four in-patient medical surgical units in two Midwestern hospitals. All nurses employed on the units providing direct patient care were asked to participate. Nurses who did not perform direct patient care were excluded. A total of 161 registered nurses (RNs) and 18 licensed practice nurses (LPNs) were eligible for study participation. Based on a power analysis (multiple regression with 11 predictors) with an α of 0.05, medium effect size ($f^2 = .15$), and power $(1 - \beta) = .80$, 123 respondents were needed for the analysis. The number of questionnaires returned was 135, with response rates for the units ranging from 69% to 82% (overall response rate of 76%). Approval for the study was obtained from the institutional review board for each institution.

3.2. Data Variables and Survey Instrument. The survey tool used to identify perceptions of communication was a modified version of Shortell's Organizational Management in the Intensive Care Unit Survey [19]. The entire survey included 44 questions asking nurses' perceptions of communication, collaboration, the environmental values present in their respective units, as well as nursing demographic information. For the purpose of this study, the questions regarding communication, environmental values, and nursing demographics were used.

3.2.1. Communication. Communication was measured by two dimensions: openness and accuracy. Communication openness refers to "the degree to which physicians or nurses are able to 'say what they mean' when speaking with members of the other group, without fear of repercussions or misunderstanding" [19, page 712]." Four questions on the survey instrument addressed the openness of communication among nurses and four additional questions considered the openness of communication between nurses and physicians. Each item was measured by a 7-point Likert scale with anchors 1 (strongly disagree) to 7 (strongly agree). Communication accuracy refers to the "degree to which nurses and physician believe in the accuracy of the information conveyed to them by the other party [19]." Four questions on the survey instrument addressed the accuracy of communication among nurses and four additional questions considered accuracy of communication between nurses and physicians. Each item was measured by a 7-point Likert scale (1, strongly disagree, to 7, strongly agree). Validity and reliability of the instrument had been previously reported [19]. Reliability estimations in this study also supported consistency in the items: open communication among nurses ($\alpha = 0.89$) and between nurses and physicians ($\alpha = .92$), accuracy of communication among nurses ($\alpha = .79$) and between nurses and physicians ($\alpha = .84$).

3.2.2. Nursing Characteristics. Nursing characteristics included in this study were education, years of experience, and self-reports of expertise. Level of education was measured categorically with the following options being present: diploma, associate's degree, bachelor's degree master's degree, or higher. Nursing experience was measured through a single-item question: How many years have you been

TABLE 1: Homogeneity test by unit characteristics ($n = 135$).

	Unit A M (SD)	Unit B M (SD)	Unit C M (SD)	Unit D M (SD)	F/χ^2	P
Experience as nurses (years)	15.86	12.81	8.37	11.24	2.741	.046
Expertise level	7.28	7.02	6.79	6.76	.490	.690
Educational level	N (%)	N (%)	N (%)	N (%)		
Diploma/Associate	23 (57.5)	16 (48.5)	18 (56.3)	16(55.2)	.671	.880
BSN and over	17(42.5)	17(51.5)	14 (43.8)	13 (44.8)		

working in your current job category? The final measure of nursing expertise required the nurses to identify their perceived level of expertise on a 10-point scale with anchors novice (1) to expert (10). Respondents were asked to circle the number on the scale that best reflects his/her level of expertise. Other nursing characteristics included in the study were job category (e.g., LPN or RN), unit of employment, and shift worked (e.g., day, evening, night, or rotating).

3.2.3. Environmental Values. The previous literature has identified environmental values as important precursors to the development of effective communication and collaborative relationships, including trust, respect, power equity, and time availability. Questions related to each of these values was developed and measured by a single question on a 7-point Likert scale with anchors strongly agree (1) to strongly disagree (7). Data from this study supported a highly positive correlation between the four factors, as noted by the following correlation values: trust and respect ($r = .82$), trust and time ($r = .54$), trust and status ($r = .67$), respect and time ($r = .60$), respect and status ($r = .66$), and finally time and status ($r = .62$) ($P = .001$ for each bivariate association). This supported the development of an overall environmental value variable, which was the combined average of each of the unit value items (per nurse). Reliability estimation for the environmental value variable was considered well above the acceptable range ($\alpha = 0.88$).

3.3. Procedure. Prior to distribution of the survey, nurses were presented with a 10-minute overview of the study. This overview was given to each unit at four different times of the day, in an effort to attain maximum participation. Upon completion of the in-service, each nurse received a copy of the survey. A reminder was placed in each nurse's mailbox two weeks after the initial survey distribution in an effort to increase response rate. A secure box was also placed in the nursing lounge of each unit for completed surveys.

3.4. Analysis. Data were analyzed with SPSS 18.0. Descriptive statistics were used to examine the demographics of nurses; analysis of variance (ANOVA) and chi-square tests were performed to test homogeneity of unit characteristics. To identify the difference in communication between nursing characteristics, *t*-tests were performed. Hierarchical multiple regression analysis was conducted to identify predictors of openness and accuracy of communication. A test for

multicollinearity was conducted using tolerance and VIF; no multicollinearity was identified. Residual analysis identified a normal distribution, linearity of residual, and homoscedasticity of errors. A significant value below 0.05 was considered statistically significant.

4. Findings

Nursing respondents ($n = 135$) were split nearly equally between Hospital A ($n = 74$, 55%) and Hospital B ($n = 61$, 45%). The majority of the nurses were RNs ($n = 119$, 88%) while 15 were LPNs (11%). Seventy-three (54.1%) nurses had earned an associate/diploma degree and 58 (43%) had a baccalaureate degree. Sixty-eight nurses worked the day shift and 43 nurses worked the night shift. Work experience as nurses was on average 12.30 years, ranging from 6 weeks to 46 years. Self-rating of expertise level was 6.98, with a range of 1 (novice) to 10 (expert).

Comparisons of nurse educational level, work experiences, and expertise levels by study units revealed no difference in educational level and expertise level (Table 1). A significant difference in work experiences was noted, with Unit A having the highest work experiences as nurses, followed by Unit B ($P = .046$).

4.1. Differences in the Perception of Communication. As noted in Table 2, nurses (e.g. RNs and LPNs) perceived communication to be more open among nurses than between nurses and physicians ($t = 10.227$, $P < .001$). However, nurses perceived that communication was more accurate with physicians than with nurses ($t = 2.18$, $P = .031$).

When comparing openness and accuracy of communication between job category (e.g., RN and LPN) (Table 2), LPNs perceived significantly higher levels of open communication with nurses than did RNs ($P = .042$). In contrast, RNs noted higher levels of accuracy of communication among nurses than did their LPN counterparts ($P < .001$). No significant difference between LPNs and RNs was noted in openness and accuracy of communication with physicians.

4.2. Predictors of Openness of Communication. Hierarchical multiple regression analysis was conducted to identify the variables which predicted openness of communication (Table 3). Individual nursing characteristics were entered in Step 1, explaining 8.4% of the variation in open communication among nurses (nonsignificant). After entry of the

TABLE 2: Differences in openness and accuracy of communication.

(a)

	Within nursing Mean (SD)	Between DR and RN Mean (SD)	t	P
Open communication	5.74 (1.00)	4.45 (1.30)	10.227	.000
Accuracy of communication	2.68 (.80)	2.82 (.91)	2.18	.031

(b)

	RN ($n = 119$) M (SD)	LPN ($n = 135$) M (SD)	t	P
Open communication with nurses	5.75 (1.01)	6.32 (0.7)	−2.051	.042
Open communication with physicians	4.44 (1.30)	4.60 (1.48)	−.432	.667
Accuracy of communication with nurses	3.29 (0.59)	2.56 (0.4)	4.542	.000
Accuracy of communication with physicians	3.28 (0.65)	3.04 (0.51)	1.350	.179

TABLE 3: Hierarchical multiple regression analysis predicting openness of communication ($n = 135$).

	Open communication among nurses				Open communication between nurses and physicians			
	β	$t(P)$	β	$t(P)$	β	$t(P)$	β	$t(P)$
Constant	5.542	.000	4.983	.000	3.007	.000	0.361	.375
LPN(RN = 0)	0.637	.042	0.325	.245	0.141	.724	−0.47	.072
Education	0.14	.419	0.018	.908	0.454	.049	0.189	.197
Nights(day = 0)	0.021	.914	−0.098	.572	0.033	.897	−0.119	.475
Evenings	−0.49	.087	−0.473	.061	−0.315	.400	−0.477	.048
Rotating	−0.6	.137	−0.213	.553	0.052	.922	−0.036	.916
Expertise	0.006	.917	0.001	.982	0.08	.302	−0.029	.569
Experience	0.009	.891	−0.035	.567	0.071	.425	0.125	.035
Environment			0.274	.000			0.797	.000
Unit B (Unit A = 0)			0.13	.537			0.088	.659
Unit C			−0.594	.009			0.397	.064
Unit D			−0.578	.011			0.493	.022
$F(P)$		1.580 (.148)		5.225 (.000)		1.481 (.180)		19.396 (.000)
R^2		.084		.331		.079		.646
$\triangle R^2$		.084		.247		.079		.567

unit and environmental value variables (Step 2), the total variance explained by the model was 33.1% ($F = 5.25$, $P < .001$). Only environmental values ($P < .001$) and unit ($P = .009$ and $P = .011$) were significant predictors of open communication among nurses. Specifically, the more positive the environmental values (e.g., high trust, respect, etc.), the greater the perception of communication openness among nurses. In addition, unit was a significant predictor, such that nurses on Units C and D noted lower levels of communication openness than the referent group (Unit A).

A second analysis, with dependent variable open communication between nurses and physicians, was computed with independent variables job category, education, shift, experience, and expertise entered in Step 1. Only education level was predictive of open communication between nurses and physicians. Specifically, higher education levels were associated with greater perceptions of communication openness with physician colleagues. In Step 2, the environmental values and unit variables were entered (Table 3). The final model explained 64.6% of the variance ($F = 19.396$, $P < .001$). The significant predictors of open communication with physician included the evening shift ($P = .048$), years of experience as a nurse ($P = .035$), environmental values ($P < .001$), and unit (unit 4, $P = .022$). Education levels were

TABLE 4: Hierarchical multiple regression analysis predicting accuracy of communication ($n = 135$).

	Accuracy communication among nurses				Accuracy communication between nurses and physicians			
	β	$t(P)$	β	$t(P)$	β	$t(P)$	β	$t(P)$
constant	2.385	.000	2.952	.000	2.798	.000	3.34	.000
LPN (RN = 0)	−0.994	.000	−0.801	.001	−0.217	.416	0.007	.977
Education	−0.059	.663	0.024	.855	−0.055	.721	0.058	.678
Nights (Day = 0)	0.493	.002	0.549	.000	0.562	.001	0.647	.000
Evenings	0.295	.184	0.311	.142	0.408	.104	0.4	.080
Rotating	0.693	.027	0.577	.057	1	.005	0.724	.028
Expertise	0.03	.520	0.044	.319	−0.025	.629	−0.016	.744
Experience	−0.02	.705	−0.008	.880	−0.009	.883	0.024	.675
Environment			−0.202	.000			−0.241	.000
Unit B (unit A = 0)			−0.098	.583			−0.116	.544
Unit C			0.121	.517			0.375	.065
Unit D			0.1	.600			0.399	.055
$F(P)$	5.026 (.000)		5.345 (.000)		2.790 (.010)		5.235 (.000)	
R^2	.231		.342		.141		.334	
ΔR^2	.231		.111		.141		.193	

no longer a significant predictor. Nurses working the evening shift perceived lower openness of communication compared to day shift nurses. Nurses with more years of experience noted higher levels of openness in communication ($B = .125$, $P = .035$). In addition, a more positive environment was predictive of greater openness in communication ($B = .797$, $P < .001$).

4.3. Predictors of Accuracy of Communication. Hierarchical multiple regression analysis was also used to identify the variables which predicted accuracy of communication (Table 4). Individual nursing characteristics entered in Step 1 explained 23% of the variance in accuracy of communication among nurses ($F = 5.03$, $P < .001$). An additional 11.1% of variation was explained with the inclusion of the unit and the environmental value variables entered in Step 2. The final model ($F = 5.345$, $P < .001$) explained 34.2% of the variance in accuracy of communication (among nurses). Job category (e.g., LPN) ($P = .001$), shift ($P < .001$) (e.g., night), and environmental values ($P < .001$) were significant predictors. Specifically, LPNs perceived less accuracy in communication among the nursing staff than their RN counterparts. Nurses working night shift identified greater accuracy in communication than their day shift colleagues. A more positive environment was associated with less accuracy in communication among nurses.

Another analysis, with dependent variable accuracy of communication between nurses and physicians, was computed with the following independent variables: job category, education, shift, expertise, years of experience, environmental values, and unit. The first model (Step 1) included the nursing characteristics variables and explained 14.1% of the variance in the dependent variable ($F = 2.80$, $P = .01$). The unit and environmental values variables, entered in

Step 2, explained an additional 19.3%, for a total of 33.4% of variance explained ($F = 5.235$, $P < .001$). Significant predictors included shift (night, $P < .001$, and rotating, $P = .028$) and environmental values ($P < .001$). Specifically, nursing staff working night and rotating shifts identified greater accuracy in communication between nurses and physicians than did day shift nurses. In addition, a work environment with greater trust, respect, time, and status equity was predictive of lower accuracy of communication between nurses and physicians ($P < .001$).

5. Discussion

This study sought to identify the relationship between individual nursing characteristics and perceptions of communication with the healthcare team. Findings revealed a significant relationship between some of these variables. Overall, nurses (both RNs and LPNs) reported greater openness among nurses than between nurses and physicians. In contrast, they reported communication between nurses and physicians to be more accurate than among the nursing team.

Significant variation in perceptions of openness and accuracy of communication were identified between RNs and LPNs. RNs identified significantly more accurate communication among nurses whereas LPNs identified significantly greater communication openness. This may in part be related to the role expectations of the LPN and RN. The LPN, due to licensure restrictions, must be assigned to an RN, and therefore frequent interaction among the nurse dyad (RN-LPN) is required. Due to an increase in interactions with RNs, LPNs may note greater inaccuracies in communication among the team. RNs—in contrast to LPNs—can work autonomously due to his/her greater scope of practice, and therefore, do not rely on communication from others to determine patient care needs.

Experience level was also predictive of communication. Specifically, years of experience of the nurse was significantly related to openness of communication among nurses and physicians. This may be in part due to the need for frequent interaction for antecedents of effective communication, including trust and respect, to develop [17]. Also, nurses with greater years of experience may be viewed as having greater expertise among physician colleagues, especially in an acute care environment where physician colleagues may rotate monthly. Higher levels of education were associated with greater perceptions of nurse-physician communication, but when the environment was considered, this was non-significant. This sheds some light on the importance of the context of the environment.

Unit of employment was predictive of openness and accuracy of communication. This may be related to the fact that Unit C and D had the lowest average for years of experience and self-reported expertise, which was shown to predict openness in communication between nurses and physicians. Nurse shift was also significantly associated with perceptions of communication openness and accuracy. Specifically, night shift nurses identified greater levels of accuracy of communication among nurses, and between nurses and physicians compared to nurses on the day shift; in contrast, evening shift nurses identified lower levels of communication openness than the day shift. These findings may be related to the presence of physicians on these shifts. At night, less staff (both nursing and medical) are present, which may result in a greater need to work together to ensure optimal care delivery; communication must be more accurate for timely implementation of appropriate interventions.

The values present in the environment were predictive of all four outcome variables (e.g., openness/accuracy of communication among and between nurses and physicians). As expected, when positive values, such as trust, respect, and status equity, are present on the environment, openness in communication among the healthcare team ensues. This finding is similar to other studies [16, 17] which have noted the impact of these variables on effective communication. Work environments that foster trust, respect, status equity, and time availability create an atmosphere were communication can flourish. Interestingly, the same values that fostered open communication seem to reduce accuracy in communication. According to the study findings, greater presence of the work environment values was associated with less accuracy in communication. One potential reason for this may be that staff working in a positive environment (e.g., trust and respect present) is more willing to state their opinions about patient care needs; Jones and George found trust among team members fostered greater willingness to share information freely among the team [20]. In contrast team members who do not feel valued or believe information may be used inappropriately are less willing to share pertinent information [21]. In such an environment (e.g., low trust and respect), staff may be less likely to share their thoughts, and instead state only facts that are fully supported.

There are two noteworthy limitations of this study. The data for this study came from four acute care units located in one of two Midwestern Hospitals, thus generalizability is limited to similar medical-surgical acute care units. In addition, the survey captured *perceptions* as opposed to *actual* communication patterns. Therefore, the actual accuracy and openness of communication was not measured. To study actual communication patterns would involve an extensive observational study and would be very complex and costly.

6. Conclusions

Communication among the healthcare team is critical for optimal patient care. When communication is not open and accurate, medical errors result. Findings from this study identified nursing characteristics (e.g., experience, unit, shift worked) and the environmental context as essential for open communication. Understanding the environment (e.g., presence or absence of trust, respect, status equity, and time availability) is a foundational step that must occur before implementing any strategies aimed at improving communication. A failure to understand the environment may in part explain why no one strategy has been shown to consistently improve nurse-physician communication [18]. Further research is needed to determine the best strategies for developing trust and respect among the healthcare team. For example, the development of trust requires consistent interaction. Current work environments where staff—both nursing and physicians—rotate, create less opportunity for interaction.

One potential strategy for increasing interactions among the healthcare team would be through consistent team nursing (e.g., nurses on a team work the same shifts/days). This would result in frequent interactions where the antecedents to effective communication (e.g., trust/respect) could develop among the nursing team, and subsequently with other members of the healthcare team.

Another possible strategy for improving communication among the healthcare team includes multidisciplinary education. According to a position paper on interdisciplinary education and practice from the American Association of Colleges of Nursing (AACN), programs and curricula must be developed that incorporate opportunities for collaborative learning and decision making [22]. Educating nurses and physicians together may result in greater role clarity, shared decision making, and more positive attitudes towards collaboration.

Additional strategies for improving communication include encouraging open dialogue, collaborative rounds, and engagement on interdisciplinary committees [23]. This can provide opportunities for discussing problem areas and collaboratively determining strategies to reduce miscommunication. Regardless of strategies implemented, all healthcare professionals have a common commitment to serving the patient and assisting them in reaching their optimal level of functioning. This can result when communication among the healthcare team is open and accurate.

References

[1] E. J. Dunn, P. D. Mills, J. Neily, M. D. Crittenden, A. L. Carmack, and J. P. Bagian, "Medical team training: applying crew resource management in the veterans health administration," *Joint Commission Journal on Quality and Patient Safety*, vol. 33, no. 6, pp. 317–325, 2007.

[2] K. M. Sutcliffe, E. Lewton, and M. M. Rosenthal, "Communication failures: an insidious contributor to medical mishaps," *Academic Medicine*, vol. 79, no. 2, pp. 186–194, 2004.

[3] Joint Commission. Sentinel event data root causes by event type: 2004-fourth quarter, 2010, http://www.jointcommission.org/Sentinel_Event_Statistics/.

[4] D. Rucker, B. O'Connor, and J. Buxbaum, "Reducing errors/improving care," in *HIMSS Symposium and Exhibition*, San Diego, Calif, USA, 2006.

[5] S. Chant, T. Jenkinson, J. Randle, and G. Russell, "Communication skills: some problems in nursing education and practice," *Journal of Clinical Nursing*, vol. 11, no. 1, pp. 12–21, 2002.

[6] A. B. Hamric and L. J. Blackhall, "Nurse-physician perspectives on the care of dying patients in intensive care units: collaboration, moral distress, and ethical climate," *Critical Care Medicine*, vol. 35, no. 2, pp. 422–429, 2007.

[7] M. Kramer and C. Schmalenberg, "Securing "good" nurse/physician relationships," *Nursing Management*, vol. 34, no. 7, pp. 34–38, 2003.

[8] D. K. Boyle and C. Kochinda, "Enhancing collaborative communication of nurse and physician leadership two intensive care units," *Journal of Nursing Administration*, vol. 34, no. 2, pp. 60–70, 2004.

[9] M. Krairiksh and M. K. Anthony, "Benefits and outcomes of staff nurses' participation in decision making," *Journal of Nursing Administration*, vol. 31, no. 1, pp. 16–23, 2001.

[10] W. A. Knaus, E. A. Draper, D. P. Wagner, and J. E. Zimmerman, "An evaluation of outcome from intensive care in major medical centers," *Annals of Internal Medicine*, vol. 104, no. 3, pp. 410–418, 1986.

[11] S. M. Shortell, J. E. Zimmerman, D. M. Rousseau et al., "The performance of intensive care units: does good management make a difference?" *Medical Care*, vol. 32, no. 5, pp. 508–525, 1994.

[12] M. Manojlovich, "Linking the practice environment to nurses' job satisfaction through nurse-physician communication," *Journal of Nursing Scholarship*, vol. 37, no. 4, pp. 367–373, 2005.

[13] P. A. Miller, "Nurse-physician collaboration in an intensive care unit," *American Journal of Critical Care*, vol. 10, no. 5, pp. 341–350, 2001.

[14] B. J. Foley, C. C. Kee, P. Minick, S. S. Harvey, and B. M. Jennings, "Characteristics of nurses and hospital work environments that foster satisfaction and clinical expertise," *Journal of Nursing Administration*, vol. 32, no. 5, pp. 273–282, 2002.

[15] B. A. Mark, J. Salyer, and T. T. H. Wan, "Professional nursing practice: impact on organizational and patient outcomes," *Journal of Nursing Administration*, vol. 33, no. 4, pp. 224–234, 2003.

[16] C. Schmalenberg, M. Kramer, C. R. King et al., "Excellence through evidence: securing collegial/collaborative nurse-physician relationships, part 1," *Journal of Nursing Administration*, vol. 35, no. 10, pp. 450–458, 2005.

[17] K. R. Simpson, D. C. James, and G. E. Knox, "Nurse-physician communication during labor and birth: implications for patient safety," *Journal of Obstetric, Gynecologic, and Neonatal Nursing*, vol. 35, no. 4, pp. 547–556, 2006.

[18] J. A. Seago, "Professional communication," in *Patient Safety and Quality: An Evidence-Based Handbook for Nurses*, R. Hughes, Ed., Agency for Healthcare Research and Quality, Rockville, Md, USA, 2008.

[19] S. M. Shortell, D. M. Rousseau, R. R. Gillies, K. J. Devers, and T. L. Simons, "Organizational assessment in intensive care units (ICUs): construct development, reliability, and validity of the ICU nurse-physician questionnaire," *Medical Care*, vol. 29, no. 8, pp. 709–726, 1991.

[20] G. R. Jones and J. M. George, "The experience and evolution of trust: implications for cooperation and teamwork," *Academy of Management Review*, vol. 23, no. 3, pp. 531–546, 1998.

[21] D. Bandow, "Time to create sound teamwork," *The Journal of Quality and Participation*, vol. 24, no. 2, pp. 41–47, 2001.

[22] American Association of Colleges of Nursing (AACN). AACN position paper: interdisciplinary education and practice; March 1995.

[23] M. O'Daniel and A. Rosenstein, "Professional communication and team collaboration," in *Patient Safety and Quality: An Evidence-Based Handbook for Nurses*, R. Hughes, Ed., Agency for Healthcare Research and Quality, Rockville, Md, USA, 2008.

19

Social Support Associated with Quality of Life in Home Care Patients with Intractable Neurological Disease in Japan

Tomoko Nishida,[1] Eriko Ando,[2] and Hisataka Sakakibara[3]

[1] Department of Nursing, Sugiyama Jogakuen University, 17-3 Hoshigaoka-Motomachi, Chikusa-Ku, Nagoya 464-8662, Japan
[2] Division of Health, Bureau of Health and Welfare, 1-1 Sannomaru 3-Chome, Naka-Ku, Nagoya 460-8508, Japan
[3] Department of Nursing, Nagoya University Graduate School of Medicine, 1-1-20 Daiko-Minami, Higashi-Ku, Nagoya 461-8673, Japan

Correspondence should be addressed to Tomoko Nishida, t-nishida@sugiyama-u.ac.jp

Academic Editor: Linda Moneyham

The aim of the present study was to investigate what kinds of social supports contribute to the higher quality of life (QOL) of home care patients with intractable neurological disease. We investigated the World Health Organization Quality of Life-BREF (WHOQOL-BREF) and social supports to 74 patients with intractable neurological disease in a city of the Aichi prefecture, Japan. Association between WHOQOL and social supports was examined using multiple logistic regression analyses adjusting activities of daily living (ADL). High WHOQOL scores were associated with "attending patient gatherings held by the public health center," "having someone who will listen empathically to anxieties or troubles," and ADL. Physical health was associated with ADL, while psychological well-being was related to "having a hobby," "having someone who will listen," and "having a hospital for admission in emergencies." Patients not having someone who will listen were more likely to participate in the gatherings. The present findings suggest that having someone who will provide emotional support is important for home care patients with neurological diseases. Patient gatherings held by the public health center were expected to provide patients with emotional support.

1. Introduction

Some chronic progressive degenerative neurological diseases without a cure are called "intractable neurological diseases" in Japan, where patients are provided with welfare services such as support for patient's care and subsidization. The diseases include Parkinson's disease, spinocerebellar degeneration, multiple sclerosis, and amyotrophic lateral sclerosis (ALS). They develop degenerative changes and progressively lead to motor paralysis, sensory impairment, involuntary movement, and muscle weakness/atrophy and increasing levels of physical disability [1]. Thereby the patients suffer not only medical and economical problems but also psychological difficulties. It is shown that the diseases have a significant impact on psychological well-being and quality of life (QOL) of patients as well as their physical well-being [2–6].

Many studies have investigated the factors affecting the QOL of patients with intractable neurological disease [7–10]. Social support was one of the effective factors for QOL and well-being of the patients. A strong positive correlation was found between social support and QOL among patients with MS [11]. Social support had an association with lower depression in patients with Parkinson's disease [12]. On the other hand, some studies reported that negative or unsatisfied social support could produce higher psychological distress [13, 14]. It is, hence, important to examine which social supports are helpful for patients with intractable neurological disease.

Social support is composed of material support, informational support, emotional support, and so forth. Especially emotional support is very important. Sympathy, comfort, and affection from a familiar person may be as necessary as useful information and actual help. The patients receive various supports to live at home from their family, friends, medical professionals, and volunteers. In Japan, public health departments also provide patients with support services, such as information about medical care and welfare, giving advice about the troubles of patients and their family and making an occasion to have contacts with patients. The aim of the present study was to investigate what kinds of social supports contribute to the QOL of home care patients with intractable neurological disease. We investigated the concrete social support by familiar persons, professionals, and public institutions to find some supportive measures to improve the QOL of home-care patients.

2. Methods

2.1. Subjects and Survey Methods. The present subjects were recruited from home care patients with neuromuscular diseases living in an area of A city in Japan who were entitled to receive public welfare services for the specified thirteen intractable neurodegenerative and neuromuscular diseases in 2005: Parkinson's disease, spinocerebellar degeneration, ALS, multiple sclerosis, multiple system atrophy, myasthenia gravis, Huntington's disease, adrenoleukodystrophy, subacute sclerosing panencephalitis, neurofibromatosis type 1 and 2, prion disease, amyloidosis, and moyamoya disease. The patients who had been in the hospital, had mental deficiency, and were underage were excluded from the study. This left 120 patients eligible of the subjects as in the present study.

Requests for participation in this survey were first sent by post to these 120 people together with certificates of informed consent. Eighty-nine people (74%) returned the certificates of consent for participation, and then an anonymous self-completed questionnaire form was delivered to them and collected by post. There were surveys that were not answered completely. We excluded these from the analysis. Seventy-four people (62%) completed questionnaires, which were used for analysis in this survey. The survey period was from November 2005 until June 2006. This study was approved by the Ethics Committee of Nagoya University School of Medicine.

2.2. Survey Contents. The Japanese version of the WHOQOL-BREF was used for QOL measurements of the home patients with intractable neurological diseases. The WHOQOL-BREF is widely used in many countries to assess the QOL of both healthy people and those with some disease, and its reliability and validity have been demonstrated [15]. The Japanese version of the WHOQOL-BREF is a 26-item, self-administered questionnaire developed by Tazaki and Nakane [16]. The WHOQOL-BREF consists of two general questions (on assessment of living quality and satisfaction with health) and four domains: physical health (7 items), psychological well-being (6 items), social relationships (3 items), and environment (8 items). Responses to all the items are made on a scale of 1 to 5. In the tallying process, three items of the 26 questions are negative questions, and so the response scale is reversed for tallying. Then, the total scores of WHOQOL-BREF and each domain are transformed into a 4-to-20. The higher scores indicate a higher perceived QOL.

Six items were evaluated for activities of daily living (ADL): walking, eating, toileting, changing clothes, bathing, and going out. Each item was evaluated on a 4-point scale: "Can do myself," "Can do with a little difficulty," "Need partial assistance," and "Need complete assistance." According to the responses, the subjects were classified into three groups. People who responded "Can do myself" or "Can do with a little difficulty" to all 6 items were classified in an independent group. People who did not respond "Need complete assistance" to any question but responded "Need partial assistance" to at least 1 item were classified in a low-level care group, and those who responded "Need complete assistance" to at least 1 item were classified in a high-level care group.

In addition to the above, the survey included questions on the disease name under treatment, medical consultation status, frequency of talking with others, frequency of going out, having/not having a hobby, and social supports. Social supports consisted of four dimensions: personal support (having/not having a caregiver, having/not having a person who will listen empathically to anxieties or troubles, and having/not having someone who helps you whenever you are in trouble), community support (join/does not join self-help patient groups and attend/does not attend patient gatherings held by the public health center), medical support (uses/does not use home-visit nursing or rehabilitation service, has/does not have a hospital which will admit you when your condition suddenly changes, and has received/has not received consultations with medical professionals, an easy-to-understand explanation about their diseases, and up-to-date information during medical visits).

2.3. Statistical Analysis. The subjects were divided into a high-score group and low-score group based on the median value of the total WHOQOL-BREF score and four domain scores. Survey items associations with the QOL were examined using multiple logistic regression analyses in which QOL score (high versus low) was the dependent variable. First, each survey item was included in the logistic regression analyses adjusting for sex, age, and ADL. Second, survey items that tended to be related ($P < 0.10$) were included in the logistic regression analyses, adjusting for sex, age, and ADL. Same analyses were conducted with each of the total WHOQOL and the 4 domains (physical health, psychological well-being, social relationships, and environment). A chi-square test was used to analyze the relation between survey items and the factors related to QOL in multiple logistic regression analysis. P values of < 0.05 were considered statistically significant. These statistical analyses were completed with the statistical software package SPSS 14.0J for Windows.

3. Results

The characteristics of the 74 people in this survey are shown in Table 1. There were 38 males (51.4%) and 36 females (48.6%), with ages of 22–80 years and a mean age of 63.9 ± 12.0 (mean ± standard deviation, SD) years. The number of

TABLE 1: Characteristics of patients with intractable neurological diseases (N = 74).

Age	63.9 ± 12.0
Sex	
Male	38 (51.4)
Female	36 (48.6)
Disease name	
Parkinson's disease	42 (56.8)
Amyotrophic lateral sclerosis	3 (4.1)
Spinocerebellar	10 (13.5)
Multiple sclerosis	7 (9.5)
Multiple system atrophy	4 (5.4)
Myasthenia gravis	3 (4.1)
Other	5 (6.8)
Age at disease onset	55.9 ± 13.6
Duration of illness (years)	7.95 ± 5.49
Living status	
Alone	6 (8.1)
With family	68 (91.9)
Caregiver	
Family members	45 (60.8)
Home care workers	7 (9.5)
Not having caregiver	22 (29.7)
ADL	
Independent group	37 (50.0)
Low-level care group	15 (20.3)
High-level care group	22 (29.7)
WHOQOL-BREF	
Total WHOQOL score	11.6 ± 2.4
Physical health (domain 1)	11.2 ± 3.2
Psychological well-being (domain 2)	11.5 ± 3.3
Social relationships (domain 3)	12.0 ± 3.2
Environment (domain 4)	12.0 ± 2.3

Data are expressed as frequency (%) and mean ± standard deviation (SD).

years under medical treatment was 0–28, with a mean of 8.0 ± 5.5 years. Patients with Parkinson's disease accounted for more than half of the subjects (42 patients, 56.8%), followed by 10 patients (13.5%) with spinocerebellar degeneration, and 7 patients (9.5%) with multiple sclerosis. In terms of ADL, 37 of the patients (50.0%) were in the independent group, 15 (20.3%) were in the low-level care group, and 22 (29.7%) were in the high-level care group.

The Cronbach reliability coefficient for all questions on the WHOQOL-BREF was 0.93. The coefficients for each of its domains were physical health (domain 1) 0.83, psychological well-being (domain 2) 0.89, social relationships (domain 3) 0.74, and environment (domain 4) 0.80. These confirm the good internal consistency of the instrument. The mean of the total WHOQOL-BREF score was 11.6 ± 2.4; the physical health (domain 1) score was 11.2 ± 3.2; psychological well-being (domain 2) score was 11.5 ± 3.3; social relationships (domain 3) score was 12.0 ± 3.2; environment (domain 4) score was 12.0 ± 2.3.

Based on the median value of 11.6 in the total WHOQOL-BREF score, the subjects were divided into a high-score group (n = 35) and a low-score group (n = 39). Logistic regression analyses adjusting for age, sex, and ADL (Table 2) showed significant differences between the two groups in ADL (odds ratio (OR) 2.19, 95% confidence interval (CI) 1.19–4.01), *having a hobby* (OR 3.17, 95% CI 1.30–10.64), *having a person who will listen empathically to anxieties or troubles* (OR 3.29, 95% CI 1.02–10.62), and *attending patient gatherings held by the public health center* (OR 3.83, 95% CI 1.19–12.34). The high QOL score was associated with frequency of going out (OR 1.98, 95% CI 0.97–4.05), though not statistically significant. To clarify factors closely related to QOL score, a multiple logistic regression analysis was conducted with regards to all these factors. As shown in Table 3, significant associations were encountered between the high QOL score and *attending gatherings held by the public health center* (OR 6.07, 95% CI 1.37–26.88) and *having someone who will listen empathically to anxieties or troubles* (OR 6.38, 95% CI 1.31–30.99), in addition to ADL (OR 2.17, 95% CI 1.06–4.43).

Similarly, multiple logistic regression analyses were conducted after adjusting for age, sex, and ADL for each of the 4 domains (Table 4). High physical health (domain 1) was associated with ADL (OR 2.57, 95% CI 1.27–5.20) and *having a person who will listen empathically to anxieties or troubles* (OR 3.42, 95% CI 0.98–11.92). High psychological well-being (domain 2) was associated with *having a hobby* (OR 5.78, 95% CI 1.31–25.52), *having a person who will listen empathically to anxieties or troubles* (OR 8.79, 95% CI 1.17–65.93), *having a hospital for admission* (OR 7.66, 95% CI 1.16–50.36), and *attending patient gatherings held by the public health center* (OR 5.00, 95% CI 0.95–26.32). High social relationships (domain 3) were associated with *not using home-visit nursing or rehabilitation service* (OR 0.04, 95% CI 0.01–0.30) and *having a person who will listen empathically to anxieties or troubles* (OR 4.17, 95% CI 1.04–16.64). High environment (domain 4) was associated with *having a hospital for admission* (OR 5.57, 95% CI 1.29–24.00) and *having a hobby* (OR 3.64, 95% CI 1.10–12.08).

The present study showed an association between the total QOL score and the items of "*having someone who will listen empathically to anxieties and troubles*" and "*attending patient gatherings held by the public health center.*" The characteristics of the factor were further investigated in Table 5. People having someone who will listen empathically to anxieties and troubles were also more likely to have someone who would help them (P < 0.001). In their relations with medical institutions, they tended to understand the explanations given by their doctors about their disease (P = 0.054) and to receive up-to-date information during medical visits (P = 0.086). They also tended to enjoy a hobby (P = 0.070). On the other hand, people not having someone who will listen tended to join self-help patient groups (P = 0.056) and attending patient gatherings held by the public health center (P = 0.058). There was no difference in living with family or not and the severity of ADL. Thirty-five replied "spouse" about the person who will listen empathically to anxieties or troubles, and 17 replied "other member

TABLE 2: Factors related to the total WHOQOL score (Low-score and high-score groups).

	Low-score group (N = 39)	High-score group (N = 35)	Adjusted sex, age, and ADL		
			OR	95% CI	P value
Living status					
Alone	2 (5.1)	4 (11.4)	0.59	0.08–4.21	0.600
With family	37 (94.9)	31 (88.6)			
ADL					
Independent group	17 (43.6)	5 (14.3)			
Low-level care group	8 (20.5)	7 (20.0)	2.19	1.19–4.01	0.011
High-level care group	14 (35.9)	23 (65.7)			
Hobby					
Not having	25 (64.1)	11 (32.4)	3.71	1.30–10.64	0.015
Having	14 (35.9)	23 (67.6)			
Frequency of going out					
Less than one time/week	12 (30.8)	3 (8.6)			
One time/week	7 (17.9)	5 (14.3)	1.98	0.97–4.05	0.060
Two times or more/week	20 (51.3)	27 (77.1)			
A person who will listen empathically to anxieties or troubles					
Not having	18 (47.4)	8 (23.5)	3.29	1.02–10.62	0.046
Having	20 (52.6)	26 (76.5)			
Someone who helps you whenever you are in trouble					
Not having	6 (15.4)	4 (11.4)	1.60	0.35–7.26	0.542
Having	33 (84.6)	31 (88.6)			
Self-help patient group					
Not join	33 (84.6)	26 (76.5)	1.76	0.49–6.24	0.385
Join	6 (15.4)	8 (23.5)			
Patient gatherings held by the public health center					
Not attending	31 (79.5)	20 (57.1)	3.83	1.19–12.34	0.025
Attending	8 (20.5)	15 (42.9)			
Up-to-date information during medical visits					
Not receiving	21 (53.8)	16 (45.7)	1.32	0.47–3.69	0.602
Receiving	18 (46.2)	19 (54.3)			
A hospital which will admit you when your condition suddenly changes					
Not having	14 (35.9)	6 (17.6)	2.31	0.71–7.56	0.165
Having	25 (64.1)	28 (82.4)			
An easy-to-understand explanation about their diseases					
Not receiving	7 (17.9)	7 (20.0)	0.61	0.17–2.20	0.447
Receiving	32 (82.1)	28 (80.0)			
Consultations with medical professionals during medical visits					
Not receiving	14 (35.9)	12 (35.3)	1.69	0.55–5.21	0.362
Receiving	25 (64.1)	22 (64.7)			
Home-visit nursing or rehabilitation service					
Not using	29 (74.4)	32 (91.4)	0.49	0.11–2.19	0.352
Using	10 (25.6)	3 (8.6)			
Home care services					
Not using	33 (84.6)	28 (80.0)	2.70	0.61–11.92	0.190
Using	6 (15.4)	7 (20.0)			

Data are expressed as frequency (%), odds ratio (OR), and 95% confidential interval (CI) of logistic regression analysis.
Odds ratio shows relation with the total QOL score (low-score and high-score groups) and each factor after adjusting for sex, age, and ADL, using multiple logistic regression analysis.
P value by multiple logistic regression analysis.

TABLE 3: Correlates of the total WHOQOL score (low- and high-score groups).

| | Multiple adjustment | | |
	OR	95% CI	P value
ADL	2.17	1.06–4.43	0.033
Hobby	2.25	0.69–7.37	0.179
Frequency of going out	1.78	0.81–3.94	0.152
A person who will listen empathically to anxieties or troubles	6.38	1.31–30.99	0.022
Patient gatherings held by public health center	6.07	1.37–26.88	0.018

Data are expressed by involving odds ratio (OR) and 95% confidential interval (CI) of logistic regression analysis.
Odds ratio shows value turned on sex, age, ADL, a person who will listen empathically to anxieties or trouble, frequency of going out, not attending/attending patient gatherings held by the public health center, and not having/having hobby.
P value by multiple logistic regression analysis.

TABLE 4: Correlates of each domain of WHOQOL-BREF score (low- and high-score groups).

| | Adjusted sex, age, and ADL | | Multiple adjustment | |
	OR[a] (95% CI)	P value	OR[b] (95% CI)	P value
Physical health (domain 1)				
ADL			2.57 (1.27–5.20)	0.009
A person who will listen empathically to anxieties or troubles			3.42 (0.98–11.92)	0.053
Psychological well-being (domain 2)				
ADL	—	—	1.60 (0.72–3.59)	0.249
Hobby	8.47 (2.44–29.47)	0.001	5.78 (1.31–25.52)	0.021
A person who will listen empathically to anxieties or troubles	3.42 (0.98–11.90)	0.054	8.79 (1.17–65.93)	0.034
A hospital which will admit you when your condition suddenly changes	3.34 (0.92–12.08)	0.066	7.66 (1.16–50.36)	0.034
Frequency of going out	2.10 (0.98–4.50)	0.057	1.87 (0.72–4.86)	0.196
Patient gatherings held by the public health center	3.18 (1.01–9.98)	0.048	5.00 (0.95–26.32)	0.058
Social relationships (domain 3)				
ADL	—	—	0.57 (0.24–1.39)	0.219
A person who will listen empathically to anxieties or troubles	4.76 (1.57–14.37)	0.006	4.17 (1.04–16.64)	0.043
Someone who helps you whenever you are in trouble	5.27 (1.17–23.81)	0.031	3.15 (0.53–18.72)	0.208
Home-visit nursing or rehabilitation service	0.04 (0.01–0.27)	0.001	0.04 (0.01–0.30)	0.001
Environment (domain 4)				
ADL	—	—	0.53 (0.26–1.08)	0.082
A hospital which will admit you when your condition suddenly changes	4.49 (1.36–14.76)	0.013	5.57 (1.29–24.00)	0.021
Up-to-date information during medical visits	2.31 (0.86–6.19)	0.097	2.62 (0.75–9.11)	0.131
Hobby	2.46 (0.93–6.53)	0.070	3.64 (1.10–12.08)	0.035
Self-help patient group	3.07 (0.84–11.20)	0.089	4.07 (0.88–18.93)	0.073

Data are expressed as odds ratio (OR) and 95% confidential interval (CI) of logistic regression analysis.
[a] Odds ratio shows relation with each domain of WHOQOL-BREF and each factor after adjusting for sex, age, and ADL.
[b] Odds ratio shows relation with each domain and the factors that tend to be related ($P < 0.10$) when adjusting for sex, age, and ADL.
P value by multiple logistic regression analysis.

of their family" (including multiple answers). Nine replied "friends or other person." Patients who had attended patient gatherings held by the public health center also tended to join self-help patient groups ($P = 0.004$). There were no differences in other items.

4. Discussion

The present study showed that the total WHOQOL of home care patients with intractable neurological disease was associated with "attending patient gatherings held by the public health center" and "having someone who will listen

empathically to anxieties or troubles" as well as ADL. ADL was associated with physical health, while "having someone who will listen" was related with psychological well-being. Earlier studies have shown an association between QOL of patients with neurological diseases and the severity of ADL [4, 17]. Although the present study showed a similar relation between the total WHOQOL score and ADL, the relationship with ADL was found in the physical domain, but not in the psychological domain. The present findings may suggest that emotional support such as "having someone who will listen empathically to anxieties or troubles" is important for home care patients with intractable neurological diseases, regardless of the severity of ADL.

TABLE 5: Relation with a person who will listen empathically to anxieties or troubles with the use of welfare resources and medical institutions.

	Have no person who will listen		Have person who will listen		P value
	n	%	n	%	
Living status					
Alone	1	3.8	5	10.9	0.408
With family	25	96.2	41	89.1	
Hobby					
Not having	17	65.4	18	40.0	0.070
Having	9	34.6	27	60.0	
Patient gatherings held by the public health center					
Not attending	14	53.8	36	78.3	0.058
Attending	12	46.2	10	21.7	
Someone who helps you whenever you are in trouble					
Not having	9	34.6	1	2.2	<0.001
Having	17	65.4	45	97.8	
Self-help patient group					
Not join	18	69.2	40	88.9	0.056
Join	8	30.8	5	11.1	
Up-to-date information during medical visits					
Not receiving	17	65.4	19	41.3	0.086
Receiving	9	34.6	27	58.7	
An easy-to-understand explanation about their diseases					
Not receiving	8	30.8	5	10.9	0.054
Receiving	18	69.2	41	89.1	
Consultations with medical professionals during medical visits					
Not receiving	13	50.0	13	28.3	0.112
Receiving	13	50.0	33	71.7	

Data are expressed as frequency (%). P value by chi-square test.

Previous studies have reported that QOL was linked with depression, fatigue, and anxiety among patients with neurological diseases [5, 18, 19]. A study has indicated that depression was a major contributor to the QOL scores of patients with Parkinson's disease [6]. Meanwhile, an association between QOL and the existence of confiding and emotional support has been reported among people with neuromuscular disorders [20], Parkinson's disease [14], and ALS patients [21]. It is, hence, considered that emotional supports from family, friends, and health professionals are important to improve their symptoms of depression and QOL [9, 22]. In the present study, people having someone who will listen were also more likely to have someone who helps whenever he or she is in trouble. These findings suggested that the presence of someone nearby who will provide emotional as well as physical support was a key factor in the QOL of patients with neurological diseases.

Most of the patients replied "spouse" or "other member of their family" about persons who will listen empathically to anxieties or troubles. A family member is one of the most important factors affecting the QOL of patients with neuro-logical disease [23]. A previous study of ALS patients showed the importance of the presence of caring family as well as

the availability of technical aids [24]. In the present study, most patients (91.9%) had lived with family, and 60.8% had been cared for by family members. However, about one-third (35.1%) of the present patients replied "no" to a question of "having someone who will listen empathically to anxieties or troubles." These results may suggest that their family cannot necessarily be such an emotional supporter as a person who would listen empathically to anxieties of the patients, even if patients live with family. On the other hand, family caregivers may bear physical and psychological distress [25–27]. A study on family caregivers of patients with Parkinson's disease has reported an association between the caregiver's psychological burden and QOL of the patients [28]. We could not elucidate the psychological states and burden of their family, because we did not investigate their family. But family caregivers may have anxieties or troubles due to the burden of caring, and they would also need social supports.

The present results showed a close relationship between the total QOL score and "attending patient gatherings held by the public health center." Such relations were encountered in the psychological domain, though the significance was borderline ($P = 0.058$). The public health center in the city under study holds gatherings regularly for patients with neurological diseases and their family to contact and communicate with each other. On these occasions, public health nurses counsel the patients and their families. Such gatherings may be good occasions to provide patients and their family with emotional support to improve their QOL. Reversely, it was also shown that some patients not having someone who will listen were more likely to participate in the gatherings. The patients and families may attend such gatherings to seek out someone who will listen empathically to them or where they can find companionship for physical and emotional help.

In the present study, "having a hospital which will admit you when your condition suddenly changes" was associated with QOL in the psychological domain and environment domain. Previous studies have reported that anxiety about a medical institute to be accepted in emergencies was associated with QOL [29] and that patients satisfied with their medical care tended to have higher QOL [2, 29]. A study of ALS patients reported that higher patient satisfaction was related to their feeling that the physician understood their feelings [30]. For home care patients with intractable neurological diseases, having a certain hospital for admission can provide a sense of ease, as a place that can deal with sudden changes or emergencies. Medical institutions and professionals are necessary for patients as a place of refuge and people who can give medical care and provide emotional supports.

There were some limitations in this study. The present study had only 74 (62%) subjects within a limited area. These results may not adequately reflect the general conditions of home care patients with neurological diseases in Japan. Second, neurological diseases of participants in this study were of several kinds, so the findings may have been potentially affected by the kind of neurological diseases. Moreover, their QOL was assessed using the WHOQOL-BREF, a general QOL assessment, though it is used to assess the QOL of people with some disease as well. Specific assessment items may be required in the case of individual neurological diseases. Finally, this was a cross-sectional study, but longitudinal assessments will also be warranted since neurological diseases gradually lead to deterioration.

5. Conclusion

The present study found that the QOL of home care patients with intractable neurological disease was associated with "attending patient gatherings held by the public health center" and "having someone who will listen empathically to anxieties or troubles" as well as ADL. The present findings suggested that having someone who will provide emotional support was important for home care patients with neurological diseases. Furthermore, patient gatherings held by the public health center were expected to provide patients with emotional support. The patients and their families may attend such gatherings to seek out someone who will listen empathically to them or where they can find companionship for physical and emotional help. Public health nurses may be able to use the gatherings to provide emotional support to patients.

Conflict of Interests

There are no conflict of interests to disclose.

References

[1] D. L. Kasper, E. Braunwald, S. Hauser et al., *Harrison's Principles of Internal Medicine*, McGraw-Hill, New York, NY, USA, 16th edition, 2004.

[2] Global Parkinson's Disease Survey Steering Committee, "Factors impacting on quality of life in Parkinson's disease: results from an international survey," *Movement Disorders*, vol. 17, no. 1, pp. 60–67, 2002.

[3] M. S. Hirayama, S. Gobbi, L. T. B. Gobbi, and F. Stella, "Quality of life (QoL) in relation to disease severity in Brazilian Parkinson's patients as measured using the WHOQOL-BREF," *Archives of Gerontology and Geriatrics*, vol. 46, no. 2, pp. 147–160, 2008.

[4] K. H. Karlsen, E. Tandberg, D. Årsland, and J. P. Larsen, "Health related quality of life in Parkinson's disease: a prospective longitudinal study," *Journal of Neurology Neurosurgery and Psychiatry*, vol. 69, no. 5, pp. 584–589, 2000.

[5] A. Schrag, F. Geser, M. StampferKountchev et al., "Health-related quality of life in multiple system atrophy," *Movement Disorders*, vol. 21, no. 6, pp. 809–815, 2006.

[6] J. Sławek, M. Derejko, and P. Lass, "Factors affecting the quality of life of patients with idiopathic Parkinson's disease-a cross-sectional study in an outpatient clinic attendees," *Parkinsonism and Related Disorders*, vol. 11, no. 7, pp. 465–468, 2005.

[7] M. B. Bromberg, "Assessing quality of life in ALS," *Journal of Clinical Neuromuscular Disease*, vol. 9, no. 2, pp. 318–325, 2007.

[8] L. Dennison, R. Moss-Morris, and T. Chalder, "A review of psychological correlates of adjustment in patients with multiple sclerosis," *Clinical Psychology Review*, vol. 29, no. 2, pp. 141–153, 2009.

[9] K. S. Malcomson, L. Dunwoody, and A. S. Lowe-Strong, "Psychosocial interventions in people with multiple sclerosis: a review," *Journal of Neurology*, vol. 254, no. 1, pp. 1–13, 2007.

[10] J. Marinus, C. Ramaker, J. J. van Hilten, and A. M. Stiggelbout, "Health related quality of life in Parkinson's disease: a systematic review of disease specific instruments," *Journal of Neurology Neurosurgery and Psychiatry*, vol. 72, no. 2, pp. 241–248, 2002.

[11] C. Schwartz and R. Frohner, "Contribution of demographic, medical, and social support variables in predicting the mental health dimension of quality of life among people with multiple sclerosis," *Health and Social Work*, vol. 30, no. 3, pp. 203–212, 2005.

[12] Y. Cheng, C. Liu, C. Mao, J. Qian, K. Liu, and G. Ke, "Social support plays a role in depression in Parkinson's disease: a cross-section study in a Chinese cohort," *Parkinsonism and Related Disorders*, vol. 14, no. 1, pp. 43–45, 2008.

[13] L. H. Goldstein, L. Atkins, S. Landau, R. G. Brown, and P. N. Leigh, "Longitudinal predictors of psychological distress and self-esteem in people with ALS," *Neurology*, vol. 67, no. 9, pp. 1652–1658, 2006.

[14] J. Simpson, K. Haines, G. Lekwuwa, J. Wardle, and T. Crawford, "Social support and psychological outcome in people with Parkinson's disease: evidence for a specific pattern of associations," *British Journal of Clinical Psychology*, vol. 45, no. 4, pp. 585–590, 2006.

[15] The WHOQOL Group, "Development of the World Health Organization WHOQOL-BREF quality of life assessment," *Psychological Medicine*, vol. 28, no. 3, pp. 551–558, 1998.

[16] M. Tazaki and M. Nakane, *WHOQOL26 Guidance*, Kaneko-Shobo, Tokyo, Japan, 1997.

[17] T. Iizuka, Y. Ogata, M. Minowa, and T. Fujita, "A follow-up study on effects of ADL deterioration on QOL in patients with neurological intractable diseases," *Nippon Kōshū Eisei Zasshi*, vol. 46, no. 8, pp. 595–603, 1999.

[18] V. Janardhan and R. Bakshi, "Quality of life in patients with multiple sclerosis: the impact of fatigue and depression," *Journal of the Neurological Sciences*, vol. 205, no. 1, pp. 51–58, 2002.

[19] A. Vignola, A. Guzzo, A. Calvo et al., "Anxiety undermines quality of life in ALS patients and caregivers," *European Journal of Neurology*, vol. 15, no. 11, pp. 1231–1236, 2008.

[20] L. H. Goldstein, L. Atkins, and P. N. Leigh, "Correlates of quality of life in people with motor neuron disease (MND)," *Amyotrophic Lateral Sclerosis and other Motor Neuron Disorders*, vol. 3, no. 3, pp. 123–129, 2002.

[21] K. Okamoto, T. Kihira, T. Kondo et al., "Changing QOL in ALS patient and examination concerning the related factor," *Kosei no Shihyo*, vol. 52, no. 5, pp. 29–33, 2005 (Japanese).

[22] J. E. McLeod and D. M. Clarke, "A review of psychosocial aspects of motor neurone disease," *Journal of the Neurological Sciences*, vol. 258, no. 1-2, pp. 4–10, 2007.

[23] M. A. Lee, R. W. Walker, A. J. Hildreth, and W. M. Prentice, "Individualized assessment of quality of life in idiophatic Parkinson's disease," *Movement Disorders*, vol. 21, no. 11, pp. 1929–1934, 2006.

[24] M. Hecht, T. Hillemacher, E. Gräsel et al., "Subjective experience and coping in ALS," *Amyotrophic Lateral Sclerosis and Other Motor Neuron Disorders*, vol. 3, no. 4, pp. 225–232, 2002.

[25] A. Gauthier, A. Vignola, A. Calvo et al., "A longitudinal study on quality of life and depression in ALS patient-caregiver couples," *Neurology*, vol. 68, no. 12, pp. 923–926, 2007.

[26] M. Miyashita, Y. Narita, A. Sakamoto et al., "Care burden and depression in caregivers caring for patients with intractable neurological diseases at home in Japan," *Journal of the Neurological Sciences*, vol. 276, no. 1-2, pp. 148–152, 2009.

[27] R. A. Ray and A. F. Street, "Caregiver bodywork: family members' experiences of caring for a person with motor neurone disease," *Journal of Advanced Nursing*, vol. 56, no. 1, pp. 35–43, 2006.

[28] P. Martínez-Martín, J. Benito-León, F. Alonso et al., "Quality of life of caregivers in Parkinson's disease," *Quality of Life Research*, vol. 14, no. 2, pp. 463–472, 2005.

[29] S. Kodera, K. Tanji, A. Watanabe et al., "Intractable disease Patient's QOL and relation between medical treatment and health needs," *Kosei no Shihyo*, vol. 51, no. 15, pp. 1–7, 2004 (Japanese).

[30] A. Chiò, A. Montuschi, S. Cammarosano et al., "ALS patients and caregivers communication preferences and information seeking behaviour," *European Journal of Neurology*, vol. 15, no. 1, pp. 51–60, 2008.

20

Living with Uncertainty: Older Persons' Lived Experience of Making Independent Decisions over Time

Agneta Breitholtz,[1,2] **Ingrid Snellman,**[3] **and Ingegerd Fagerberg**[1,4]

[1] *Department of Neurobiology, Care Sciences and Society (NVS), Karolinska Institutet, 141 83 Huddinge, Sweden*
[2] *School of Health, Care and Social Welfare, Mälardalen University, P.O. Box 883, 721 23 Västerås, Sweden*
[3] *School of Health, Care and Social Welfare, Mälardalen University, P.O. Box 325, 631 05 Eskilstuna, Sweden*
[4] *Department of Health Care Sciences, Ersta Sköndal University College, P.O. Box 11189, 100 61 Stockholm, Sweden*

Correspondence should be addressed to Agneta Breitholtz; agneta.breitholtz@mdh.se

Academic Editor: Pirkko Routasalo

The aim of the study was to illuminate the meaning of older persons' independent decision making concerning their daily care. Autonomy when in care is highly valued in the western world. However, research shows that autonomy can give rise to problematic issues. The complexity of independence and dependence for older people when living at home with help has also been highlighted. In Sweden, older people are increasingly expected to live at home with help from municipal home care services, and study into this aspect of care is limited. This study is a part of an ongoing project and has a qualitative life world perspective. Audiotaped narrative interviews were conducted and analysed using a phenomenological hermeneutic method. Findings revealed a main theme: "living with uncertainty as to how to relate one's own independence and dependence with regard to oneself, and others." This involves a constant process of relating to one's independence controlled by others or oneself, and adjusting one's independence and dependence with regard to oneself and others. The conclusion is that professional carers need to acknowledge the changing vulnerability of dependent older persons over time. The implication is a relational approach to autonomy beyond the traditional individualistic approach.

1. Introduction

The care of the old, with an increasing population over 60 years old, presents a challenge worldwide [1]. In Sweden municipalities are responsible for the care of the old, and older people are now increasingly expected to live at home aided by municipal home help services. As a consequence older people's care needs have increased as well as the workload for professional carers [2]. Older people apply for support, and the help available includes laundry, cleaning, shopping, personal care, meals, and emergency alarms. Care managers assess their needs according to the Social Service Act, which requires that people's right to self-determination and integrity should be respected [3].

Autonomy when in care is highly valued in the western world and involves people's right to make their own choices without involving others [4–6]. Nevertheless, in the care of

the old this individualistic approach to autonomy is problematic due to their dependence on others in their everyday lives [4, 7–9]. However, Sandman [6] argues that it is important to recognize that people value their autonomy differently. Further, it is therefore important to distinguish between different aspects of autonomy, that is, self-determination, freedom, desire fulfilment, and independence. The most central aspect is considered self-determination and means how people make decisions in accordance with their own will. Whereas independence means how people perform or carry out decisions regardless if they decide to do it themselves or hand it over to someone else to decide. Olaison and Cedersund [10] found that in assessment meetings between care managers and older people applying for home care the focus was on fixed standard solutions based on social service practice, and older people had to negotiate within the standard solution context to make clear their individual needs.

Research into older people in need of home help and care highlights the complexity of independence and dependence. Independence for older people has both positive aspects, for example to be able to make one's own decisions, and negative aspects in terms of isolation and underestimating one's needs [11]. In a study [12] with older people of their experiences of frailty and followed over time, findings show the complexity of how they balanced between autonomy and dependence. The findings of Hammarström and Torres [13] show the complexity of older people's striving for self-determination at the same time as accepting their dependency. However, Welford et al. [14] reveals in a concept analysis of autonomy for older people in residential care that professional carers can improve older people's autonomy in caring relationships and create the opportunity for them to be involved in decision making based on their own abilities.

Studies into older people's independent decision making using municipal home help services appear to be rare. Nevertheless research shows the complexity of the balance between independence and dependence for older people in home help care. In addition the findings in Breitholtz et al. [15] study reveal that the older persons struggled for the opportunity versus resigning themselves to losing the opportunity to make their own decisions. This was further understood as the older persons are not being treated as individuals, not having their needs met, and their life situation being stressful. These findings were considered important and inspired us to further deepen the understanding of the older persons' lived experiences of making independent decisions. This study is a part of an on-going project adopting a qualitative and life world perspective [16] to illuminate the meaning of older person's independent decision making and of their professional carers to enable this. Accordingly, the focus is on the meaning of the lived experiences. The aim of this study was to illuminate the meaning of older persons' independent decision making concerning their daily care.

2. Materials and Methods

2.1. Participants. The participants were seven older persons who had been part of the project from the start and who are presented elsewhere [15]. The inclusion criteria were aged 70 or more, both men and women, being able to speak and understand Swedish, and varied levels of care needs and still living alone at home with daily help from municipal home help services. In addition they were cognitively screened prior to enrolment and before data collection for this present study according to MMSE [17], requiring a score of at least 24 out of 30. Before data collection commenced staff managers phoned the old people to ask if they were still interested in participating and being cognitively screened again. After they had been screened and given their verbal consent to continue participating they were phoned by the first author and an appointment for a second interview was set up. Participants were between 80 and 91 years old, with four from one municipality and three from another, and with one man and six women. They still lived alone at home with professional carers visiting between one to six times a day. The domestic help provided consisted of tasks such as preparing meals, cleaning, washing up and making up beds, and care help with such matters as personal hygiene.

2.2. Data Collection. In order to deepen the meaning and understanding of the participating older persons' lived experiences of independent decision making, they were each interviewed three times in October and November 2009 and January 2010. The interviews were conducted during and after one of the participating older persons' professional carer, they were paired with, participated in an educational programme. The same [15] open-ended interview guide was used with open questions such as the following. Can you tell me what it is like when professional carers help you with your daily care? Can you tell me how you experience the opportunity to make your own decisions about your daily care when a professional carer is helping you? To deepen the understanding follow-up questions were asked such as the following. Can you tell me more about what you thought about that? Can you tell me some more about how you felt? Participants were encouraged to narrate as freely as possible about their lived experiences of making independent decisions. The interviews were conducted in the older person's homes and lasted between 40 to 65 minutes.

2.3. Data Analysis. Data analysis followed the phenomenological hermeneutic methodological stages: naïve reading, structural analysis, and comprehensive understanding with a dialectic movement between explanation and understanding [18, 19]. The three interviews with each participant were first separately transcribed and read and a first naive understanding was formulated for each of them. Thereafter, all interviews were analysed as a whole to enable an in-depth understanding of the older persons lived experiences. A naïve understanding was formulated and guided the succeeding structural analysis. This analysis began with dividing the whole text into meaning units expressing one meaning and those were further condensed to formulate the essential meaning as briefly as possible. The condensed meaning units were then abstracted in an on-going process into sub-themes, themes and a main theme (see Table 1). They were further reflected upon with the naive understanding in mind, in an on-going process to validate the naïve understanding. A comprehensive understanding was formulated through reflections on the interview texts, naive understanding, main theme, themes and sub themes, the research question, authors' preunderstanding, and relevant literature to deepen the understanding [18].

2.4. Ethical Considerations. This study was approved by the Regional Ethics Committee (ref. 2008/256). Participants were informed in advance [15] that they would be paired with a professional carer, followed over time and cognitively screened again prior to their continued participation. Confidentiality was assured and an informed consent was signed and collected before the first interview. They were contacted by the staff manager before data collection for this study and asked if they still wanted to participate. This procedure was chosen primarily to obtain a declaration that the older persons receiving municipal home help service still wanted

TABLE 1: Examples of the structural analysis.

Meaning units	Condensed meaning units	Subtheme	Theme	Main theme
Yes, they come with me and sometimes they have to go on their own if I am not well and I have to stay home. Well sometimes I go by myself.... Well it is like you look forward to something at the beginning of the week then you go shopping. But I am not allowed to really.... I am happy with the way it is.... Well I go along with the way things are. Well I wait for Friday as if it is something special	To not be able to go out and shop for oneself and to be dependent on professional carers help imply that one's wishes will be limited. It does not feel good but it will work	Neglecting one's own need to allow for the needs of others	Adjusting one's own independence and dependence with regard to oneself and others	Living with uncertainty as to how to relate one's own independence and dependence with regard to oneself and others
If the professional carer does not have the time then she tells me. Then I have to understand that she will have to rush off somewhere else. There could be other people lying on the floor needing help to get up, so that is what comes first	To accept that the professional carer says that she does not have the time to help. There may be other caretakers who need her help urgently which she must attend to first			
Well there are some who are a little bit faster but she is rarely here but that doesn't really matter. Well they sometimes are in a hurry like that.... It is not often they take their time. It is different; all girls are different and do different things. Well you know who is who and who is better than the other but you never say anything because each of them does things their way. Well I would not do it that way, but we all are different I get the help I should have anyway...	All professional carers are different; some are more stressed than others. One does not always agree with their ideas. To accept as long as they do what they should	Withholding one's thoughts		
Usually you can tell by looking at people what they want themselves and what they would think if you get too close or like that. If you ask someone about a personal matter they will tell you, if they do not like it, of course they would. But it happens so rarely so I cannot recall, you really notice on people how open they are. Well then you avoid that of course, remembering those you can't talk to anyhow or about anything. Others I can talk to about anything as if they were one's daughter coming to visit	Some professional carer is more difficult to get contact with than others. It is important to know who want to open or distance themselves. To learn gradually wish of them, it is possible to talk to or not			

to participate and that their health had not declined since the first interview was conducted in spring 2009.

3. Findings

3.1. Naïve Understanding. Making independent decisions is conditional on the other people involved in the organization. One's life is a part of that organization that includes all the people being involved, and one tries to understand how one fits in. To make it smoother for all persons involved, one complies and sets aside one's own needs and wishes. One's own ability to express needs and wishes are limited by the fact that the decisions and regulations within the organization are outside one's own control and that of professional carers. To expect the arrival of a particular professional carer is both joyful when they show up but also disappointing if they do not. The endless wait for them to come limits one's own freedom or induces feelings of fear of being left alone and not being able to take care of oneself in one's own home. Deciding for oneself is to have the opportunity to participate in one's own care and a trustful relationship with professional carers, giving and taking with each other. The wish is to be independent and professional carers are an extended arm no matter who provides the help. Yet one's own dependency

TABLE 2: Subthemes, themes, and main theme.

Sub-themes	Theme	Main theme
Relying on others to manage one's life	One's independence lies in the hands of others	Living with uncertainty as to how to relate to independence and dependence with regard to oneself and others
Deciding for oneself is beyond one's reach		
Waiting for others to come		
Deciding for oneself when to become involved	One's independence lies in one's own hands	
Managing oneself with professional carers as an extended arm		
Handing over the decisions to others		
Giving and taking in the relationship with professional carers		
Neglecting one's own needs to allow for the needs of others	Adjusting one's own independence and dependence with regard to oneself and others	
Withholding one's thoughts		

changes over time and it feels safe to hand over responsibility to a professional carer to decide about one's daily care. It may involve an implicit struggle and a wish that the responsibility should rest in their hands, but it is not taken for granted that they acknowledge one's spoken or unspoken needs. The ability to receive help from one's surroundings makes one feel less dependent on one's professional carers. Not wanting to be a bother to one's relatives makes oneself feel more dependent on professional carers.

3.2. *Structural Analysis.* The findings from the structural analysis are presented in a main theme following themes and their subthemes (see Table 2).

3.2.1. *Living with Uncertainty as to How to Relate One's Own Independence and Dependence with regard to Oneself and Others.* Making independent decisions in daily care over a period of time involves "Living with uncertainty as to how to relate one's own independence and dependence with regard to oneself and others." Being aware of one's own vulnerability to dependence on others and still wanting to be independent presents a life-changing situation, as one tries to comprehend one's everyday life. This comprehension involves relating to one's own independence and dependence on others, but this raises uncertainty because one's dependence changes over time and is affected by circumstances within the organizations and professional carers' working conditions. It makes it complicated and one has to live with uncertainty every day since one never knows who is going to come. Although one has a particular professional carer who provides special attention over a period of time, there is still no guarantee that one's needs and wishes will be fulfilled, and one is still uncertain when this person will come. Being uncertain makes one dependent on others such as relatives and other people in

the organization, and one tries to comprehend how to make it work for all persons involved.

3.2.2. *One's Independence Lies in the Hands of Others.* When *relying on others to manage one's life* one has to strive for independence with the help of others. Feeling independent depends on what help one may get from professional carers and close friends and family. On the one hand being able to get help from relatives, friends, or the private sector facilitates a decreased independence on one's professional carers. On the other hand, one's desire to not burden relatives induces an increased dependence on professional carers.

> Well, I just told her that we only can have one lamp on in the bathroom. Directly she says, but then I can help you I can fix that for you she said. Well at that time I had already had my breakfast so she didn't have to make any breakfast for me. Afterwards when I had taken the shower and my foot was fixed, well she reckoned she had the time to fix it for me. But otherwise I never ask for help like that, because I have my children who help me with many things. I usually try to let them fix things like this for me. But otherwise it is no problem for me to ask for help with things and I get it done.

Independence is relying on the willingness of others to help, and this is something one tries to handle to organize life in the best interest of all persons involved.

Deciding for oneself is beyond one's reach when others are making decisions about one's needs and without having the opportunity to express one's wishes due to the time-pressured working of professional carers. One has no opportunity to arrange their work schedules, and one therefore, has to accept that one may have to meet different people every time. One's own needs and wishes are not fulfilled when one has to follow their work schedules without the opportunity to express what would be appropriate for oneself.

> *Well they just bring what I want, but I do not like though that they are not allowed to heat in a pot nor in a frying pan. They are only allowed to heat food up in the microwave. It becomes quite monotonous. They are not allowed to fry eggs or anything like that. There is a lot that you would like to have that can only be fried, but they are not allowed to do that. Well, it is just that you have to have stuff that goes in the microwave and it's not good, an omelette would be nice. No, they are not allowed under any circumstances. Well, it would feel like a relief because I could shop differently than I do now.*

Care managers assess one's needs and professional carers have to follow their decisions with no opportunity for oneself or them to change these. Having to ask care managers for support on every single help need complicates everyday life.

Waiting for others to come not knowing at what time professional carers will arrive limits one's freedom to live in accordance with one's life plans. It prevents one from making plans for everyday life, when you are sitting and waiting for them. Even though one can leave home it is not good knowing someone is there while one is out. Not knowing when they show up can also induce a feeling of limited freedom and of being disturbed trying to live one's life, but also a fear of being abandoned and not being able to take care of oneself.

> *... It is tough very very tough, well phew.... That is really the worst part of it, being in the bed well, because then I am vulnerable. That is why I tell them every time when they leave, make sure the door is locked. Because it would be awful if someone broke in, well there would be absolutely nothing you could do... ugh....*

Expecting and waiting for a particular carer that one trusts is a joyful experience, but disappointing if they do not turn up. One just waits and gets ready for someone in particular to come who can fulfil one's wishes and needs.

3.2.3. One's Independence Lies in One's Own Hands. Deciding for oneself when to become involved and having the opportunity to decide, when expressing one's wishes for encouraging and responsive professional carers, is good. It is also good having control over situations, knowing the best way to carry out chores for one's own personal well-being, and making one's own decisions in line with one's wishes when one has different alternatives to choose from. Not being restricted in one's own private home allows one to be free to decide.

> *... I do not want anything more on the table than this, one newspaper, perhaps a crossword and then the medicine that is what I want, and those pens as well. They do not care a bit, and say that my table is a mess, they never do care. But, I just tell*

them, I want this stuff, that's it. But no one has ever said something like that, like someone has said do not have it this way, put it this way or that way instead. No they couldn't do that....

Arriving at the best solutions with professional carers allows one to decide. When they have time to listen to one's wishes it enables one to decide for oneself in cooperation with them, like being asked if there is something more one needs help with or feeling free to ask for more help.

When *managing oneself with professional carers as an extended arm*, although being dependent, the help given infuses a feeling of independence. It does not matter which one of them turns up since they are all equal. One can take care of oneself, just having them as an extended arm performing chores one is not capable of alone.

> *... I do not see any difference between the girls, they do exactly what I tell them. They just stand next to me watching when I step into the shower, all of them do. Then when I sit there washing, which I want to do myself, they leave and make up the bed. Then I just call out and tell them to help me wash my back, which they do. Then they leave and do whatever they have to do, like washing the dishes. I do not know what they are doing since it is only washing the dishes and making the bed they are supposed to do in the morning. Well, it feels good, I just call out and tell them to come.*

Receiving help is just like doing it oneself, seeing professional carers as an extended arm. It is oneself who has control over the situation and one either tells them what to do or they already know. Sometimes nothing needs to be said, perhaps just a brief chat, and just get help with daily chores, and then they can leave.

Handing over the decisions to others when one's independence changes over time feels reassuring, although the wish is to be as independent as possible. To be as independent as possible yet dependent in any given situation when one has a professional carer standing by as support is the ideal. It is easier to be offered help by those who take the initiative. When the body fails to perform as it should it feels safe to hand over the responsibility to a reliable professional carer who knows exactly where one's belongings are.

> *Well, it was like this morning when she went into the closet in the hallway and found my pillowcases, which the others couldn't find because I did not know where I had put them. Consequently they were put on a shelf a little bit higher up were they couldn't find them. Now it turned out that the one who had taken care of the laundry and put it away had put it in another place. But she picked it out. Well it is my home, but I do not look after it all on my own, since we are so happy together so she can do whatever she wants here. She knows how to put the clothes away, and she does it without me asking her. If I want a particular pair of trousers she knows in which closet to look and she picks them out for me.*

One needs to be aware of one's varying vulnerability in life, and one's ability to take care of oneself differs from time to time. In a changing life situation, it feels reassuring to be cared for by a professional carer one can trust, to remind oneself of one's value as a human being.

Giving and taking in the relationship with professional carers when one has a mutual relationship with them increases the opportunities to decide for oneself. It feels good to have contact with those one can discuss one's personal interests with. To get help from those who encourage one to manage things infuses confidence and one feels more independent. A mutual and trusting relationship takes time to develop and one needs to be devoted.

> *...Of course she has learned because she has been here so many times with me in different situations. We do not only talk about how she helps me but we have private chats as well. How life goes for her and how life has been for me, so there is a very good communication between us. Well it seems quite natural together with her....*

To give and take in the relationship is comforting and to feel respect for one another shows a willingness to make it easier for each other. Being persuaded for one's own good by a professional carer one trusts makes it easier rather than more difficult to fulfil one's wishes.

3.2.4. Adjusting One's Own Independence and Dependence with regard to Oneself and Others. Neglecting one's own need to allow for the needs of others when one sees and hears professional carers in a hurry and knowing that there are other caretakers in more need of their attention and care is also a situation to consider. One must also realise what they are authorized to do and allow for this when trying to persuade oneself to manage, as long as one gets help with the most urgent chores.

> *No, but I see by looking at them that they are busy. No, but then I think it may be why I do not ask for help. No, I don't because if I need help with something it may not be so urgent. If it is, I ask them and then they help me. But otherwise you can just see by looking at the different way they react.*

When feeling a sense of loyalty towards professional carers and other caretakers one's own needs are not so important compared to theirs. When seeing that they are stressed one feels that one does not want to bother them and accept the fact that there is no time. Although some small talk with them would be appreciated one still has no expectations and in some instances they are not even allowed to sit down and talk.

Withholding one's thoughts how the professional carers perform their task implies a struggle taking place. One wants professional carers to understand, but even though one's own needs and wishes are not fulfilled one still says nothing. If they do things without asking it may be difficult to sort it out afterwards. It is hard correcting their mistakes while it is easier just to let it go even though one is not happy about it.

> *It is bad, when for example, they have done the laundry and hung up the clothes which have been in the washing machine; they never ask where to put it, they just put it anywhere. Then I do not know where it is. I do not know if it is me being stupid, but I do not want to push them too much either. Well, I think that I can correct it later.*

One observes the professional carers and their different ways of working while some of them take their time others just rush around and then leave. One goes along with it and has thoughts of being nice and gentle and hoping to get one's own needs and wishes fulfilled. One tries to adjust to their personalities and adopt what one thinks is an appropriate approach. This is something one gradually finds strategies for.

4. Comprehensive Understanding and Reflections

The findings with the same group of older persons [15] revealed that they struggled for the opportunity versus resigning themselves to losing the opportunity to make their own decisions. In this present study, the findings reveal a changed understanding of older persons' independent decision making as a life situation involving living with uncertainty over time. Older persons are aware of their own vulnerability and dependence but still want to be independent. They try to comprehend everyday life and this involves a movement, a dynamic process over time changing from day to day which makes them more vulnerable. Ricœur et al. [20] states that the starting point for reflection is via objectives and opens up the world for humans to acknowledge their needs and desires and what is lacking. It opens up as a sign to offer for others to recognize in mutuality even in the isolation of suffering (pages 18-19). In the present study the findings reveal that older persons adjusting own independence and dependence with regard to oneself and others, implying that there may be a struggle in wanting professional carers to understand their needs. This is further understood as an "implicit struggle" means that the old open up and invite professional carers to enter into a mutual understanding, wanting them to recognize their exposed situation along with their suffering. Accordingly when the professional carers fail to acknowledge this invitation and their needs it makes the older persons vulnerable.

As patients become more dependent increased attention is needed to enhance their well-being [21]. Autonomy is highly valued in the western care context [4–6]. Sandman [6] suggests that it is important to distinguish between four different aspects of autonomy as they can be valued differently by people, and there is no easy norm to follow. The central aspect, *self-determination*, means how people decide and act in accordance with their own will and thus make decisions. *Freedom* is an aspect of having different valuable alternatives to choose from, while *desire fulfilment* is an aspect of actual outcomes of decisions. *Independence* is an aspect of involvement and accomplishment to do things themselves. When the old have to relate to when their independence lies the in hands of others they have reduced self-determination, freedom, desire fulfilment and independence due to internal and external organizational circumstances. On the other hand, when independence lies in their own hands they have the opportunity to be involved and to have freedom, desire fulfilment, and independence. Older persons' dependency changes over time like circumstances in organizations and professional carers working conditions. This complicates everyday life and they have to live with uncertainty since they never know how things will be. Research shows that the ageing process makes things one is surrounded by in the home be seen in a different way and that routines provide continuity for older persons to live independently [22]. Accordingly attention needs to be paid to how older persons perceive everyday life and the importance of continuity for them. In a study, findings show that frail older people living at home with help experienced little support for their efforts in their everyday life [23]. Agich [4] argues that dependent older people have to accept being placed in the hands of others, relying on others to recognize their needs and help them. In this study, it was found that when older persons' independence lies in the hands of others it was interpreted as professional carers not recognizing their everyday life, which results in a routinized care. They also adjust to their independence and dependence, are aware of their dependency, and accept the situation. This is in line with the findings of Anderberg and Berglund [24] who found that when communication failed between the old and professional carers in nursing homes the old hid their vulnerability in order to be accepted. Ricœur et al. [20] point out that it is human limitations that make man fallible and fragility provides the opportunity for evil to arise (page 146). When autonomy is so highly valued in today's society it is easy to say that dependency is negative. Instead perhaps, the focus should change to help vulnerable older people and see their dependence as something human. Professional carers should acknowledge older peoples' changing vulnerability in everyday care and not just focus on independence and respect for self-determination. However, findings reveal that mutual caring relationships increase the opportunities for older persons to decide in accordance with their own needs, to be free to decide whether or not they want to hand over to professional carers to decide for them, or to decide for themselves or together with their carers. Nevertheless they are still uncertain because they never know when they will arrive. Dependence becomes accepted if patients feel free to be dependent in a mutual understanding with nurses [25]. This underlines a care with a person-centered perspective [26] and a change from an individualistic approach on autonomy towards a relational to focus on interdependence [4, 9, 27] to enable shared-decision making [28]. This relational perspective could be useful for professional carers to help vulnerable older people in caring encounters [29] to make their own decisions [6].

5. Methodological Considerations

In a life world perspective, it is important to have varied characteristics and experience amongst the participants [16] which was achieved. Participants were interviewed three times each and data material was therefore considered rich and enabled a deepened understanding. First interview texts were transcribed and read separately for each participant (three interviews each) and a first naïve understanding was formulated. Thereafter, all interviews were analysed as a whole to enable an in-depth understanding of older persons' lived experiences over time. Lindseth and Norberg (2004) stress that interpretations have different meanings and there is not only one single truth possible. The meaning in this study of older persons lived experiences is one of the conceivable meanings, found by the authors as most useful. The findings in this study present knowledge that creates a foundation for other groups of older people dependent on help, if the reader decontextualizes the interpretation into their own context [18].

6. Conclusions and Implications for Practice

Professional carers have to acknowledge that the life situation of older persons involves an existence of living with uncertainty over time as to how they relate to their own independence and dependence as regards themselves and others. Older persons are aware of their dependence but still want to be independent. It is suggested that one should focus on seeing older persons as interdependent in the caring encounter through a relational approach on autonomy, that it is important to help dependent older persons and to acknowledge their changing vulnerability over time. Respect for older people's right to self-determination should not just be a norm to be followed at the risk of leaving them to fend for themselves'. There is a need to pay attention to continuity and the routines essential for older persons, in order to understand their everyday lives when they are being cared for by municipal home help services. The implications for practice are a care of the old which focuses on a relational approach on autonomy beyond the traditional individualistic and a person-centered practice. It makes it easier for older people to have a professional carer they trust which acknowledges their vulnerability and that their independency and dependency changes over time. Further research is needed on how professional carers can improve older people's independent decision making in the relationship through a relational approach to autonomy focusing on interdependence.

Conflict of Interests

The authors declare that there is no conflict of interests.

Acknowledgments

The authors would like to thank the older persons who participated in this study and Michael Cole for linguistic revision. This study has received Grants from Mälardalen University, School of Health, Care and Social Welfare, the Swedish Society of Nursing (SSF), Uppsala Hemsysterskolas Fund, and the Solstickan foundation.

References

[1] World Health Organization, "Ageing and life course," World Health Organization, 2011, http://www.who.int/ageing/en/index.html.

[2] Socialstyrelsen, "Care and social services for the elderly. Progress report 2008. Efforts and support to persons with impairments. Individual and care of the elderly," Socialstyrelsen, Stockholm, Sweden, 2008, http://www.socialstyrelsen.se.

[3] Government Offices of Sweden, "Elderly care in Sweden," Ministry of Health and Social Affairs, Stockholm, Sweden, 2011, http://www.sweden.gov.se/sb/d/15473/a/183501.

[4] G. J. Agich, *Dependence and Autonomy in Old Age: An Ethical Framework for Long-Term Care*, Cambridge University Press, New York, NY, USA, 2nd edition, 2003.

[5] T. L. Beauchamp and J. F. Childress, *Principles of Biomedical Ethics*, Oxford University Press, New York, NY, USA, 6th edition, 2009.

[6] L. Sandman, "On the autonomy turf. Assessing the value of autonomy to patients," *Medicine, Health Care, and Philosophy*, vol. 7, no. 3, pp. 261–268, 2004.

[7] G. Becker, "The oldest old: autonomy in the face of frailty," *Journal of Aging Studies*, vol. 8, no. 1, pp. 59–76, 1994.

[8] B. J. Collopy, "Autonomy in long term care: some crucial distinctions," *Gerontologist*, vol. 28, supplement, pp. 10–17, 1988.

[9] B. McCormack, "Autonomy and the relationship between nurses and older people," *Ageing and Society*, vol. 21, no. 4, pp. 417–446, 2001.

[10] A. Olaison and E. Cedersund, "Assessment for home care: negotiating solutions for individual needs," *Journal of Aging Studies*, vol. 20, no. 4, pp. 367–380, 2006.

[11] D. Plath, "Independence in old age: the route to social exclusion?" *British Journal of Social Work*, vol. 38, no. 7, pp. 1353–1369, 2008.

[12] C. Nicholson, J. Meyer, M. Flatley, and C. Holman, "The experience of living at home with frailty in old age: a psychosocial qualitative study," *International Journal of Nursing Studies*, 2012.

[13] G. Hammarström and S. Torres, "Being, feeling and acting: a qualitative study of Swedish home-help care recipients' understandings of dependence and independence," *Journal of Aging Studies*, vol. 24, no. 2, pp. 75–87, 2010.

[14] C. Welford, K. Murphy, M. Wallace, and D. Casey, "A concept analysis of autonomy for older people in residential care," *Journal of Clinical Nursing*, vol. 19, no. 9-10, pp. 1226–1235, 2010.

[15] A. Breitholtz, I. Snellman, and I. Fagerberg, "Older people's dependence on caregivers' help in their own homes and their lived experiences of their opportunity to make independent decisions," *International Journal of Older People Nursing*, 2012.

[16] K. Dahlberg, H. Dahlberg, and M. Nyström, *Reflective Lifeworld Research*, Studentlitteratur, Lund, Sweden, 2nd edition, 2008.

[17] M. F. Folstein, S. E. Folstein, and P. R. McHugh, "'Mini mental state'. A practical method for grading the cognitive state of patients for the clinician," *Journal of Psychiatric Research*, vol. 12, no. 3, pp. 189–198, 1975.

[18] A. Lindseth and A. Norberg, "A phenomenological hermeneutical method for researching lived experience," *Scandinavian Journal of Caring Sciences*, vol. 18, no. 2, pp. 145–153, 2004.

[19] P. Ricoeur, *Interpretation Theory : Discourse and the Surplus of Meaning*, Texas Christian University Press, Fort Worth, Tex, USA, 7th edition, 1976.

[20] P. Ricœur, *Fallible Man*, Fordham University Press, New York, NY, USA, Revised edition, 1986.

[21] D. C. Thomasma, "Freedom, dependency, and the care of the very old," *Journal of the American Geriatrics Society*, vol. 32, no. 12, pp. 906–914, 1984.

[22] Å. Alftberg, *What is aging? An ethnological study of aging, body and materiality [thesis]*, Lunds University, Lund, Sweden, 2012.

[23] C. Nicholson, J. Meyer, M. Flatley, C. Holman, and K. Lowton, "Living on the margin: understanding the experience of living and dying with frailty in old age," *Social Science & Medicine*, vol. 75, no. 8, pp. 1426–1432, 2012.

[24] P. Anderberg and A. L. Berglund, "Elderly persons' experiences of striving to receive care on their own terms in nursing homes," *International Journal of Nursing Practice*, vol. 16, no. 1, pp. 64–68, 2010.

[25] G. Strandberg, A. Norberg, and L. Jansson, "An exemplar of a positive perspective of being dependent on care," *Scholarly Inquiry for Nursing Practice*, vol. 14, no. 4, pp. 327–346, 2000.

[26] B. McCormack, "A conceptual framework for person-centred practice with older people," *International Journal of Nursing Practice*, vol. 9, no. 3, pp. 202–209, 2003.

[27] M. A. Verkerk, "The care perspective and autonomy," *Medicine, Health Care, and Philosophy*, vol. 4, no. 3, pp. 289–294, 2001.

[28] L. Sandman, B. B. Granger, I. Ekman, and C. Munthe, "Adherence, shared decision-making and patient autonomy," *Medicine, Healthcare and Philosophy*, vol. 15, no. 2, pp. 115–127, 2011.

[29] I. Snellman, *Human professionalism: a philosophical investigation of the significance of the authentic encounter for the well-being of the patient [thesis]*, Uppsala University, Uppsala, Sweden, 2001.

21

Epigenetic Mechanisms Shape the Biological Response to Trauma and Risk for PTSD: A Critical Review

Morgan Heinzelmann and Jessica Gill

National Institute of Nursing Research, National Institutes of Health, Bethesda, MD 20814, USA

Correspondence should be addressed to Morgan Heinzelmann; morgan.heinzelmann@nih.gov

Academic Editor: Debra E. Lyon

Posttraumatic stress disorder (PTSD) develops in approximately one-quarter of trauma-exposed individuals, leading us and others to question the mechanisms underlying this heterogeneous response to trauma. We suggest that the reasons for the heterogeneity relate to a complex interaction between genes and the environment, shaping each individual's recovery trajectory based on both historical and trauma-specific variables. Epigenetic modifications provide a unique opportunity to elucidate how preexisting risk factors may contribute to PTSD risk through changes in the methylation of DNA. Preexisting risks for PTSD, including depression, stress, and trauma, result in differential DNA methylation of endocrine genes, which may then result in a different biological responses to trauma and subsequently a greater risk for PTSD onset. Although these relationships are complex and currently inadequately described, we provide a critical review of recent studies to examine how differences in genetic and proteomic biomarkers shape an individual's vulnerability to PTSD development, thereby contributing to a heterogeneous response to trauma.

1. Introduction

Up to 90% of individuals experience a traumatic event at some time during their lives, yet most recover and suffer from no long-term ramifications; however, a subset of individuals develop posttraumatic stress disorder (PTSD) and are at high risk for health decline [1–4]. This heterogeneous response suggests that preexisting factors might influence how people respond to traumatic situations. We suggest that a more comprehensive examination of biomarkers that approximate PTSD risk would be of great value. Biomarker discovery in PTSD has been hindered by the lack of prospective studies in traumatized individuals, resulting in an insufficient understanding of the preexisting risk factors for PTSD onset as well as the mechanistic pathways that underlie this risk. Without this knowledge, we are unable to identify traumatized individuals at risk for PTSD development and, therefore, unable to implement effective, preventive interventions. Yet, additional biological analysis methods have become available, and these new strategies will be useful in addressing this critical issue. Specifically, the use of whole-genome gene expression and epigenetic modifications (DNA methylation)

provide an opportunity to explore more than candidate biomarkers, to identify novel mechanisms related to PTSD risk, and to pinpoint genetic pathways that may be implicated in both risk and resilience to trauma.

A traumatic event places individuals at high risk for developing PTSD, resulting in rates of PTSD between 18% and 36% in trauma-exposed patients [1–4]; as mentioned above, most trauma-exposed individuals recover and do not develop PTSD. PTSD is viewed as a disorder of dysregulation of fear and processing of stimuli associated with trauma, and it is characterized by three main clusters of symptoms: reexperiencing, avoidance, and hyperarousal. Reexperiencing symptoms include distressing recollections or dreams of the event, flashbacks, and intense psychological and physiological reactivity to internal and external cues; avoidance symptoms include evasion of any thoughts or feelings of people and places that remind the individual of the traumatic event, decreased interest in participating in activities, and emotional numbing; and hyperarousal symptoms include problems falling or staying asleep, irritability or anger, hypervigilance, and exaggerated startle reflex. It has become increasingly clear that environmental influences early in development remain pervasive into adulthood, a relationship that is attributed to an interaction of gene function and environment. Both genetic and environmental factors are critical to developmental processes, and even minor changes in either type of factor can result in trajectories of resilience or vulnerability [5]; however, it is the interaction between these factors that may provide the most vital information to understanding the heterogeneous response to trauma. Epigenetic modifications occur in response to an environmental factor and include DNA methylation, acetylation, and histone modification which alter DNA accessibility and chromatin structure, thereby regulating activity of the gene in a long-lasting manner. Because the risk for PTSD onset is influenced by environmental factors that predate trauma exposure, epigenetics may provide novel insights into the heterogeneous response to a trauma. Large epidemiological studies link pretrauma risks including previous depression, stressors, and traumatic events to a greater risk for PTSD onset following trauma exposure [6], suggesting that these factors may contribute to variability of individuals in response to a trauma.

The support for the mediating link of epigenetic modifications and PTSD vulnerability is reported in preclinical studies. Specifically, preclinical models illustrate these complex relationships and link epigenetic modifications in neurons to psychological vulnerability following stressors. In rats, the offspring of the high caring mothers (i.e., high licking) exhibit the reduced methylation of the glucocorticoid receptor gene [7] and endocrine regulation of a subsequent stressor [8]. In contrast, in non-human primates, offspring that face early adversity exhibits endocrine dysregulation [9] as well as reductions in neuronal plasticity in the prefrontal cortex that persist into adulthood [10]. Early stressors in humans have also been linked to epigenetic modifications, including increased methylation of the glucocorticoid promoter in hippocampal neurons of suicide completers with histories of early childhood maltreatment [11]. Cord blood collected from mothers with high levels of depression and anxiety during the third trimester displays similar glucocorticoid methylation differences, which are linked to a dysregulation of the endocrine system [12]. In studies of rats who exhibit PTSD-like behavior, there is evidence of increased methylation of stress response genes including brain-derived neurotrophic factor [13] and nuclear protein phosphate-1 [14] in neurons, which result in the onset of PTSD-like behavior [15]. These preclinical studies provide insights into the heterogeneous response to trauma and stress and suggest that epigenetic modifications in neurons result in the onset of PTSD [16, 17].

We suggest that the heterogeneous response to trauma relates to complex interactions between genes and the environment, shaping each individual's recovery trajectory based on both historical and trauma specific variables (see Figure 1). One of the major environmental factors linked to epigenetic changes is stress, which is a critical factor in the pathogenesis of PTSD. There is robust evidence linking PTSD onset to epigenetic changes following stress; yet this evidence is only starting to accumulate from the clinical studies. Recent advances in laboratory analyses and biostatistical methods provide new opportunities to determine the mechanisms of PTSD onset; however, many of these advances are not yet applied. Additionally, current studies are limited by our inability to determine pretrauma epigenetic status as well as our restriction to peripheral blood samples in clinical samples. Here, we provide a critical review of recent studies to examine how differences in genetic and proteomic biomarkers may underlie the vulnerability of the individual to develop PTSD, and how this field of study may provide fundamental insights into the identification of individuals at risk for PTSD development following trauma and the development of novel, interventional strategies.

2. Methods

In order to obtain a comprehensive pool of prospective studies investigating peripheral biomarkers of PTSD following trauma, PubMed, OVID/MEDLINE, the Cochran Database, Embase, Scopus, CINAHL, and PsychInfo were systematically searched using the following National Library of Medicine Medical Subject Headings (MeSH) "posttraumatic stress disorder," "genes," "cytokines," "neuropeptides," and "inflammation." Additionally, each key word was cross-referenced with each other in each of the various databases. The search extended to the literature published between 2000 and 2013, and studies were included in the review if they (1) were primary research articles, (2) were published in English, (3) were conducted in humans, and (4) examined epigenetic modifications (i.e., DNA methylation), gene expression, or a proteomic biomarker that was linked to PTSD risk following a trauma. The following components and variables of interest were appraised to provide an overall synthesis of the available literature: study purpose, design, methods, sample size, demographics, type of trauma, severity of injuries sustained (mild, moderate, and severe), type of biological sample collected, and times of collection following trauma. We were able to locate 6 clinical studies that examined epigenetic modifications (i.e., DNA methylation), 9 studies of gene expression, and 14 studies that used a proteomic biomarker to examine the risk for PTSD onset (3 pediatric and 9 adult studies). All studies were reviewed and are presented in Tables 1, 2, and 3.

2.1. Epigenetics. Clinical studies are restricted to examining epigenetic modifications in samples of peripheral blood, but these studies do provide some key insights into how these molecular changes relate to PTSD risk (see Table 1). Specifically, these studies implicate insufficient regulation of inflammatory activity and reduced neurotransmitter activity in PTSD risk. In support of this, studies in chronic PTSD-affected patients report hypermethylation of inflammatory initiator genes (toll-like receptors 1 & 3, IL-8, chemokine ligand 1, and others) and demethylation of inflammatory regulatory genes (FK506 binding protein-5 [FKBP5]) [18]. In a subsequent study, Ressler et al. (2011) linked these molecular-genetic mechanisms to higher concentrations of inflammatory cytokines in patients with chronic PTSD [19]. Together, these association studies suggest that observations by us and others of excessive inflammation in chronic PTSD [20, 21] likely relate to these DNA methylation differences;

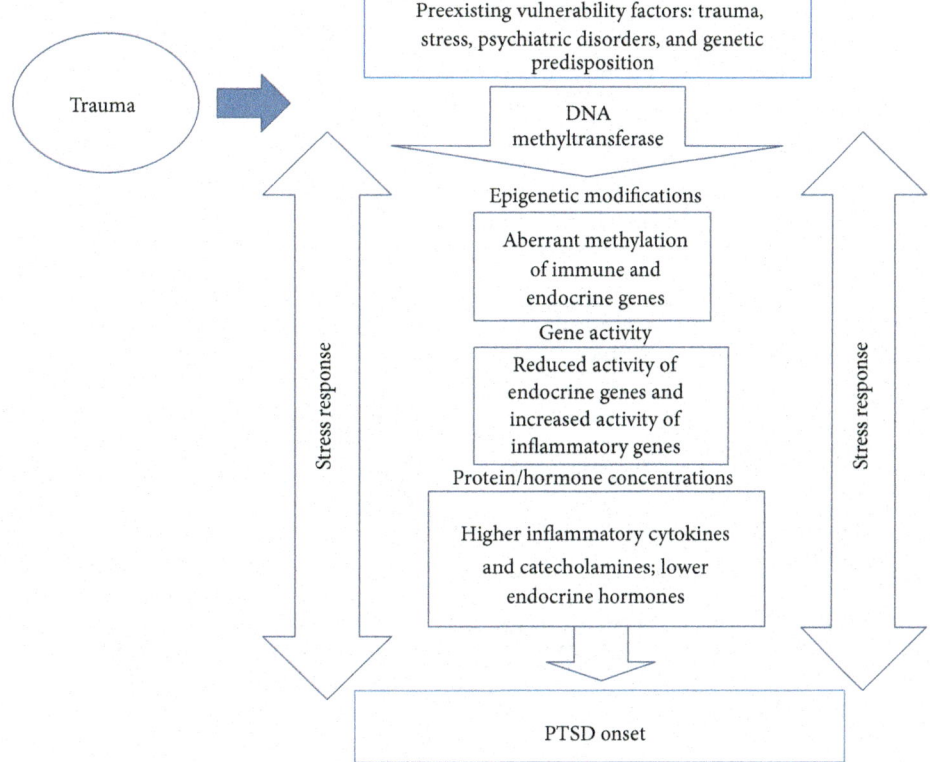

FIGURE 1: Epigenetic mechanisms of PTSD onset.

however, their cross-sectional designs prohibit linking these molecular differences to PTSD vulnerability.

In contrast, a recent study measured DNA methylation and reported that postdeployment hypomethylation of LINE-1 was associated with PTSD onset following deployment [25]. The authors of this report postulate that LINE-1, a regulator of stress response in the immune system, may represent an adaptive response to combat stress that protects against PTSD; yet additional studies are needed in more generalized samples that include women and various traumatic events. In addition, this study did not determine predeployment factors such as previous PTSD, depression, or trauma that contributed to precombat methylation differences, resulting in an inability to understand how the interactions between genes and environment prior to trauma underlies PTSD risk.

Other studies suggest that differential methylation of neurotransmitter genes is linked to PTSD onset. In two studies using samples of civilians from the Detroit Neighborhood Health Study, neurotransmitter genes were implicated in the risk for PTSD development. In one study that examined the serotonin transporter gene (SLC6A4), methylation levels were modified by the effect of the number of traumatic events on PTSD after controlling for SLC6A4 genotype, such that persons with more traumatic events were at increased risk for PTSD, but only at lower methylation levels. At higher methylation levels, individuals who reported more traumatic events were protected from this disorder, suggesting that the

serotonin transporter gene may also be important in trauma-related resilience [22]. In a study using the same patient sample, the candidate gene MAN2C1 showed a significant methylation × trauma experience interaction such that those with both higher MAN2C1 methylation and greater exposure to traumatic events showed an increase in risk of lifetime PTSD [24]. Although these studies provide unique insights into risks for PTSD based on DNA methylation, trauma, and psychiatric-related symptoms, these studies used cross-sectional design and did not include definitive diagnoses determined through a clinical interview.

Although not epigenetic in nature, previous studies that examine genetic inheritance provide further evidence of genetic underpinnings in endocrine modulating genes in the risk for PTSD. In brief, previous studies link single nucleotide polymorphisms (SNPs) of FKBP5, a negative regulator of GCR sensitivity to a greater risk for PTSD onset [29, 49, 50]. Current findings indicate that genetic predisposition differences in another key inflammatory gene, corticotrophin-releasing hormone type 1 receptor gene (CRHR1), increase PTSD onset in children who were abused at an early age [51]. With pediatric injury patients, a longitudinal study identified one SNP significantly related to acute PTSD symptoms as well as trajectory of symptoms over time [52]. These findings are meaningful in terms of genetic and environmental interplay producing risk for PTSD; however, current studies do not explicate the link between baseline epigenetics in immune

TABLE 1: Epigenetics studies.

Study	Analysis method	Sample	Findings
Uddin et al., 2010 [18]	DNA methylation; >14,000 genes	100 individuals from DNHS (PTSD = 23)	PTSD had greater methylation of toll-like receptors 1 and 3, IL-8, and others compared to controls and had a greater overall number of uniquely methylated genes.
Koenen et al., 2011 [22]	DNA methylation and genotype; SLC6A4	100 individuals from DNHS (PTSD = 23)	Neither genotype nor methylation of SLC6A4 was associated with PTSD; however, when controlling with genotype, lower methylation levels were associated with increased risk for developing PTSD among individuals with more traumatic events.
Ressler et al., 2011 [19]	DNA methylation; 44 SNPs of PACAP and PAC1	64 individuals, primarily African American (PTSD = 24)	An SNP in ADCYAP1R1, rs2267735, predicted PTSD diagnosis and symptoms in women; methylation of this gene was also associated with PTSD.
Smith et al., 2011 [23]	DNA methylation; global and site specific	110 African Americans (PTSD = 50)	Global methylation was increased in subjects with PTSD, as compared to control subjects or subjects with a history of childhood trauma; CpG sites in TPR, CLEC9A, APC5, ANXA2, and TLR8 were differentially methylated in subjects with PTSD.
Uddin et al., 2011 [24]	DNA methylation; 33 candidate genes	100 individuals from DNHS (PTSD = 23)	One candidate gene, MAN2C1, showed significantly higher methylation in subjects with lifetime PTSD.
Rusiecki et al., 2012 [25]	DNA methylation; LINE-1 and Alu	150 service members (PTSD = 75)	LINE-1 was hypomethylated in PTSD versus controls postdeployment and hypermethylated postdeployment versus predeployment in controls; Alu was hypermethylated in PTSD versus controls predeployment.

regulatory genes and the risk for PTSD onset following a trauma. Yet, taking these studies together with studies that examine gene function, there is evidence that a combination of genetic and environmental factors contributes to psychological vulnerability following a trauma by shaping an individual's neuronal and biological stress response, warranting future prospective studies to determine these important temporal relationships [53].

2.2. Gene Expression. Nine studies have also used gene expression analysis of peripheral blood to examine the mechanisms of PTSD, providing additional insights into the complex biological processes underlying PTSD onset. Gene expression involves processes that alter the ultimate product of the gene, which is most often the production of proteins. Current studies using gene expression analysis methods also support the role of insufficient inflammatory regulation in the risk for PTSD onset, by implicating higher expression of inflammatory genes and lower expression of genes that regulate inflammatory processes (see Table 2). In a recent cross-sectional study of PTSD patients, a reduction in the transcriptional activity of genes that regulate inflammation including FKBP5 and IL18 and STAT pathways was reported in an urban sample of primarily African American participants [30]. Reductions in gene expression of STAT5B and MHC II class receptor genes in participants who developed PTSD following the 9-11 terrorist attacks were also reported [29]. Also, in a sample of participants who developed PTSD following 9-11, reduced FKBP5 gene expression was most related to PTSD severity in regression analysis as well as a reduction in STAT5B, a direct inhibitor of GR, and a major histocompatibility complex (MHC) class II gene expression;

however, significant differences were related to PTSD symptom severity and not a definitive diagnosis of PTSD [27]. Lastly, in a recent study of 12 women with PTSD related to child abuse, increased glucocorticoid receptor sensitivity in monocytes was linked to increased NF-κB activity; however, this study did not use a whole-genome analysis like the other reviewed studies, but instead a DNA binding ELISA in mononuclear cells [31]. Thus, together, these studies suggest that reduced gene expression of immune regulatory genes is associated with PTSD but is limited to small sample sizes and cross-sectional design.

In contrast, two recent studies provide vital insights into how gene expression differences contribute to PTSD onset through the use of a prospective design in male service members who are evaluated prior to and then following deployment. In a study of 448 male soldiers, predeployment high glucocorticoid receptor numbers and low FKBP5 mRNA expression were associated with increased risk for a high level of PTSD symptoms [32]. In a similar sample, a high level of PTSD symptoms after deployment was independently associated with a high DEX sensitivity of T-cell proliferation before deployment, but only in individuals who reported PTSD symptoms without depressive symptoms [33]. These studies link alterations in gene expression to functional immune cell changes. Importantly, these studies also link preexisting biological differences in cell function and gene expression to the risk for PTSD onset following a trauma. These studies are limited by their use of gene expression analysis of only predetermined target genes, restricting our ability to identify novel biological targets for PTSD risk and to understand how known risks relate to less well known genes related to PTSD risk. Although these studies have some limitations, they provide fundamental information regarding

TABLE 2: Gene expression studies.

Study	Analysis method	Sample	Findings
Zieker et al., 2007 [26]	Pre-selected stress-immune genes, whole-blood	16 individuals (PTSD = 8)	In PTSD, upregulated (4): glutamate transported, IGF-2; downregulated (14): IL-18, IL-16, colony stimulating factor.
Yehuda et al., 2009 [27]	Whole blood gene expression	35 individuals exposed to 9/11 (PTSD = 15)	FKBP5, STAT5B, and MHC class II showed reduced expression in individuals with PTSD.
Neylan et al., 2011 [28]	CD14+ monocyte; gene expression	67 ± trauma-exposed individuals (PTSD = 34)	In PTSD patients, three monocyte genes were underexpressed in men but not in women.
Sarapas et al., 2011 [29]	Genome-wide gene expression	40 individuals exposed to 9/11 (PTSD = 20)	PTSD patients showed a reduction in gene expression of STAT5B and nuclear factor I/A.
Mehta et al. 2011 [30]	Whole-blood gene expression and SNP of FKBP5	211 low income (PTSD = 75)	With FKBP5 SNP added to interaction with PTSD, there was a reduction in 32 genes including IL-18 and STAT pathway.
Pace et al., 2012 [31]	Nuclear factor-κB activity in peripheral blood	36 women (PTSD = 12)	Increased nuclear factor-κB activity was associated with women with PTSD as compared to controls.
van Zuiden et al., 2012 [32]	GR number; FKBP5, GILZ, and SGK1 mRNA expression	448 military personnel (PTSD = 35)	Predeployment high GR number, low FKBP5 mRNA expression, and high GILZ expression predicted PTSD development.
van Zuiden et al., 2012 [33]	GC sensitivity of leukocytes	526 military personnel (PTSD = 46)	Predeployment sensitivity of GCRs on leukocytes predicted development of PTSD.
Matić et al., 2013 [34]	GR function and expression using PCR	347 ± war trauma-exposed individuals (PTSD = 113)	Lower GR sensitivity in PBMCs and low gene-expression of GR were found in PTSD patients.

TABLE 3: Proteomic studies.

Pediatric studies	Sample	Collection; followup	Outcome	Results
Delahanty et al., 2005 [35]	58 ED patients	ED; 6 wks	Diagnosis	High cortisol and epinephrine predicted acute PTSD symptoms.
Ostrowski et al., 2007 [36]	54 ED patients	ED; 6 wks, 7 mos	Diagnosis	High cortisol predicted acute PTSD symptoms and PTSD onset in boys.
Pervanidou et al., 2007 [37]	56 MVA patients (9 = PTSD)	ED; 1, 6 mos	Diagnosis	High cortisol and IL-6 predicted PTSD onset.
Adult studies	Sample	Collection; followup	Outcome	Results
Resnick et al., 1995 [38]	37 rape survivors (19 = PTSD)	ED; 17–157 days	Diagnosis	Low cortisol in previously assaulted women predicted PTSD onset.
Yehuda et al., 1998 [39]	20 rape survivors (11 = PTSD)	ED; 27–157 days	Diagnosis	Cortisol and MHPG did not predict PTSD onset.
Delahanty et al., 2000 [40]	99 MVA patients (9 = ASD)	ED; 1 mo	Diagnosis	Low cortisol predicted acute PTSD symptoms.
Bonne et al., 2003 [41]	21 ED patients (8 = PTSD)	1 wk; 6 mos	Diagnosis	Cortisol did not predict PTSD onset.
Heinrichs et al., 2005 [42]	43 firefighters (7 = PTSD at 2 yrs)	Training; 6, 9, 12, 24 mos	Symptom report	Cortisol and CA did not predict PTSD onset.
McFarlane et al., 1997 [43]	40 MVA patients (7 = PTSD)	ED; 2, 10 days and 6 mos	Diagnosis	Low cortisol predicted PTSD onset.
Ehring et al., 2008 [44]	53 MVA patients (5 = PTSD)	ED; 2 wks, 6 mos	Diagnosis	Low cortisol predicted PTSD onset.
Shalev et al., 2008 [45]; Videlock et al., 2008 [46]	155 ED patients (31 = PTSD)	ED; 10 days, and 1, 5 mos	Diagnosis	Cortisol, ACTH, GR, and NE did not predict PTSD onset.
Cohen et al., 2011 [47]	48 orthopedic patients, 13 HC	At hospitalization; 1 mo	Symptom report	High IL-8 and low TGF-β predicted acute PTSD symptoms.
van Zuiden et al., 2011 [48]	68 service members, (34 = PTSD)	Prior; following deployment	Symptom report	High GR predicted PTSD onset.

the mechanisms of PTSD onset. Specifically, these studies report that it is likely an accumulation of preexisting factors that result in differential gene activity and vulnerability to develop PTSD following trauma exposure.

2.3. Proteomics. Studies of proteomic biomarkers of PTSD risk have been undertaken for far longer than studies that use genetic analyses; yet they have been limited by many methodological issues. These issues include an inability to control for timing of the sample collection, with most proteins exhibiting substantial circadian variation, the impact of the physical consequences of trauma, and differences in the timing between the occurrence of the trauma and the biological sample. Despite these limitations, these studies provide some vital insights into the biological mechanisms underlying PTSD vulnerability. Proteins play important roles in both intracellular processes and intercellular communication, thereby contributing to the orchestration of responses to traumatic events. Thus, proteins should be considered as possible PTSD biomarkers. Studies of acutely traumatized individuals suggest that high concentrations of inflammatory proteins are linked to PTSD onset. Here, we review 14 studies that collect a biological sample within the acute period following a trauma and use this biomarker to approximate PTSD risk (see Table 3).

In children following a motor vehicle accident (MVA), high concentrations of IL-6 twenty four hours after the MVA predicted PTSD onset at six months [37]; however, these elevations were no longer evident in those children who developed PTSD. Similar findings are reported in a study of adults hospitalized for orthopedic injuries, reporting that high concentrations of IL-6 as well as IL-8 related to the risk acute stress disorders symptoms; however, this study did not link these biomarkers to the risk for PTSD onset [47]. IL-8 is a mediator of the innate immune system, with higher concentrations indicating a greater immune challenge. In contrast, low concentrations of IL-8 predicted high PTSD symptoms following the earthquakes in China, whereas high IL-6 predicted anxiety and depression symptoms but was not specific to PTSD [54]. The Song et al. [54] study differs from the other two studies as biomarker collection was within months, not hours of the trauma, and many of the participants did not sustain physical injuries. A benefit of the Song study was the evaluation of cooccurring depression with PTSD, which is a limitation of the other prospective studies. In studies of chronic PTSD, cooccurring depression is associated with higher concentrations of IL-6 [20, 55]. Therefore, inflammation in the acute recovery period may be very detrimental to psychological recovery as high concentrations of inflammatory cytokines exert central effects including the induction of "sickness behavior" [56–60]. In addition, inflammatory cytokines increase blood brain barrier disruption [61–63] and alter metabolism of serotonin [64–67], all of which contributes to neuronal vulnerability despite of the excessive central inflammatory actions, including overactivation of microglia [68–70]. Together, these studies suggest that increased concentrations of inflammatory cytokines relate to the risk for PTSD onset.

There is also evidence that endocrine dysregulation relates to PTSD risk; however, this risk may relate to previous trauma. In three studies of children recruited from emergency departments, high cortisol measured in the urine predicted acute stress symptoms at six weeks following the trauma; however, in the Ostrowski et al. (2007) study high cortisol predicted PTSD onset in boys only [36]. This is of interest as studies of adult women report that it is low cortisol concentrations that predict PTSD onset [39]. Resnick et al. (1995) support this finding in a similar sample but reports that this relationship only relates to those women who report a trauma prior to the rape [38]. In samples of men and women following an MVA, low cortisol concentrations are also linked to PTSD risk [40, 44]; however, the role of previous trauma is not reported in these studies. Other studies do not link cortisol concentrations to PTSD risk [39, 41, 42, 45, 46]. In a unique study of service members prior to and following deployment, concentrations of cortisol were not related to PTSD risk; however, greater glucocorticoid binding in mononuclear cells prior to deployment predicted PTSD onset, suggesting that systems that regulate cortisol activity relate to PTSD risk [48].

ANS dysregulation contributes to PTSD vulnerability [71, 72]; however, current biomarker studies that measure catecholamines or metabolites have not supported this relationship. Studies that examined catecholamine concentrations from blood samples did not significantly differ in studies of adults [39, 46] or children [35, 37]. Studies of concentrations of catecholamines using urine samples also did not show significant findings in adults [35, 40, 42, 46] or in children [35]. Therefore, ANS dysregulation may relate to PTSD risk yet this is not supported in biomarkers studies; this discrepancy may be related to the high degree of turnover of catecholamines in circulation, in which current studies may not be able to capture. Future studies that are able to approximate ANS dysregulation will be important as catecholamines influence immune and endocrine function, and also neuronal circuitry required to psychologically cope with trauma [73].

3. Conclusions

In this review, we provide a comprehensive examination of the biomarkers that contribute to PTSD risk. We suggest that epigenetic modifications shape the resulting proteomic response of the individual through differential gene activity, thereby contributing to the heterogeneous response to trauma and differential risk for PTSD onset. Additional studies are needed to elucidate these relationships and to design technological methods to use these biomarkers to identify trauma patients at the highest risk for PTSD onset. Preventative interventions would be of great value in patients at the highest risk for PTSD to prevent chronic symptomatology. In addition, these studies may inform the development of novel interventions including pharmacological agents that are better able to prevent the onset of PTSD.

Addressing this issue is critical, as delivering effective, preventive interventions for PTSD could save the USA up to 180 million dollars each year in health care costs [74–79] and the lives of up to 9,000 individuals from suicide [80–83]. Health care providers have an opportunity to reduce the risk for PTSD onset as up to 3 million adults seek immediate medical care for traumatic injuries each year [84], resulting in the onset of PTSD in almost 1 million of Americans annually [1, 4, 85–87]. However, even in this group, there is a high level of interindividual response variability to traumatic injuries, suggesting that a biomarker that is able to approximate PTSD risk would be of great value in directing preventive measures. Preventing PTSD is paramount and would reduce the substantial morbidity and health-related mortality associated with this devastating disorder [2, 85].

References

[1] D. S. Davydow, W. J. Katon, and D. F. Zatzick, "Psychiatric morbidity and functional impairments in survivors of burns, traumatic injuries, and ICU stays for other critical illnesses: a review of the literature," *International Review of Psychiatry*, vol. 21, no. 6, pp. 531–538, 2009.

[2] D. Zatzick, "Posttraumatic stress, functional impairment, and service utilization after injury: a public health approach," *Seminars in Clinical Neuropsychiatry*, vol. 8, no. 3, pp. 149–157, 2003.

[3] J. A. Coplan, "Rotational motion of the knee: a comparison of normal and pronating subjects," *Journal of Orthopaedic and Sports Physical Therapy*, vol. 10, no. 9, pp. 366–369, 1989.

[4] D. F. Zatzick, D. C. Grossman, J. Russo et al., "Predicting posttraumatic stress symptoms longitudinally in a representative sample of hospitalized injured adolescents," *Journal of the American Academy of Child and Adolescent Psychiatry*, vol. 45, no. 10, pp. 1188–1195, 2006.

[5] R. Jaenisch and A. Bird, "Epigenetic regulation of gene expression: how the genome integrates intrinsic and environmental signals," *Nature Genetics*, vol. 33, supplement, pp. 245–254, 2003.

[6] N. Breslau, "Epidemiologic studies of trauma, posttraumatic stress disorder, and other psychiatric disorders," *Canadian Journal of Psychiatry*, vol. 47, no. 10, pp. 923–929, 2002.

[7] I. C. G. Weaver, N. Cervoni, F. A. Champagne et al., "Epigenetic programming by maternal behavior," *Nature Neuroscience*, vol. 7, no. 8, pp. 847–854, 2004.

[8] D. Liu, J. Diorio, B. Tannenbaum et al., "Maternal care, hippocampal glucocorticoid receptors, and hypothalamic-pituitary-adrenal responses to stress," *Science*, vol. 277, no. 5332, pp. 1659–1662, 1997.

[9] M. M. Sanchez, "The impact of early adverse care on HPA axis development: nonhuman primate models," *Hormones and Behavior*, vol. 50, no. 4, pp. 623–631, 2006.

[10] F. Fumagalli, R. Molteni, G. Racagni, and M. A. Riva, "Stress during development: impact on neuroplasticity and relevance to psychopathology," *Progress in Neurobiology*, vol. 81, no. 4, pp. 197–217, 2007.

[11] P. O. McGowan, A. Sasaki, A. C. D'Alessio et al., "Epigenetic regulation of the glucocorticoid receptor in human brain associates with childhood abuse," *Nature Neuroscience*, vol. 12, no. 3, pp. 342–348, 2009.

[12] T. F. Oberlander, J. Weinberg, M. Papsdorf, R. Grunau, S. Misri, and A. M. Devlin, "Prenatal exposure to maternal depression,

[13] T. L. Roth, P. R. Zoladz, J. D. Sweatt, and D. M. Diamond, "Epigenetic modification of hippocampal *Bdnf* DNA in adult rats in an animal model of post-traumatic stress disorder," *Journal of Psychiatric Research*, vol. 45, no. 7, pp. 919–926, 2011.

[14] K. Koshibu, J. Gräff, and I. M. Mansuy, "Nuclear protein phosphatase-1: an epigenetic regulator of fear memory and amygdala long-term potentiation," *Neuroscience*, vol. 173, pp. 30–36, 2011.

[15] F. Tian, A. M. Marini, and R. H. Lipsky, "Effects of histone deacetylase inhibitor Trichostatin A on epigenetic changes and transcriptional activation of *Bdnf* promoter 1 by rat hippocampal neurons," *Annals of the New York Academy of Sciences*, vol. 1199, pp. 186–193, 2010.

[16] E. Vanderbilt-Adriance and D. S. Shaw, "Neighborhood risk and the development of resilience," *Annals of the New York Academy of Sciences*, vol. 1094, pp. 359–362, 2006.

[17] E. Vanderbilt-Adriance and D. S. Shaw, "Conceptualizing and re-evaluating resilience across levels of risk, time, and domains of competence," *Clinical Child and Family Psychology Review*, vol. 11, no. 1-2, pp. 30–58, 2008.

[18] M. Uddin, A. E. Aiello, D. E. Wildman et al., "Epigenetic and immune function profiles associated with posttraumatic stress disorder," *Proceedings of the National Academy of Sciences of the United States of America*, vol. 107, no. 20, pp. 9470–9475, 2010.

[19] K. J. Ressler, K. B. Mercer, B. Bradley et al., "Post-traumatic stress disorder is associated with PACAP and the PAC1 receptor," *Nature*, vol. 470, no. 7335, pp. 492–497, 2011.

[20] J. Gill, D. Luckenbaugh, D. Charney, and M. Vythilingam, "Sustained elevation of serum interleukin-6 and relative insensitivity to hydrocortisone differentiates posttraumatic stress disorder with and without depression," *Biological Psychiatry*, vol. 68, no. 11, pp. 999–1006, 2010.

[21] C. S. de Kloet, E. Vermetten, A. R. Rademaker, E. Geuze, and H. G. M. Westenberg, "Neuroendocrine and immune responses to a cognitive stress challenge in veterans with and without PTSD," *European Journal of Psychotraumatology*, vol. 2012, article 3, 2012.

[22] K. C. Koenen, M. Uddin, S. C. Chang et al., "*SLC6A4* methylation modifies the effect of the number of traumatic events on risk for posttraumatic stress disorder," *Depression and Anxiety*, vol. 28, no. 8, pp. 639–647, 2011.

[23] A. K. Smith, K. N. Conneely, V. Kilaru et al., "Differential immune system DNA methylation and cytokine regulation in post-traumatic stress disorder," *American Journal of Medical Genetics B*, vol. 156, no. 6, pp. 700–708, 2011.

[24] M. Uddin, S. Galea, S. C. Chang et al., "Gene expression and methylation signatures of MAN2C1 are associated with PTSD," *Disease Markers*, vol. 30, no. 2-3, pp. 111–121, 2011.

[25] J. A. Rusiecki, L. Chen, V. Srikantan et al., "DNA methylation in repetitive elements and post-traumatic stress disorder: a case-control study of US military service members," *Epigenomics*, vol. 4, no. 1, pp. 29–40, 2012.

[26] J. Zieker, D. Zieker, A. Jatzko et al., "Differential gene expression in peripheral blood of patients suffering from post-traumatic stress disorder," *Molecular Psychiatry*, vol. 12, no. 2, pp. 116–118, 2007.

[27] R. Yehuda, G. Cai, J. A. Golier et al., "Gene expression patterns associated with posttraumatic stress disorder following exposure to the world trade center attacks," *Biological Psychiatry*, vol. 66, no. 7, pp. 708–711, 2009.

[28] T. C. Neylan, B. Sun, H. Rempel et al., "Suppressed monocyte gene expression profile in men versus women with PTSD," *Brain, Behavior, and Immunity*, vol. 25, no. 3, pp. 524–531, 2011.

[29] C. Sarapas, G. Cai, L. M. Bierer et al., "Genetic markers for PTSD risk and resilience among survivors of the world trade center attacks," *Disease Markers*, vol. 30, no. 2-3, pp. 101–110, 2011.

[30] D. Mehta, M. Gonik, T. Klengel et al., "Using polymorphisms in *FKBP5* to define biologically distinct subtypes of posttraumatic stress disorder: evidence from endocrine and gene expression studies," *Archives of General Psychiatry*, vol. 68, no. 9, pp. 901–910, 2011.

[31] T. W. Pace, K. Wingenfeld, I. Schmidt, G. Meinlschmidt, D. H. Hellhammer, and C. M. Heim, "Increased peripheral NF-κB pathway activity in women with childhood abuse-related posttraumatic stress disorder," *Brain, Behavior, and Immunity*, vol. 26, no. 1, pp. 13–17, 2012.

[32] M. van Zuiden, E. Geuze, H. L. Willemen et al., "Glucocorticoid receptor pathway components predict posttraumatic stress disorder symptom development: a prospective study," *Biological Psychiatry*, vol. 71, no. 4, pp. 309–316, 2012.

[33] M. van Zuiden, C. J. Heijnen, M. Maas et al., "Glucocorticoid sensitivity of leukocytes predicts PTSD, depressive and fatigue symptoms after military deployment: a prospective study," *Psychoneuroendocrinology*, vol. 37, no. 11, pp. 1822–1836, 2012.

[34] G. Matić, D. V. Milutinović, J. Nestorov et al., "Lymphocyte glucocorticoid receptor expression level and hormone-binding properties differ between war trauma-exposed men with and without PTSD," *Progress in Neuro-Psychopharmacology and Biological Psychiatry*, vol. 43, pp. 238–245, 2013.

[35] D. L. Delahanty, N. R. Nugent, N. C. Christopher, and M. Walsh, "Initial urinary epinephrine and cortisol levels predict acute PTSD symptoms in child trauma victims," *Psychoneuroendocrinology*, vol. 30, no. 2, pp. 121–128, 2005.

[36] S. A. Ostrowski, N. C. Christopher, M. H. M. Van Dulmen, and D. L. Delahanty, "Acute child and mother psychophysiological responses and subsequent PTSD symptoms following a child's traumatic event," *Journal of Traumatic Stress*, vol. 20, no. 5, pp. 677–687, 2007.

[37] P. Pervanidou, G. Kolaitis, S. Charitaki et al., "Elevated morning serum interleukin (IL)-6 or evening salivary cortisol concentrations predict posttraumatic stress disorder in children and adolescents six months after a motor vehicle accident," *Psychoneuroendocrinology*, vol. 32, no. 8-10, pp. 991–999, 2007.

[38] H. S. Resnick, R. Yehuda, R. K. Pitman, and D. W. Foy, "Effect of previous trauma on acute plasma cortisol level following rape," *The American Journal of Psychiatry*, vol. 152, no. 11, pp. 1675–1677, 1995.

[39] R. Yehuda, H. S. Resnick, J. Schmeidler, R. K. Yang, and R. K. Pitman, "Predictors of cortisol and 3-methoxy-4-hydroxyphenylglycol responses in the acute aftermath of rape," *Biological Psychiatry*, vol. 43, no. 11, pp. 855–859, 1998.

[40] D. L. Delahanty, A. J. Raimonde, and E. Spoonster, "Initial posttraumatic urinary cortisol levels predict subsequent PTSD symptoms in motor vehicle accident victims," *Biological Psychiatry*, vol. 48, no. 9, pp. 940–947, 2000.

[41] O. Bonne, D. Brandes, R. Segman, R. K. Pitman, R. Yehuda, and A. Y. Shalev, "Prospective evaluation of plasma cortisol in recent trauma survivors with posttraumatic stress disorder," *Psychiatry Research*, vol. 119, no. 1-2, pp. 171–175, 2003.

[42] M. Heinrichs, D. Wagner, W. Schoch, L. M. Soravia, D. H. Hellhammer, and U. Ehlert, "Predicting posttraumatic stress symptoms from pretraumatic risk factors: a 2-year prospective follow-up study in firefighters," *The American Journal of Psychiatry*, vol. 162, no. 12, pp. 2276–2286, 2005.

[43] A. C. McFarlane, M. Atchison, and R. Yehuda, "The acute stress response following motor vehicle accidents and its relation to PTSD," *Annals of the New York Academy of Sciences*, vol. 821, pp. 437–441, 1997.

[44] T. Ehring, A. Ehlers, A. J. Cleare, and E. Glucksman, "Do acute psychological and psychobiological responses to trauma predict subsequent symptom severities of PTSD and depression?" *Psychiatry Research*, vol. 161, no. 1, pp. 67–75, 2008.

[45] A. Y. Shalev, E. J. Videlock, T. Peleg, R. Segman, R. K. Pitman, and R. Yehuda, "Stress hormones and post-traumatic stress disorder in civilian trauma victims: a longitudinal study—part I: HPA axis responses," *International Journal of Neuropsychopharmacology*, vol. 11, no. 3, pp. 365–372, 2008.

[46] E. J. Videlock, T. Peleg, R. Segman, R. Yehuda, R. K. Pitman, and A. Y. Shalev, "Stress hormones and post-traumatic stress disorder in civilian trauma victims: a longitudinal study—part II: the adrenergic response," *International Journal of Neuropsychopharmacology*, vol. 11, no. 3, pp. 373–380, 2008.

[47] M. Cohen, T. Meir, E. Klein, G. Volpin, M. Assaf, and S. Pollack, "Cytokine levels as potential biomarkers for predicting the development of posttraumatic stress symptoms in casualties of accidents," *International Journal of Psychiatry in Medicine*, vol. 42, no. 2, pp. 117–131, 2011.

[48] M. van Zuiden, E. Geuze, H. L. D. M. Willemen et al., "Pre-existing high glucocorticoid receptor number predicting development of posttraumatic stress symptoms after military deployment," *The American Journal of Psychiatry*, vol. 168, no. 1, pp. 89–96, 2011.

[49] D. Mehta and E. B. Binder, "Gene *x* environment vulnerability factors for PTSD: the HPA-axis," *Neuropharmacology*, vol. 62, no. 2, pp. 654–662, 2012.

[50] J. A. Boscarino, P. M. Erlich, S. N. Hoffman, M. Rukstalis, and W. F. Stewart, "Association of FKBP5, COMT and CHRNA5 polymorphisms with PTSD among outpatients at risk for PTSD," *Psychiatry Research*, vol. 188, no. 1, pp. 173–174, 2011.

[51] C. F. Gillespie, J. Phifer, B. Bradley, and K. J. Ressler, "Risk and resilience: genetic and environmental influences on development of the stress response," *Depression and Anxiety*, vol. 26, no. 11, pp. 984–992, 2009.

[52] A. B. Amstadter, N. R. Nugent, B. Z. Yang et al., "Corticotrophin-releasing hormone type 1 receptor gene (CRHR1) variants predict posttraumatic stress disorder onset and course in pediatric injury patients," *Disease Markers*, vol. 30, no. 2-3, pp. 89–99, 2011.

[53] S. L. Szanton and J. M. Gill, "Facilitating resilience using a society-to-cells framework: a theory of nursing essentials applied to research and practice," *Advances in Nursing Science*, vol. 33, no. 4, pp. 329–343, 2010.

[54] Y. Song, D. Zhou, Z. Guan, and X. Wang, "Disturbance of serum interleukin-2 and interleukin-8 levels in posttraumatic and non-posttraumatic stress disorder earthquake survivors in Northern China," *NeuroImmunoModulation*, vol. 14, no. 5, pp. 248–254, 2007.

[55] J. Gill, M. Vythilingam, and G. G. Page, "Low cortisol, high DHEA, and high levels of stimulated TNF-α, and IL-6 in

women with PTSD," *Journal of Traumatic Stress*, vol. 21, no. 6, pp. 530–539, 2008.

[56] S. Bonaccorso, V. Marino, A. Puzella et al., "Increased depressive ratings in patients with hepatitis C receiving interferon-α-based immunotherapy are related to interferon-α-induced changes in the serotonergic system," *Journal of Clinical Psychopharmacology*, vol. 22, no. 1, pp. 86–90, 2002.

[57] G. A. Bonanno and A. D. Mancini, "The human capacity to thrive in the face of potential trauma," *Pediatrics*, vol. 121, no. 2, pp. 369–375, 2008.

[58] L. Capuron, J. F. Gumnick, D. L. Musselman et al., "Neurobehavioral effects of interferon-α in cancer patients: phenomenology and paroxetine responsiveness of symptom dimensions," *Neuropsychopharmacology*, vol. 26, no. 5, pp. 643–652, 2002.

[59] L. Capuron, G. Neurauter, D. L. Musselman et al., "Interferon-α-induced changes in tryptophan metabolism: relationship to depression and paroxetine treatment," *Biological Psychiatry*, vol. 54, no. 9, pp. 906–914, 2003.

[60] M. C. Wichers, G. Kenis, G. H. Koek, G. Robaeys, N. A. Nicolson, and M. Maes, "Interferon-α-induced depressive symptoms are related to changes in the cytokine network but not to cortisol," *Journal of Psychosomatic Research*, vol. 62, no. 2, pp. 207–214, 2007.

[61] T. H. Wu and C. H. Lin, "IL-6 mediated alterations on immobile behavior of rats in the forced swim test via ERK1/2 activation in specific brain regions," *Behavioural Brain Research*, vol. 193, no. 2, pp. 183–191, 2008.

[62] M. Maes, M. Kubera, and J. C. Leunis, "The gut-brain barrier in major depression: intestinal mucosal dysfunction with an increased translocation of LPS from gram negative enterobacteria (leaky gut) plays a role in the inflammatory pathophysiology of depression," *Neuro endocrinology letters*, vol. 29, no. 1, pp. 117–124, 2008.

[63] S. J. Campbell, R. M. J. Deacon, Y. Jiang, C. Ferrari, F. J. Pitossi, and D. C. Anthony, "Overexpression of IL-1β by adenoviral-mediated gene transfer in the rat brain causes a prolonged hepatic chemokine response, axonal injury and the suppression of spontaneous behaviour," *Neurobiology of Disease*, vol. 27, no. 2, pp. 151–163, 2007.

[64] A. Pierucci-Lagha, J. Covault, H. L. Bonkovsky et al., "A functional serotonin transporter gene polymorphism and depressive effects associated with interferon-α treatment," *Psychosomatics*, vol. 51, no. 2, pp. 137–148, 2010.

[65] S. Su, J. Zhao, J. D. Bremner et al., "Serotonin transporter gene, depressive symptoms, and interleukin-6," *Circulation: Cardiovascular Genetics*, vol. 2, no. 6, pp. 614–620, 2009.

[66] A. Schäfer, M. Scheurlen, J. Seufert et al., "Platelet serotonin (5-HT) levels in interferon-treated patients with hepatitis C and its possible association with interferon-induced depression," *Journal of Hepatology*, vol. 52, no. 1, pp. 10–15, 2010.

[67] M. C. Wichers, G. H. Koek, G. Robaeys, R. Verkerk, S. Scharpé, and M. Maes, "IDO and interferon-α-induced depressive symptoms: a shift in hypothesis from tryptophan depletion to neurotoxicity," *Molecular Psychiatry*, vol. 10, no. 6, pp. 538–544, 2005.

[68] J. T. Järvelä, S. Ruohonen, T. K. Kukko-Lukjanov, A. Plysjuk, F. R. Lopez-Picon, and I. E. Holopainen, "Kainic acid-induced neurodegeneration and activation of inflammatory processes in organotypic hippocampal slice cultures: treatment with cyclooxygenase-2 inhibitor does not prevent neuronal death," *Neuropharmacology*, vol. 60, no. 7-8, pp. 1116–1125, 2011.

[69] J. T. Yu, C. H. Lee, K. Y. Yoo et al., "Maintenance of anti-inflammatory cytokines and reduction of glial activation in the ischemic hippocampal CA1 region preconditioned with lipopolysaccharide," *Journal of the Neurological Sciences*, vol. 296, no. 1-2, pp. 69–78, 2010.

[70] C. D. Munhoz, B. García-Bueno, J. L. Madrigal, L. B. Lepsch, C. Scavone, and J. C. Leza, "Stress-induced neuroinflammation: mechanisms and new pharmacological targets," *Brazilian Journal of Medical and Biological Research*, vol. 41, no. 12, pp. 1037–1046, 2008.

[71] R. A. Bryant, J. E. Marosszeky, J. Crooks, and J. A. Gurka, "Elevated resting heart rate as a predictor of posttraumatic stress disorder after severe traumatic brain injury," *Psychosomatic Medicine*, vol. 66, no. 5, pp. 760–761, 2004.

[72] R. A. Bryant, A. G. Harvey, R. M. Guthrie, and M. L. Moulds, "A prospective study of psychophysiological arousal, acute stress disorder, and posttraumatic stress disorder," *Journal of Abnormal Psychology*, vol. 109, no. 2, pp. 341–344, 2000.

[73] J. H. Krystal and A. Neumeister, "Noradrenergic and serotonergic mechanisms in the neurobiology of posttraumatic stress disorder and resilience," *Brain Research*, vol. 1293, pp. 13–23, 2009.

[74] E. A. Walker, W. Katon, J. Russo, P. Ciechanowski, E. Newman, and A. W. Wagner, "Health care costs associated with posttraumatic stress disorder symptoms in women," *Archives of General Psychiatry*, vol. 60, no. 4, pp. 369–374, 2003.

[75] M. D. Marciniak, M. J. Lage, E. Dunayevich et al., "The cost of treating anxiety: the medical and demographic correlates that impact total medical costs," *Depression and Anxiety*, vol. 21, no. 4, pp. 178–184, 2005.

[76] S. Priebe, J. J. Gavrilovic, A. Matanov et al., "Treatment outcomes and costs at specialized centers for the treatment of PTSD after the war in former Yugoslavia," *Psychiatric Services*, vol. 61, no. 6, pp. 598–604, 2010.

[77] M. L. O'Donnell, M. Creamer, P. Elliott, and C. Atkin, "Health costs following motor vehicle accidents: the role of posttraumatic stress disorder," *Journal of Traumatic Stress*, vol. 18, no. 5, pp. 557–561, 2005.

[78] R. Kimerling, J. Alvarez, J. Pavao, K. P. MacK, M. W. Smith, and N. Baumrind, "Unemployment among women: examining the relationship of physical and psychological intimate partner violence and posttraumatic stress disorder," *Journal of Interpersonal Violence*, vol. 24, no. 3, pp. 450–463, 2009.

[79] A. Nandi, S. Galea, M. Tracy et al., "Job loss, unemployment, work stress, job satisfaction, and the persistence of posttraumatic stress disorder one year after the september 11 attacks," *Journal of Occupational and Environmental Medicine*, vol. 46, no. 10, pp. 1057–1064, 2004.

[80] H. C. Wilcox, C. L. Storr, and N. Breslau, "Posttraumatic stress disorder and suicide attempts in a community sample of urban American young adults," *Archives of General Psychiatry*, vol. 66, no. 3, pp. 305–311, 2009.

[81] D. J. Stein, W. T. Chiu, I. Hwang et al., "Cross-national analysis of the associations between traumatic events and suicidal behavior: findings from the WHO world mental health surveys," *PloS ONE*, vol. 5, no. 5, Article ID e10574, 2010.

[82] J. L. Gradus, P. Qin, A. K. Lincoln et al., "Posttraumatic stress disorder and completed suicide," *The American Journal of Epidemiology*, vol. 171, no. 6, pp. 721–727, 2010.

[83] J. R. Cougle, H. Resnick, and D. G. Kilpatrick, "PTSD, depression, and their comorbidity in relation to suicidality: cross-sectional and prospective analyses of a national probability

sample of women," *Depression and Anxiety*, vol. 26, no. 12, pp. 1151–1157, 2009.

[84] S. B. Vyrostek, J. L. Annest, and G. W. Ryan, "Surveillance for fatal and nonfatal injuries—United States, 2001," *Morbidity and Mortality Weekly Report: Surveillance Summaries*, vol. 53, no. 7, pp. 1–57, 2004.

[85] D. Zatzick, G. J. Jurkovich, F. P. Rivara et al., "A national US study of posttraumatic stress disorder, depression, and work and functional outcomes after hospitalization for traumatic injury," *Annals of Surgery*, vol. 248, no. 3, pp. 429–437, 2008.

[86] N. Breslau, "Trauma and mental health in US inner-city populations," *General Hospital Psychiatry*, vol. 31, no. 6, pp. 501–502, 2009.

[87] D. Zatzick, J. Russo, D. C. Grossman et al., "Posttraumatic stress and depressive symptoms, alcohol use, and recurrent traumatic life events in a representative sample of hospitalized injured adolescents and their parents," *Journal of Pediatric Psychology*, vol. 31, no. 4, pp. 377–387, 2006.

22

Toothbrush Contamination: A Review of the Literature

Michelle R. Frazelle[1] and Cindy L. Munro[1, 2]

[1] School of Nursing, Virginia Commonwealth University, 1100 East Leigh Street, Richmond, VA 23298-0567, USA
[2] School of Nursing, University of South Florida, 12901 Bruce B Downs Boulevard, Tampa, FL 33612, USA

Correspondence should be addressed to Michelle R. Frazelle, frazellemr@vcu.edu

Academic Editor: Mary George

Toothbrushes are commonly used in hospital settings and may harbor potentially harmful microorganisms. A peer-reviewed literature review was conducted to evaluate the cumulative state of knowledge related to toothbrush contamination and its possible role in disease transmission. A systematic review was conducted on adult human subjects through three distinct searches. The review resulted in seven experimental and three descriptive studies which identified multiple concepts related to toothbrush contamination to include contamination, methods for decontamination, storage, design, and environmental factors. The selected studies found that toothbrushes of healthy and oral diseased adults become contaminated with pathogenic bacteria from the dental plaque, design, environment, or a combination of factors. There are no studies that specifically examine toothbrush contamination and the role of environmental factors, toothbrush contamination, and vulnerable populations in the hospital setting (e.g., critically ill adults) and toothbrush use in nursing clinical practice.

1. Introduction

Toothbrushes play an essential role in oral hygiene and are commonly found in both community and hospital settings. Toothbrushes may play a significant role in disease transmission and increase the risk of infection since they can serve as a reservoir for microorganisms in healthy, oral-diseased and medically ill adults [1]. Contamination is the retention and survival of infectious organisms that occur on animate or inanimate objects. In healthy adults, contamination of toothbrushes occurs early after initial use and increases with repeated use [2, 3]. Toothbrushes can become contaminated from the oral cavity, environment, hands, aerosol contamination, and storage containers. Bacteria which attach to, accumulate, and survive on toothbrushes may be transmitted to the individual causing disease [4, 5]. In the hospital setting, toothbrushes are commonly used for oral care by nurses. There is a need for standardized nursing guidelines to prevent toothbrush contamination, which may increase the risk of infections from potentially pathogenic microorganisms and is clinically relevant for assessing the risks and benefits of oral care and informing nursing practice. This review of peer-reviewed literature was conducted to evaluate the cumulative state of knowledge related to toothbrush contamination, its possible role in disease transmission, and in preparation for a research study related to toothbrush contamination in critically ill adults.

2. Methods

A systematic review of the scientific literature was conducted. There were no relevant articles available in print prior to 1977. Articles published from 1977 to 2011, on human subjects and using the English language were obtained. The review included studies that evaluated toothbrush contamination in healthy and oral-diseased adults, guidelines for toothbrush and oral care in both healthy and medically ill persons, hospitalized and nonhospitalized patients, and interventions for reducing contamination of toothbrushes. Experimental and nonexperimental designs were included in the review. The following databases were searched: Pub Med (clinical inquiries and MESH), CINAHL, Cochrane Library, National Guidelines Clearinghouse, Web of Science, and Google Scholar. Key search terms used in the review were *toothbrush, tooth brushing, colonization, bacterial contamination, contamination, oral hygiene, oral health, nursing practice,*

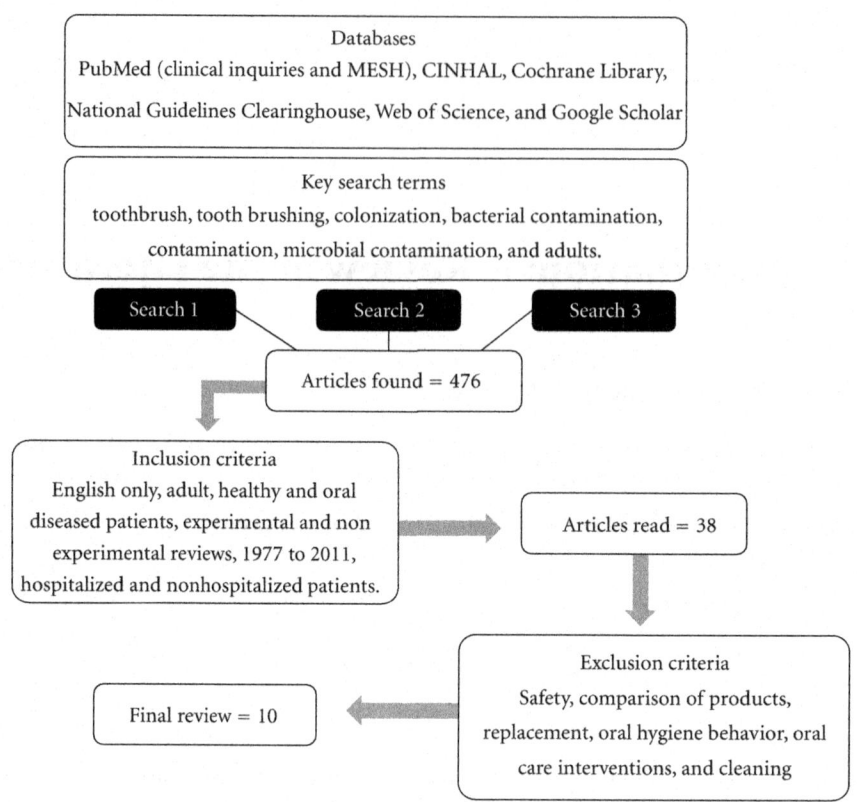

FIGURE 1: Literature search process.

TABLE 1: Results of Search 1.

Database	Initial number of articles located
PubMed	26
CINAHL	16
Cochrane Library	10
National Guidelines Clearinghouse	None
Web of Science	22
Google Scholar	376

microbial contamination, and *adults.* This search strategy was verified by a health sciences librarian. A total of three separate searches were conducted in a systematic fashion using the inclusion and exclusion criteria and search terms. The first search (search 1) identified articles in the selected databases and complete copies of articles that were considered to have met the inclusion criteria were obtained for further review (Table 1). Articles were excluded if they did not meet the inclusion criteria listed above, were conducted on a pediatric population, were duplicates from other databases, or only explored antibacterial methods.

The second search (search two) included articles identified through cited articles and were reviewed following the same criteria. There were a total of 23 new articles identified through the second search. A third search (search three) was conducted one year after the first search in order to

capture any recently published articles. There were three new articles identified in the third search. After a review of the abstracts for the articles obtained through the three searches, a total of 88 relevant articles were identified for further evaluation. After inclusion criteria were applied, 38 articles were selected; after exclusion criteria were applied, ten articles were retrieved to be read in their entirety and included in this review (Figure 1).

3. Results

A comprehensive summary of the studies is listed in Table 2. Studies that were reviewed included: seven experimental and three descriptive studies. The selected studies are grouped by setting in vivo, in vitro, and studies that combined both types of settings. The sample sizes ranged from 3 to 103 with the majority of studies having a sample size under 30. Overall, the studies evaluated several perspectives related to toothbrush contamination to include: contamination, methods for decontamination, storage, design, and environmental factors.

3.1. Contamination. All of the studies examined toothbrush contamination and found significant bacterial retention and survival on toothbrushes after use [6, 7]. Glass found that toothbrushes from both healthy patients and patients with oral disease contained potentially pathogenic bacteria and viruses such as *Staphylococcus aureus, E. coli, Pseudomonas,*

TABLE 2: Studies Selected.

Study	Purpose	Design	Sample	Results
In vitro studies				
Bunetel et al. (2000) [8]	Does retention and survival of microorganisms on toothbrushes pose a threat to patients at risk of infection?	Experimental	$N = 3$ toothbrush types with two series of experiments	Contamination of toothbrushes occurs early in the life of the brush and tends to increase with repeated use.
Dayoub et al. (1977) [18]	To determine the degree of bacterial contamination of toothbrushes after contamination and storage in vented containers or in air.	Experimental	$N = 103$ toothbrushes	The numbers of bacteria on toothbrushes stored in room air after use decrease more quickly than on brushes in containers.
Glass and Jensen (1994) [9]	To evaluate toothbrush design and UV sanitation on microbial growth.	Experimental	$N = 72$ toothbrushes	UV sanitizing kills bacteria; viruses can survive on toothbrushes for 24 hours; toothbrush design, color, opacity, and bristle arrangement are a major factor in retaining microorganisms.
In vivo studies				
Efstratiou et al. (2007) [14]	To examine the contamination and the survival rate of periodontopathic and cariogenic species on new toothbrushes with antibacterial properties after a single use in periodontic patients.	Experimental	$N = 10$ patients; 4 toothbrushes per patient.	Immediately after brushing, the toothbrushes harbored a significant number of microorganisms with no difference between the types of toothbrushes. The antibacterial toothbrush did not limit bacterial contamination.
Mehta et al. (2007) [10]	To determine the extent of bacterial contamination of toothbrushes after use, evaluate the efficacy of chlorhexidine and Listerine in decontamination, and effectiveness of covering the toothbrush head with a cap.	Experimental	$N = 10$ patients	Toothbrushes become contaminated during use; retention of moisture and the presence of organic matter may promote bacterial growth. Toothbrush contamination may lead to colonization and infection. Caps increase bacterial growth. Chlorhexidine was more effective than Listerine.
Quirynen et al. (2003) [15]	To evaluate the effects of coated tuffs and toothpaste on toothbrush contamination.	Experimental	$N = 8$ patients	Toothbrushes become contaminated and toothpaste reduced bacterial growth in toothbrushes.
Taji and Rogers (1998) [11]	To investigate the microbial contamination of toothbrushes.	Descriptive	$N = 10$ patients	Most toothbrushes were contaminated.
Verran and Leahy-Gilmartin (1996) [13]	To evaluate toothbrush contamination using a range of selective and nonselective media.	Descriptive	$N = 28$ toothbrushes	Used toothbrushes supported a wide variety of microorganisms. All media showed growth.
Combination of both in vitro and in vivo studies				
Caudry et al. (1995) [5]	To demonstrate, quantitatively, the presence of microorganisms adherent to toothbrush bristles.	Experimental	$N = 20$ toothbrushes	Toothbrushes, in normal use, are heavily contaminated by microorganisms and the bacteria are extremely adherent to the bristles.

TABLE 2: Continued.

Study	Purpose	Design	Sample	Results
Glass and Lare (1986) [6]	Do toothbrushes harbor pathogenic microorganisms and if there is a correlation between contaminated brushes and the presence of disease.	Descriptive	$N = 30$ toothbrushes	Toothbrushes can harbor pathogenic microorganisms.

and herpes simplex virus [1]. Glass also found toothbrushes contaminated with herpes simplex virus 1 in numbers sufficient to cause an infection in the patient [1]. Bunetel et al. found that toothbrushes used by patients with existing oral disease quickly became contaminated [8]. This study also found a significant relationship between repeated use and bacterial retention on toothbrushes and that the oral cavity can be inoculated from a contaminated toothbrush. Several of the studies found that toothbrushes were contaminated before use [5, 9]. Caudry et al. found that toothbrushes are heavily contaminated with normal use [5]. Mehta et al. found that 70% of the toothbrushes in their study became heavily contaminated with pathogenic microorganisms after use [10]. Studies by both Taji and Rogers [11] and Glass [12] found extensive toothbrush contamination after use except in cases where an oral antiseptic, such as mouthwash, was used immediately prior to brushing. Verran and Leahy-Gilmartin found that toothbrushes supported many different bacteria and the amount of growth was varied [13].

3.2. Decontamination. Several studies included in this review explored decontamination techniques for contaminated toothbrushes. Bunetel et al. found that toothpaste, mouthwash, and oral antiseptics all decrease microbial load on toothbrushes [8]. Caudry et al. examined toothbrushes in healthy adults as well as possible options for disinfection [5]. Their study found that the toothbrushes became heavily contaminated after use. Soaking the toothbrush in Listerine for 20 minutes prior to and after brushing decreased the microbial load. The use of antimicrobial coated toothbrushes in adults with oral disease was explored by Efstratiou et al. as a means to prevent toothbrush contamination [14]. This study, however, found that coating the bristles with triclosan did not change bacterial growth but the use of toothpaste did. Glass and Jensen explored ultraviolet light as a means of decontamination and found this method to be effective at reducing the bacterial load on toothbrushes [9]. The use of coated tufts and toothpaste was investigated in adult patients with oral disease. Quirynen et al. found that coated tuffs did not inhibit contamination but use of toothpaste did reduce contamination [15]. Mehta et al. found that an overnight immersion in chlorhexidine gluconate was highly effective in decreasing toothbrush contamination and chlorhexidine was more effective than Listerine in reducing the microbial load of bacteria [10]. Sato et al. found that rinsing toothbrushes with tap water resulted in continued high levels of contamination and biofilm [16]. Warren et al. found that the use of regular and triclosan-containing

toothpaste resulted in lower toothbrush contamination than no toothpaste use [17].

3.3. Storage and Environment. Toothbrushes can become contaminated through contact with the environment, and bacterial survival is affected by toothbrush storage containers. Dayoub et al. found that toothbrushes placed in closed containers and exposure to contaminated surfaces yielded higher bacterial counts than those left open to air [18]. Mehta et al. found that the use of a cap for toothbrush storage increased bacteria survival [10]. Glass found that increased humidity in the environment increased bacterial survival on toothbrushes [12]. In addition, Glass found that bacteria survived more than 24 hours when moisture is present [12].

3.4. Design. Toothbrushes are manufactured in a variety of styles. Toothbrush bristles range from soft to hard with different cluster patterns and plastic shapes while toothbrush handles included different plastic shapes and decorative moldings. Different toothbrush design elements were examined by some of the studies. Bunetel et al. found that bacteria become trapped inside the bristles of the toothbrush and bacterial survival is dependent upon the bacteria (aerobic versus anaerobic) and toothbrush design [8]. In addition, the researchers found that solid handles had less bacteria retention and that as the surface area increased, so did the microbial load. Efstratiou et al. found that filament type affected bacterial retention [14]. Toothbrushes with bristles that are frayed and arranged closely together trapped and retained more bacteria [19]. This finding was also echoed in a study by Glass [1] that explored the level of bacterial retention based on toothbrush brand, color and bristle pattern. Contamination was the lowest in soft and round, clear, two bristle row toothbrushes. Glass also found that pathogenic bacteria adhere to plastic after short exposure times [1]. Caudry et al. found that bacteria strongly adhere to the bristles [5]. Mehta et al. found that the retention of moisture and oral debris in the bristles increased bacterial survival [10].

4. Conclusions

Due to the limited number of publications specifically related to toothbrush contamination, it was necessary to conduct a preliminary evaluation of the majority of identified articles for this review. For example, several of the articles combined an in vivo examination of bacterial survival on actual patient's toothbrushes and then conducted an in vitro autoinoculation experiment to examine decontamination methods on sterile toothbrushes in the laboratory. This made database searching and identification of articles for the review more challenging. The selected studies all found that toothbrushes of healthy and oral diseased adults become contaminated with potentially pathogenic bacteria from the dental plaque, design, environment, or a combination of factors. The trend identified in the literature is to evaluate methods to reduce toothbrush contamination or toothbrush design rather than evaluating the process related to how the toothbrush initially becomes contaminated, is stored, or is disinfected.

In a vulnerable population such as critically ill adults, pathogenic contamination may increase the risk of infection and mortality. Although some interventions such as chlorhexidine, toothpaste, mouthwash, and ultraviolet sanitizers reduce bacterial survival, oral hygiene practices in the hospital setting by nurses vary. Currently, there are no nursing guidelines related to toothbrush frequency of use, storage, and decontamination. In the hospital setting, the environment as a source of pathogenic bacteria is now a hot topic and the focus of many current infectious disease research studies. Surfaces in close contact with the patient such as bed frames, countertops, sinks, bedside tables, linens, and mattresses may act as fomites. Toothbrushes may come into contact with these surfaces prior to or after use thus increasing risk. While there is significant literature available on environmental contamination and risk for infection, no studies have specifically examined the toothbrush on more vulnerable hospital populations such as critically ill adults.

Toothbrush storage is inconsistent in both community and hospital environments and may increase exposure to pathogenic organisms. The storage conditions of toothbrushes play an important role in bacterial survival: toothbrushes stored in aerated conditions had a lower number of bacteria than those stored in plastic and bacterial growth on the toothbrush increased 70% in a moist, covered environment [10]. In clinical practice, the author has observed that there is no standardized nursing protocol for the storage or replacement of toothbrushes and that some commonly observed nursing practices include storing the toothbrush in the bath basin with other bathing/personal supplies and linens, in a paper towel, in a plastic wrapper, on the bedside table, next to the sink, and in an oral rinse cup at the bedside. These practices may impact the contamination of toothbrushes.

In this review, the majority of studies identified had small sample sizes. Studies with larger sample sizes would be beneficial in future studies. Importantly, despite multiple studies supporting toothbrush contamination and the likely relationship between contamination and disease transmission, there are no studies that specifically examine toothbrush contamination and the role of environmental factors, toothbrush contamination and vulnerable populations in the hospital setting (e.g., critically ill adults), and toothbrush use in nursing clinical practice. Additional descriptive studies to evaluate these relationships would be beneficial and informative for future research. The relationship between environmental factors, toothbrush contamination, and patient oral colonization would inform development of nursing oral care

guidelines for adults that minimize risks related to toothbrush contamination.

References

[1] R. T. Glass, "The infected toothbrush, the infected denture, and transmission of disease: a review," *Compendium*, vol. 13, no. 7, pp. 592–598, 1992.

[2] M. J. M. Bonten, M. K. Hayden, C. Nathan et al., "Epidemiology of colonisation of patients and environment with vancomycin-resistant enterococci," *The Lancet*, vol. 348, no. 9042, pp. 1615–1619, 1996.

[3] Centers for Disease Control. In CDC's National Center for Infectious Diseases, 2002, http://www.cdc.gov/oralhealth/infectioncontrol/factsheets/toothbrushes.htm.

[4] ADA.org: ADA statement on toothbrush care: cleaning, storage and replacement, 2009, http://www.ada.org/1887.aspx.

[5] S. D. Caudry, A. Klitorinos, and E. C. Chan, "Contaminated toothbrushes and their disinfection," *Journal (Canadian Dental Association)*, vol. 61, no. 6, pp. 511–516, 1995.

[6] R. T. Glass and M. M. Lare, "Toothbrush contamination: a potential health risk?" *Quintessence International*, vol. 17, no. 1, pp. 39–42, 1986.

[7] N. Grewal and K. Swaranjit, "A study of toothbrush contamination at different time intervals and comparative effectiveness of various disinfecting solutions in reducing toothbrush contamination," *Journal of the Indian Society of Pedodontics and Preventive Dentistry*, vol. 14, no. 1, pp. 10–13, 1996.

[8] L. Bunetel, S. Tricot-Doleux, G. Agnani, and M. Bonnaure-Mallet, "In vitro evaluation of the retention of three species of pathogenic microorganisms by three different types of toothbrush," *Oral Microbiology and Immunology*, vol. 15, no. 5, pp. 313–316, 2000.

[9] R. T. Glass and H. G. Jensen, "The effectiveness of a u-v toothbrush sanitizing device in reducing the number of bacteria, yeasts and viruses on toothbrushes," *Journal—Oklahoma Dental Association*, vol. 84, no. 4, pp. 24–28, 1994.

[10] A. Mehta, P. S. Sequeira, and G. Bhat, "Bacterial contamination and decontamination of toothbrushes after use," *The New York State Dental Journal*, vol. 73, no. 3, pp. 20–22, 2007.

[11] S. S. Taji and A. H. Rogers, "The microbial contamination of toothbrushes. A pilot study," *Australian Dental Journal*, vol. 43, no. 2, pp. 128–130, 1998.

[12] R. T. Glass, "Toothbrush types and retention of microorganisms: how to choose a biologically sound toothbrush," *Journal—Oklahoma Dental Association*, vol. 82, no. 3, pp. 26–28, 1992.

[13] J. Verran and A. A. Leahy-Gilmartin, "Investigations into the microbial contamination of toothbrushes," *Microbios*, vol. 85, no. 345, pp. 231–238, 1996.

[14] M. Efstratiou, W. Papaioannou, M. Nakou, E. Ktenas, I. A. Vrotsos, and V. Panis, "Contamination of a toothbrush with antibacterial properties by oral microorganisms," *Journal of Dentistry*, vol. 35, no. 4, pp. 331–337, 2007.

[15] M. Quirynen, M. De Soete, M. Pauwels, S. Gizani, B. Van Meerbeek, and D. van Steenberghe, "Can toothpaste or a toothbursh with antibacterial tufts prevent toothbrush contamination?" *Journal of Periodontology*, vol. 74, no. 3, pp. 312–322, 2003.

[16] S. Sato, V. Pedrazzi, E. H. Guimarães Lara, H. Panzeri, R. F. De Albuquerque, and I. Y. Ito, "Antimicrobial spray for toothbrush disinfection: an in vivo evaluation," *Quintessence International*, vol. 36, no. 10, pp. 812–816, 2005.

[17] D. P. Warren, M. C. Goldschmidt, M. B. Thompson, K. Adler-Storthz, and H. J. Keene, "The effects of toothpastes on the residual microbial contamination of toothbrushes," *Journal of the American Dental Association*, vol. 132, no. 9, pp. 1241–1245, 2001.

[18] M. B. Dayoub, D. Rusilko, and A. Gross, "Microbial contamination of toothbrushes," *Journal of Dental Research*, vol. 56, no. 6, article 706, 1977.

[19] M. C. Goldschmidt, D. P. Warren, H. J. Keene, W. H. Tate, and C. Gowda, "Effects of an antimicrobial additive to toothbrushes on residual periodontal pathogens," *Journal of Clinical Dentistry*, vol. 15, no. 3, pp. 66–70, 2004.

23

Primary Health Care: Comparing Public Health Nursing Models in Ireland and Norway

Anne Clancy,[1,2] Patricia Leahy-Warren,[3] Mary Rose Day,[3] and Helen Mulcahy[3]

[1] *Department of Health and Social Work, School of Nursing, Harstad University College, 9480 Harstad, Norway*
[2] *University of Tromsø, 9019 Tromso, Norway*
[3] *School of Nursing & Midwifery, Brookfield Health Sciences Complex University College Cork, Cork, Ireland*

Correspondence should be addressed to Anne Clancy; anne.clancy@hih.no

Academic Editor: Kari Glavin

Health of populations is determined by a multitude of contextual factors. Primary Health Care Reform endeavors to meet the broad health needs of populations and remains on international health agendas. Public health nurses are key professionals in the delivery of primary health care, and it is important for them to learn from global experiences. International collaboration is often facilitated by academic exchanges. As a result of one such exchange, an international PHN collaboration took place. The aim of this paper is to analyse the similarities and differences in public health nursing in Ireland and Norway within the context of primary care.

1. Introduction

The movement toward primary care as a model of health care service delivery was introduced 30 years ago and has been moving in that direction since then. It has been reiterated across international policy documents during this period [1]. The time for prevarication has passed and action is warranted. Public health nurses (PHNs) due to their public health orientation and guiding philosophy are acutely sensitive to any proposed changes in health policy underpinned by primary health care [2]. This is due to the fact that they work in the community and provide universal low threshold services guided by health promotion and disease prevention and their health outcomes are difficult to measure. Evidence indicates that a preventative approach to community-based health interventions reduces the use of acute hospital services, improves the management of chronic illnesses, and empowers clients to self-care [3]. The remit of PHNs encompasses nursing and public health; therefore, the focus is on primary, secondary, and tertiary prevention [4]. The aim of this paper is to discuss primary health and primary health care and analyse similarities and differences between Ireland and Norway in relation to geography, demography, and health status. The origins of public health nursing are presented. This is followed by an exploration of the different models

and the merits and demerits of specialists and generalists' roles and functions in both countries. The paper concludes by pulling together the salient points contributing to a greater insight to PHN practice in Ireland and Norway. The impetus for this paper came from an academic collaboration between the authors as a result of one authors' (AC) Erasmus visit to University College Cork in 2012. The European Erasmus programme promotes educational exchanges between university students and staff. Ireland and Norway are participants in this programme. This visit presented an ideal opportunity to examine the similarities and differences of public health nursing and primary care in two jurisdictions. This paper will contribute to the discourse on public health nursing in the context of primary health care internationally.

2. Primary Health Care and Primary Care

Primary health care (PHC) as defined by the WHO in 1978 [5] is essential health care based on practical, scientifically sound and socially acceptable methods. Primary health care is considered to be both a philosophy and an approach to providing health resources. The approach is usually termed primary care (PC) and in Ireland is often used synonymously with "general practice" (GP). However, whilst PC incorporates GP care, it encompasses a wide range of health and personal social services delivered by a variety of professionals and is seen as a first point of contact service [6]. Countries with more highly developed systems of primary health care tend to have lower health care costs. Norway was one of the first countries to adopt this model of health care. The organisation of primary care in Norway is decentralised to municipalities. In 1984, 430 local authorities were made responsible for financing and providing primary care services founded on social democratic values and funded by taxes and block grants [7]. It is much easier to support PHC reforms when growth in health expenditure is through prepaid systems than out of pocket expenditures [2].

In contrast, in Ireland Primary care was first proposed as a model of health care to be considered in the mid-1980s [8] but due to the poor fiscal economy, in essence, the first primary care strategy was not published until 2001. This strategy established a community-driven model designed to strengthen the capacity of services at primary care level. As a consequence, dependency on secondary can be minimized achieving increased accessibility to local primary care teams (PCTs).

Health care in Ireland is a two-tier system where public and private sectors exist. The public health care system is governed by the Health Act of 2004 [9], which established the Health Service Executive to be responsible for providing health and personal social services to everyone living in Ireland. The public health system, despite massive expenditure in recent years, has a number of on-going issues which could have an impact on primary care services. These include long waiting lists; over capacity on hospital beds; patients awaiting admission on trolleys in the A&E departments; moratorium on staff recruitment and staff shortages. Ireland's two-tier health care system has failed in many respects to delivery adequate, fair, and equitable services to meet people's needs [10]. Not all citizens in Ireland have free health care at the point of delivery as it is based on income. Many health care payment schemes operate such as the General Medical Services (GMS) card, Pay Related Social Insurance (PRSI), and drug payment scheme. About 39% of the population are covered by a medical card or a GP visit card [11]. In general, PHNs in Ireland deal with all children and adults with GMS. Eligibility for non-GMS adults is contentious but PHNs deal with these referrals on a case by case basis [12].

The reality of the number and composition of primary care teams in Ireland has yet to be realised. Approximately 600–1,000 primary care teams (PCTs) were envisaged by the primary care strategy to meet population needs [13]. Data from the Comptroller & Auditor General [14] suggest that there were 319 PCTs and 24 new primary care centres; however, Gartland [15] reported a figure of 411 teams, and a survey of general practitioners (GPs) reported that only 36% were part of a functioning PCT [16]. In Norway, the compositions of the PCTs are similar to Ireland with regard to the health care professionals involved. The large number, small size, and organisational models of Norwegian municipalities necessitate flexibility and intermunicipal collaboration in the smallest communities in order to provide functional interdisciplinary PCTs. As in Ireland, GPs work in private practices but are contracted by the municipalities to perform public

health services. PHNs provide domiciliary home visiting services to all newborns and work mainly at health clinics and school health services, whereas in Ireland, PHNs are generalists with some specialism within child health. In Ireland, 22% of areas have a dedicated school PHN [12]. Norway is currently in the throes of a new major public health reform (Act of 2011) with the primary focus on prevention and early intervention [17, 18] and governed from local municipalities. A consequence of the new reform [18] with shorter hospital stays for mothers and babies after childbirth could influence their workload. The health system in Ireland, which is governed centrally by the Health Service Executive, is also under reform. This reform also includes a move towards universal health insurance which envisages equitable access to health services. Early hospital discharge in both countries has the potential to increase the need for PHNs services.

Norway is more advanced in their health reforms, and devolution of care in the community locally within a team is a key component of PC. However, there are challenges in maintaining professional individuality so that the clinical accountability of professions is not lost. The individual contribution of distinct professions to the team decision needs to be transparent. Reports to the government on public health work focus on coordination of services and not on professional groups [18, 19], so that now the focus is even more so on professional neutrality. Due to the nature of preventive and promotive work, it is difficult to measure the effects of PHNs' work. Aging populations and lack of visibility of public health nursing in official documents provide challenges. In report no. 16, (Stortingsmelding, 2002-2003) the role of professions is toned down. This is illustrated by the following quote: "it's important to focus on what has to be done in the municipality—not on who does it" [19]. Stenvoll et al. [20] compare this report with a similar public health document from 1993 and conclude that the focus on preventive institutions, such as child health clinics and school health services as well as professions working there, has been weakened. The trend towards professional neutrality is reiterated across current government reports. Reducing the visibility of public health nursing is not conducive to professional development and can mitigate against effective primary care. Effective primary care is more dependent on the context of care than the composition of teams. It ultimately reflects on all the determinants of health. Therefore, it is necessary to examine the health contexts of both Ireland and Norway.

3. Ireland and Norway: Geography, Demography, and Health

Ireland and Norway differ in geography and economic situation but have some similarities in relation to population statistics and public health challenges. Demography and vital statistics for Ireland and Norway are presented in Table 1.

Ireland is often called the "Emerald Isle." The country is characterised by vibrant green fields, hedgerows, low plains, rugged coastlands, lakes, rivers, and islands. Climate in Ireland is mainly mild and humid, winter days are drizzly, cold, and short because of the Gulf Stream, and there is rarely snow. However artic conditions and snow in 2010

TABLE 1: Demography and vital statistics for Ireland and Norway.

	Ireland	Norway
Population	4,588,252 million	4.8 million
Over 65 years	535,393	742,000
Life expectancy	Female: 81.6 years Male: 76.8 years	Females: 83.4 years Males: 79 years
Birth rates	15.81 births/1,000 population	12.1 births/1,000 population
Infant mortality	3.2/1000 live births	3.5/1000 live births
Under 20 years	27.5%	26%
Density of population	64.95 people per square km	15 inhabitants per square km
Health spending	8.7% of GDP (under OECD average 8.9)	10% of GDP (over OECD average)

presented major challenges in Ireland for the delivery of health services. On the contrary, Norway is dominated by mountainous or high terrain, and the country is renowned for its Viking heritage, natural resources, and its long indented coastline and fjords. Climate and geography create challenges for an egalitarian provision of municipal health services and being a welfare state means, inequalities are less acceptable in Norway. The climate in the country differs from North to south, but winters are cold throughout.

Ireland is a member of the European Union (EU), is the third largest island in Europe, and is situated to the North West of Continental Europe. Politically Ireland is divided between the Republic of Ireland (ROI) (26 counties) and Northern Ireland (6 counties) which is part of the United Kingdom. Ireland has a population of 4,588,252 people; 1.2 million people live in Dublin city and county and the density of population is approximately 64.95 people per square km [21]. In Ireland, 535,393 people are aged over 65 years, but life expectancy is slightly lower for females 81.6 years and for men 76.8 years [22]. Overall the population of Ireland is relatively young, and birth rates are 15.81 births/1,000 population. Conversely Norway is not a member of the EU and borders on Russia, Sweden, and Finland. It has a similar population size of approx. 4.8 million but in contrast to Ireland, it is one of the most sparsely populated countries in Europe with only 15 inhabitants per square km. Most of the municipalities are small, and a quarter of the population lives in rural areas. Twenty-six percent of Norway's population is under 20 years of age, and birth rates are 12.1 births/1,000 population. There are 742,000 aged over 65 years in Norway, and life expectancy for females in Norway is 83.4 years and 79 years for men and these rank among the highest in the world [23]. In terms of population structure, Ireland's population is younger and still growing, whereas Norway's has stabilised and their life expectancy is much greater.

The social, economic, and environmental conditions in which people live strongly influence health. There is a strong association between environment, ill health, chronic illness, and morbidity [24]; and Ireland has many health inequalities. For example, the life expectancy for the travellers (Ireland's main minority ethnic group) is currently only 61.7 years consistent with life expectancy of general population in the 1940s in Ireland [25]. Not surprisingly, they were also less likely to report good health. Poverty levels are increasing

and in 2010, 15.8% of the population (706,500) had incomes below €10,831 [26]. Ireland has the highest proportion of children in the EU (24.5%) [24], nearly 9% of these children live in families in consistent poverty and over 18% are at risk of poverty [27]. Mental health, suicide, and poor physical health and well-being are significantly higher in lower social classes and socially deprived areas [28]. The first longitudinal study on people aged over 50 years found that older adults have excellent health. However, it also found that those unemployed had poorer health [29]. There is a growing epidemic of obesity levels in both younger and older people [22, 30, 31]. Ireland has low breast feeding rates, and the rates are more pronounced in lower socioeconomic groups. This is also the case in relation to low birth weight [32]. Current health services in Ireland favour the more well off, yet people who are less well off and socially excluded have poorer health and thus may be more in need of services [33].

Conversely Norway is one of the richest countries in the world, and there has been no increase in poverty in recent years [34]. There are fewer poor people in Norway compared with other countries, and poverty seems to be a temporary condition for most people. Immigrants from nonwestern countries are those most affected. The extensive nature of public welfare services in Norway ensures that poor people are seldom deprived of necessary living conditions [34]. Money can ensure the provision of services but cannot buy health, and Norway has a widening gap in issues of inequalities in health [35]. Norway has topped the UN's annual ranking for national achievement in health, education, and income [36]. The general health of population in Norway is good but there is still a sizeable gradient in morbidity and mortality [37]. It is well recognized that early childhood years can directly and indirectly affect health in later life, and children's living conditions are closely linked to their family's socioeconomic status [38].

Norwegian health services experience many challenges in relation to aging populations, shortened hospital stay, heightened expectations, and an increasing dependency on expertise to solve problems [39]. Psychological problems are a major challenge for public health in Norway [19], and every third adolescent that is in touch with a Norwegian PHN has psychological problems [40]. Gambling addiction often coincides with other health and social disorders, and excessive on-line gaming amongst young people provides new challenges for their health and well-being. One in four pupils in Norway who start secondary education drops out and this can impact on health and life expectancy [38]. Conversely more recent data reported that more children in Ireland leave school early than children in Norway [41], and there is greater socio-economic gradient. There is an increase in reports of teenage suicides and some of these have been linked to cyber bullying, which makes the health needs of adolescents more of a public health priority [42].

Certain population groups in Norway have special health challenges such as those with long-term social problems, people living alone, immigrants, people with mental health issues, and children and young people at risk. Research has shown that ethnic groups in Norway have suffered ethnic discrimination [43]. Similarly Ireland faces many public health challenges in relation to health inequalities, health, aging populations, chronic illness, medical advances, shorter hospital stay, social factors (living alone, isolation, and poor social networks), and economic decline [22, 25]. Both Ireland and Norway are experiencing significant public health challenges in relation to growing levels of chronic illness-related to lifestyle factors [30, 38]. The health challenges of susceptible groups are relevant to PHNs' work in the context of primary health care in both Ireland and Norway.

4. Public Health Nursing in Norway and Ireland

Community nurses in Norway were traditionally concerned with caring for the sick. School health services were introduced with the implementation of the School Act in 1860 [44], and the first mother and child health clinic was opened in 1911 [45]. The early development of Norwegian public health nursing services was influenced by the American model. In many communities, the public health nurse and doctor were the only public health professionals until the late seventies.

Norwegian PHNs are nurses with a specialist qualification in public health nursing. Their current tasks do not involve nursing care of the sick, that is, curative nursing. This care is provided by district nursing services and nurses in local institutions. PHNs in Norway are usually assigned a geographical area and provide universal services at child health clinics and school health services. They perform home visits and carry out immunisations and developmental screening; they also counsel and give advice to individuals and groups. Almost 100% of families avail of the services at child health clinics. There are 2069 PHNs employed in municipal family health clinics and school health services [46], and in Ireland there were 1702 PHNs employed in the Irish Health Service Executive [47]. Table 2 illustrates key similarities and differences related to education, organisational structure, remit, focus of care, and current challenges in public health nursing in Ireland and Norway.

PHNs in Ireland operate at the level of generalist nurses with a specialist qualification in public health nursing. Public Health Nursing similarly originated in the 1800s and because of historical links with Britain mirrored developments there. The origins of the service were more specialist in orientation,

that is, district nursing and community midwifery. The model was specifically generalist since the 1960s, and this was recognised as a strength by the Commission on Nursing [48] who recommended a continuation of generalist geographic focus. However, there has always been an acknowledgement of the specialist versus generalist debate in community nursing. A number of reviews have taken place in Ireland, the most recent [12] of which reiterates the need to reexamine the organisational model for reform. In Norway, the tendency has been to move towards a specialised role in providing services for families and the young population, which will be discussed further in the next section.

Smith describes public health nursing as a nursing speciality that combines nursing and public health principles [49]. The individual-/family-based approach is the Norwegian PHNs' strength, and PHNs have been criticised for not becoming more engaged in public health work at a community level [50]. Helseth [51] explicates, however, the continued importance of the PHN's direct contact with individuals and groups. Primary preventative child health work is carried out mainly by physicians in the USA and mainly nurses in Western Europe, including Ireland and Norway. Eliciting and attending to parental concerns is a key element of effective developmental surveillance and is in line with international best practice [52]. It is acknowledged that there are significant gains from home visiting [53] and sound reasons for the service to remain universal. Universal and targeted child health intervention programs have been shown to improve maternal and child health and reduce inequalities in health [38]. There is a continued need for a universal service that identifies and facilitates the health needs of ordinary people [54, 55]. Specific measures of service effectiveness may be lacking but in terms of efficiency in the delivery of core health checks Irish PHNs have achieved an adherence rate of between 81 and 97% with the scheduled developmental checks [56]. The primary immunisation programme which is actively promoted by PHNs achieves uptake rates over 90% in all of the reporting districts and rates of 95% in 75% of reporting districts [57]. Similarly, immunisation coverage for children in Norway is between 92 and 95% (regardless of socio-economic groupings) with an increase from 2010 [58]. Information technology has provided Norway with an efficient national immunisation registry (SYSVAK) [58]. In one small area, good public health outcomes are being achieved in both countries. However, population outcome data is limited and is not conducive to promoting the reform of the PHN role. In contrast, public health measures have been far more successful in Norway, which has high breastfeeding initiation rates of 99% and duration 80% at 6 months [59]. Ireland has been less successful with an initiation of 46% and duration of 13% at 6 months [60]. Quality and accountability in primary care have been compromised by relatively poor investment in health care informatics and technology in Ireland [61].

Reform is contingent on the implementation of the recommendations of the National Health Information Strategy [62] to implement electronic health records and unique health identifier numbers. This is a particular requirement where child health is concerned.

TABLE 2: Public health nursing: key similarities and differences between Ireland and Norway.

	Education	Organisational model	Remit	Focus of care	Challenges
Norway	1-year level 9 university postgraduate programme or 2 year Master programme	Decentralised to municipal level	Children, young people, and families	Prevention and promotion Egalitarian provision of and access to services Geographically based	Geographical conditions Issues of invisibility due to professional neutrality Funding Organisational model Implementation of the new coordination reform
Ireland	1-year level 9 university postgraduate programme	Employed by the health services executive and geographically based	All age groups (cradle to grave) regulated by the department of health policy	Preventative and curative Generalist and geographically based home visiting	Historical influences economic Organisational model Reform is overdue

Bellman and Vijeratnam [63] caution that the benefits of developmental surveillance should not only be viewed in terms of the abnormalities detected, but also in terms of the support and reassurance to parents. Public health nursing services focus on health promotion and the provision of supportive counselling services. Supportive counselling provided by PHNs has been shown to be effective [64–66]. The focus in Ireland and Norway is also on disease prevention through immunisation programs, developmental screening, and subsequent referrals to other services. Use of specialized health services by children and young people increases with the length of parents education, whereas use of PHNs primary care health services at clinics and schools is more determined by need than social status [38]. Reasons for social inequalities in health can start in childhood; each individual factor may not be important but when these social factors are added up their negative effects can be significant [67].

The school health service has insufficient capacity in many of Norway's municipalities [38]. Not all children and adolescents receive adequate psychological care. It has been put forward that PHNs lack competencies in providing mental health services for this group [40]. Norway is currently concerned with providing specialised mental health services for children, young people, and families in their own communities [18], an area that is very underresourced in Ireland [68]. Many children with mental health problems need assistance from several services, and collaboration is vital. Psychosocial problems are an important focus for PHNs and there is a need for improved collaboration with PHNs on psychosocial, medical, and child protection issues [50, 51, 69, 70]. A recent Norwegian national survey has shown that mental health services are those missed most by communal primary care professionals [71]. Emotional and mental health care in schools is not a feature of the work of PHNs in Ireland where the focus is on immunisations and screening for vision, hearing, and growth [12]. Although emotional health is acknowledged as being vitally important by the HSE [72], it was found by the ONMSD [12] that the school immunisation programme takes precedence over this and indeed there are also unmet targets in relation to screening.

Elo and Calltorp [73] developed a *health promotive and preventive action model* (HPA model) for illustrating the wide range of public health services provided by PHNs. The model was constructed in order to illustrate wherein the process of health-ill health and at what developmental stages PHNs provide health care services. An adapted HPA model (Figure 1) is used to illustrate current Norwegian and Irish public health nursing practice related to the health-ill health continuum. Norwegian PHNs' services for children and young people can be described as being health promotive, supportive, health protective, diagnostic, and therapeutic. The Irish PHNs generalist services include curative care and encompass other services not included in the Norwegian PHNs remit. All models have limitations. The HPA model provides a framework and cannot capture all factors that influence public health nursing service provision.

5. Advancing Public Health Nursing

The previous three sections explored how public health nursing in Ireland and Norway has evolved. However, its not as if future PHN service delivery models were not previously considered. For example, there has always been an acknowledgement of the specialist versus generalist debate that exercises those involved in community health nursing. The journal Public Health Nursing republished an article [74] that first appeared in 1916. This article has as a core message that the debate should not be specialist *or* generalist; rather the model should be specialist *and* generalist. Brainard [74] recognised the fact that communities have different complexities and requirements which she believed should ultimately determine the best model and that there is a place and need for both models. She used the example of general practitioner and medical specialist to argue that they supplement each other's work rather than duplicating it.

McKenna et al. [75] were the only authors to study professional and lay views of generic and specialist roles in the island of Ireland. Each jurisdiction in Ireland has very different models of nursing in the community, that is, 11 different specialist community nurses in Northern Ireland (NI) and one generalist PHN in the Republic of Ireland (ROI). Although there are not as many specialist nurses in the community, public health nursing in Norway has a long tradition of specialist practice and thus is like NI in that respect. It would appear that Norway has achieved a good specialist/generalist balance in terms of community nursing. McKenna et al.'s [75] study concluded with the view that there were too many specialists in NI and too few in

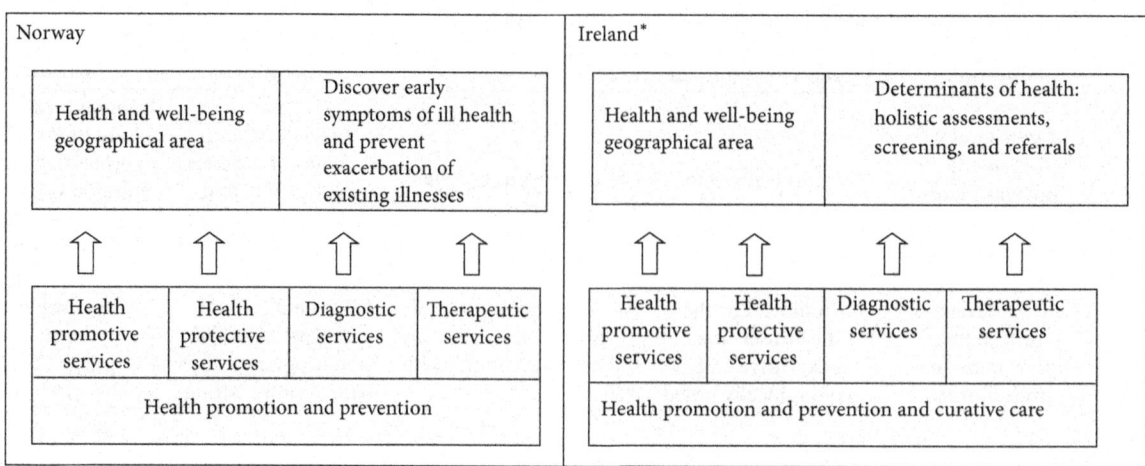

*Public health nursing services in Ireland also encompass registered nurses, home helps and care assistants. These are not part of the Norwegian model.

FIGURE 1: Adapted health promotive and preventive action model illustrating current range of services provided by PHNs in Ireland and Norway.

the ROI, and both were "heading for an imbalance" (page 544).

In the ROI it would appear that the day of imbalance has arrived as there have been recent moves to seriously consider moving public health nursing in a specialist direction [12, 47]. In response to the problem of "duplication of effort" identified by the Office of the Nursing & Midwifery Services Director [12] and the Institute of Community Health Nursing [76]; it was recommended that "consideration must be given to matching skills with the health needs of the population in a more integrated manner" (page 19). A more pressing imperative comes in the wake of a number of child protection reports which highlighted that child welfare and family needs were not prioritised. The current generalist role of PHNs is seen as serious disadvantage from a child and family perspective as the curative role constantly takes precedence [47]. This National report [47] indicated that illness-related nursing care was prioritised over child health and welfare.

The Minister for Children and Youth Affairs [47], in the task force report document, recommends that the PHNs who provide the child and family part of the service should be directly employed by the Child and Family Support Agency (CFSA). Efforts to avoid fragmenting the service could be achieved by colocating PHNs with the local health service. The precise detail of how this change in governance would be configured has yet to be explored. However, the ICHN has canvassed the views of their members in relation to four potential options and found broad support for the need to change the current method of service delivery [76].

McKenna et al. [75] found that while more specialist nurses are required in the community in the future, this has the potential to increase role conflict between nurses and other community professionals. This issue was raised previously for Norway which faces similar challenges regarding coordination and collaboration. Nevertheless, it is suggested by McKenna et al. [75] that colocation of professionals from different organisations can create an arena for staff to work across professional boundaries, to recognise their joint role as supportive professionals, and thus to enable families to find their way through the challenges they face [55, 69].

A further area of concern in Ireland is the schools service provided by PHNs. According to the ONMSD [12], there is a general lack of direction and focus in the school health programme. Local health office areas vary in relation to whether or not they have a dedicated school health nurses. The ONMSD [12] acknowledge the potential importance of schools nurses in influencing the current and future health of the school going population. However, their findings indicate "an imbalance in the activities undertaken by schools nurses, in that immunisations tend to dominate possibly at the expense of health promotion activities" [12]. While large clinical caseloads are adversely affecting delivery of valuable population health initiatives, Irish PHNs are open to redressing "the balance of their roles in this regard" [12, page 27].

In contrast, the school health service in Norway can be seen as a continuation of the clinics' services and has a focused remit in health promotive and preventative work. Unlike Ireland the Norwegian PHN has office hours at the school and is available for pupils, (primary and postprimary) school administration, and collaborators at certain times of the week. Borup and Holstein's [77] Danish study concludes that school nurses play an important role for pupils in susceptible situations. However, Clausson's [78] doctoral thesis showed that PHNs have a deep knowledge of schoolchildren's health that is not used to its full potential. This finding indicates the difficulties in getting the model right in health systems that seem to have everything in terms of funding and policy commitment. This point is just as relevant to Ireland in the Celtic tiger era where there was money and a commitment to PHC [1] but reform was not delivered.

It is much easier to support PHC reforms when growth in health expenditure is through prepaid systems than out of pocket expenditures [2]. Even though the Norwegian population enjoys good health, inequalities continue to exist in certain social groups [35, 37]. Norway's strategy to tackle social inequalities in health is to address the root causes of these inequalities. The current policy is geared specifically towards parts of the population where both the challenges and potential for improvement are greatest [79]. Equity is a specific goal that is top-down and government owned. The underpinning concept is a move from a health-specific to a coordinated strategy [17]. The strategy is to combine universal measures and general welfare with strategies that target the most vulnerable [80]. Coordination of services can, however, be time consuming and provide new challenges for PHNs regarding professional boundaries and co-location of services. Outcomes of collaboration can also be difficult to measure.

6. Conclusion

Ireland and Norway have many similarities from a geographic and demographic perspective. Both countries have similar sized populations, but economically there are vast differences in relation to poverty, life expectancy that is lower, and inequalities that are higher in Ireland. A fundamental feature of primary care relates to equity of access to health services at the point of contact for all. However, health services are more accessible to high income earners in Ireland but universal health care is proposed. Differences identified relate to policy, economics, and public health achievements. A commitment to primary care in the view of the authors requires that health services be available free at the point of access. In the case of Ireland this will require a fundamental societal shift demanding a reexamination of the concept of equality and openness to higher taxation to fund health services. Nevertheless, both countries have a strong commitment to WHO reforms towards primary care, and PHNs have been identified as key players in the delivery of PC services, particularly primary prevention. The Norwegian PHN service model is specialist and aligned with a public health agenda. Ireland has been generalist to date but there is evidence of some movement in a specialist direction. On a very basic level, Norway has far more PHNs devoted specifically to public health issues, with one client group, compared with PHNs in Ireland providing services to all client groups with a preventative and curative remit. While Norway is a wealthy country and has realised an enviable PHN model, Ireland failed to achieve that and deliver on primary care reform, when money was available. Strategy embedded in public health policy similar to Norway is necessary to ensure that Public Health Nursing in Ireland is aligned with a public health agenda. It is, however, important to remember that despite Norway's wealth and specialist PHN model, everything is not perfect and current reforms may not provide the answer to complex problems. To quote the WHO (2008) [2, page viii] "in moving forward, it is important to learn from the past and, in looking back, it is clear that we can do better in the future."

References

[1] Department of Health and Children, *Primary Care A New Direction*, Stationery Office, Dublin, Ireland, 2001.

[2] World Health Organisation, "Now More than Ever," Primary Health Care Report, WHO, Geneva, Switzerland, 2008.

[3] J. Doherty and R. Govender, "The cost-effectiveness of primary care services in developing countries: a review of the international literature," Background paper for the Disease Control Priorities Project, 2004, http://www.ncbi.nlm.nih.gov/pmc/articles/PMC2265356/.

[4] L. O. Keller, S. Strohschein, B. Lia-Hoagberg, and M. A. Schaffer, "Population-based public health interventions: practice-based and evidence-supported. Part I," *Public Health Nursing*, vol. 21, no. 5, pp. 453–468, 2004.

[5] World Health Organisation, *Primary Health Care Report of the International Conference on Primary Health Care*, WHO, Geneva, Switzerland, 1978.

[6] I. J. Aaraas, I. Hetlevik, G. Roksund, and S. Steinert, "Editorial: "caring for people where they are": addressing the double challenge of general practice at the 17th Nordic Congress of General Practice in Tromsø 2011," *Scandinavian Journal of Primary Health Care*, vol. 28, no. 4, pp. 194–196, 2010.

[7] Ministry of Health and Care Services, *Regula tion Relating to a Municipal Regular GP Scheme*, Ministry of Health, Oslo, Norway, 1982, Act no. 66 of 19th of November.

[8] Department of Health, *Health the Wider Dimensions 1987*, Stationary Office, Dublin, Ireland, 1987.

[9] Irish Statute Book Office of the Attorney General, "Health Act 2004," http://www.irishstatutebook.ie/2004/en/act/pub/0042/index.html.

[10] D. Tussing and M. Wren, *How Ireland Cares, the Case for Health Care Reform*, New Island, Dublin, Ireland, 2006.

[11] Central Statistics Office, *Quarterly National Household Study*, Government of Ireland, Dublin, Ireland, 2010.

[12] Office of the Nursing & Midwifery Services Director, *Review of Public Health Nursing*, ONMSD, Dublin, Ireland, 2012.

[13] Department of Health & Children, *Quality and Fairness a Health System for You*, Stationery Office, Dublin, Ireland, 2001.

[14] Accounts of the Public Services (APS), *Report of the Comptroller & Auditor General Government of Ireland*, Stationery Office, Dublin, Ireland, 2011.

[15] F. Gartland, "GP pull out of primary care teams," Irish Times, 7th January 2012, http://www.irishtimes.com/newspaper/ireland/2012/0107/1224309942246.html.

[16] C. Darker, C. Martin, O. 'Dowd T, O. 'Kelly F, O. 'Kelly M, and O. 'Shea B, *A National Survey of Chronic Disease Management in Primary Health Care*, Department of Public Health & Primary Care, Trinity College, Dublin, Ireland, 2011.

[17] Norwegian Ministry of health and care services, *The Norwegian Public Health Act (ACT-2011-06-24-29)*, Ministry of Health, Oslo, Norway, 2011.

[18] Norwegian Ministry of Health & Care Services, *The Coordination Reform: Proper Treatment—At the Right Place and Right Time*, Ministry of Health, Oslo, Norway, Report no. 47 to the Storting, summary in English, 2009.

[19] Norwegian Ministry of Health Ű Care Services, *A Prescription for a Healthier Norway*, Ministry of Health, slo, Norway, 2003.

[20] K. Stenvoll, K. Elvebakken, and K. Malterud, "Blir norsk forebyggingspolitikk mer individorientert?" *Tidsskrift for Den Norske Legeforening*, vol. 125, no. 5, pp. 603–605, 2005.

[21] Central Statistics Office, *Vital Statistics Census 2011*, Stationary Office, Dublin, Ireland, 2012.

[22] Department of Health, *Health in Ireland: Key Trends*, Government Stationery, Dublin, Ireland, 2011.

[23] Statistics Norway, 2012, http://www.ssb.no/befolkning/.

[24] C. M. O'Kelly, W. Cullen, S. M. O'Kelly, F. D. O'Kelly, and G. Bury, "A primary care-based health needs assessment in inner city Dublin," *Irish Journal of Medical Science*, vol. 179, no. 3, pp. 399–403, 2010.

[25] Department of Health and Children/Department of Health, *Social Services and Public Safety, All Ireland Traveller Health Study*, Government Publications, Dublin, Ireland, 2010.

[26] Central Statistics Office, *The Survey on Income and Living Conditions (SILC)*, Stationary Office, Dublin, Ireland, 2011.

[27] Combat Poverty Agency, "Child poverty in Ireland," 2012, http://www.cpa.ie/povertyinireland/statistics.htm .

[28] Public Health Alliance, *Health inequalities on the Island of Ireland*, Public Health alliance, Dublin, Ireland, 2007.

[29] V. Timonen, Y. Kamiya, and S. Maty, "Social engagement of older people adults," in *Fifty Plus in Ireland 2011*, A. Barrett, G. Savva, V. Timonen, and R. A. Kenny, Eds., pp. 51–71, Royal College of Surgeons in Ireland, Economic and Social Research Institute, Centre of Health Policy and Management, Trinity College Dublin, School of Social Work and Social Policy, Trinity College, Dublin, Ireland, 2011.

[30] Department of Health & Children, Government Publications, Dublin, Ireland, 2008.

[31] H. Cronin, C. O'Regan, and R. A. Kenny, "Physical and behavioural health of older Irish adults," in *Fifty Plus in Ireland 2011*, A. Barrett, G. Savva, V. Timonen, and R. A. Kenny, Eds., pp. 72–155, Royal College of Surgeons in Ireland, Economic and Social Research Institute, Centre of Health Policy and Management, Trinity College Dublin, School of Social Work and Social Policy, Trinity College, Dublin, Ireland, 2011.

[32] Institute of Public Health, "Health inequalities on the island: statistics," 2012, http://www.publichealth.ie/healthinequalities/healthinequalitiesontheislandstatistics.

[33] R. Layte and B. Nolan, "Equity in the Utilization of Health Care in Ireland," ESRI Working Paper 2, ESRI, Dublin, Ireland, 2000.

[34] I. L. S. Hansen, A. S. Grødem, A. B. Grønningsæter, R. A. Nielsen, and T. Fløtten, "Kunnskap om fattigdom i Norge: en oppsummering," KITH-rapport 2011:21, Fafo, Oslo, Norway, 2011.

[35] J. P. Mackenbach, V. Bos, O. Andersen et al., "Widening socioeconomic inequalities in mortality in six Western European countries," *International Journal of Epidemiology*, vol. 32, no. 5, pp. 830–837, 2003.

[36] United Nations, *Sustainability and Equity: A Better Future for All, Human Development Report Macmillan*, United Nations, New York, NY, USA, 2011.

[37] Norwegian Directorate of Health, *Norway and Health an Introduction*, Norwegian Directorate of Health,, Oslo, Norway, 2009.

[38] Norwegian Ministry of Health & Care Services, *National Strategy to Reduce Social Inequalities in Health*, Norwegian Ministry of Health & Care Services, Oslo, Norway, Report no. 20 to the Storting, 2006.

[39] O. S. Lian, "Global challenges, global solutions? A cross-national comparison of primary health care in Britain, Norway and the Czech Republic," *Health Sociology Review*, vol. 17, no. 1, pp. 27–40, 2008.

[40] H. W. Andersson and S. Steihaug, *Tilgjengelighet av Tjenester for Barn og Unge med Psykiske Problemer: Evaluering av Opptrappingsplanen for Psykisk Helse*, SINTEF Helse, Oslo, Norway, 2008.

[41] D. Byrne and E. Smyth, *No Way Back? The Dynamics of Early School Leaving*, The Liffey Press and The Economic and Social Research Institute, Dublin, Ireland, 2010.

[42] Ronan McGreevy, "Internet bullies cause long-term harm," 2012, http://www.irishtimes.com/newspaper/health/2012/1106/1224326174724.html.

[43] K. L. Hansen and T. Sørlie, "Ethnic discrimination and psychological distress: a study of Sami and non-Sami populations in Norway," *Transcultural Psychiatry*, vol. 49, pp. 26–50, 2012.

[44] B. Ellefsen, "The experience of collaboration: a comparison of health visiting in Scotland and Norway," *International Nursing Review*, vol. 49, no. 3, pp. 144–153, 2002.

[45] A. Schiøtz and M. Skaset, *Folkets Helse—Landets Styrke 1850–2003*, Universitetsforlag, Oslo, Norway, 2003.

[46] Statistics Norway, 2012, http://www.ssb.no/helsetjko/tab-2012-07-06-07.html.

[47] Department of Children and Youth Affairs, Government publications, Dublin, Ireland, 2012.

[48] Government of Ireland, *Report of the Commission on Nursing: A Blueprint for the Future*, The Stationery Office, Dublin, Ireland, 1998.

[49] L. Breslow, *Encyclopedia of Public Health*, Macmillan Reference USA, 2002.

[50] K. Glavin, S. Helseth, and L. G. Kvarme, *Fra Tanke til Handling: Metoder og Arbeidsmåter i Helsesøstertjenesten*, Akribe, Oslo, Norway, 2007.

[51] S. Helseth, "Teoretisk grunnlag for helsesøstertjenesten," in *Fra Tanke til Handling: Metoder og Arbeidsmåter i Helsesøstertjenesten*, K. Glavin, S. Helseth, and L. G. Kvarme, Eds., Akribe, Oslo, Norway, 2007.

[52] K. P. Marks, F. P. Galscoe, and M. M. Macias, "Enhancing the algorithm for developmental-behavioural surveillance and screening in children 0–5 years ," *Clinical Pediatrics*, vol. 50, no. 9, pp. 853–868, 2011.

[53] E. Hjälmhult and K. Lomborg, "Managing the first period at home with a newborn: a grounded theory study of mothers' experiences," *Scandinavian Journal of Caring Sciences*, vol. 26, no. 4, pp. 654–662, 2012.

[54] J. V. Appleton and S. Cowley, "Health visiting assessment-unpacking critical attributes in health visitor needs assessment practice: a case study," *International Journal of Nursing Studies*, vol. 45, no. 2, pp. 232–245, 2008.

[55] A. Clancy, "The ceremonial order of public health nursing consultations: an ethnographic study," *Journal of Clinical Nursing*, vol. 21, no. 17-18, pp. 2555–2566, 2012.

[56] S. Denyer and C. Cullen, *HSE Report on the Audit of the Child Health Screening and Surveillance Programme*, HSE, Dublin, Ireland, 2009.

[57] WHO, 2012 Immunization Profile, Ireland http://apps.who.int/immunization_monitoring/en/globalsummary/countryprofileresult.cfm.

[58] Norwegian Institute of Public Health, *Vaccination for Children in Norway—Fact Sheet*, Norwegian Institute of Public Health, Oslo, Norway, 2011.

[59] A. P. Häggkvist, A. L. Brantsæter, A. S. M. Grjibovski, E. Helsing, H. M. Meltzer, and M. Haugen, "Prevalence of breast-feeding in the Norwegian Mother and Child Cohort Study and health service-related correlates of cessation of full breast-feeding," *Public Health Nutrition*, vol. 13, no. 12, pp. 2076–2086, 2010.

[60] C. Begley, L. Gallagher, M. Clarke, M. Carroll, and S. Millar, *Infant Feeding Survey*, Health Service Executive, Trinity College, Dublin, Ireland, 2008.

[61] Accounts of the Public Services, *Report of the Comptroller and Auditor General*, APS, Dublin, Ireland, 2011.

[62] Department of Health and Children, *National Health Information Strategy NHIS*, Stationary Office, Dublin, Ireland, 2004.

[63] M. Bellman and S. Vijeratnam, "From child health surveillance to child health promotion, and onwards: a tale of babies and bathwater," *Archives of Disease in Childhood*, vol. 97, no. 1, pp. 73–77, 2012.

[64] A. Tinnfält, *Adolescents' perspectives: on mental health, being at risk, and promoting initiatives [Ph.D. thesis]*, Örebro University, Örebro, Sweden, 2008.

[65] A. Clancy and T. Svensson, "Perceptions of public health nursing consultations: tacit understanding of the importance of relationships," *Primary Health Care Research & Development*, vol. 11, no. 4, pp. 363–373, 2010.

[66] K. Glavin, L. Smith, R. Sørum, and B. Ellefsen, "Supportive counselling by public health nurses for women with postpartum depression," *Journal of Advanced Nursing*, vol. 66, no. 6, pp. 1317–1327, 2010.

[67] J. Elstad, *Social Inequalities in Health and Their Explanations*, The Norwegian Directorate of Health, Oslo, Norway, 2005.

[68] HSE, *Review of Adequacy for HSE Children & Families Services*, HSE, Dublin, Ireland, 2010.

[69] A. Clancy and T. Svensson, "Perceptions of public health nursing practice by municipal health officials in Norway," *Public Health Nursing*, vol. 26, no. 5, pp. 412–420, 2009.

[70] N. Hodgson, "Improving communication between health visitors and primary mental health workers," *Paediatric Nursing*, vol. 21, no. 7, pp. 34–37, 2009.

[71] A. Clancy, T. Gressnes, and T. Svensson, "Public health nursing and interprofessional collaboration in Norwegian municipalities: a questionnaire study," *Scandinavian Journal of Caring Sciences*, 2012.

[72] Health Service Executive, "Unit 9 child emotional and mental health," in *Training Programme for Public Health Nurses and Doctors*, HSE, Dublin, Ireland, 2008.

[73] S. L. Elo and J. B. Calltorp, "Health promotive action and preventive action model (HPA model) for the classification of health care services in public health nursing," *Scandinavian Journal of Public Health*, vol. 30, no. 3, pp. 200–208, 2002.

[74] A. Brainard, "The many sided opportunity of field nursing," *Public Health Nursing*, vol. 29, no. 3, pp. 283–285, 2012.

[75] H. McKenna, S. Keeney, and M. Bradley, "Generic and specialist nursing roles in the community: an investigation of professional and lay views," *Health and Social Care in the Community*, vol. 11, no. 6, pp. 537–545, 2003.

[76] Institute of Community Health Nursing, *The Future Direction of the Community Nursing Service. Moving the Focus of Care to Health Priorities and Delivering Outcomes in the Community*, ICHN, Dublin, Ireland, 2012.

[77] I. Borup and B. E. Holstein, "Schoolchildren who are victims of bullying report benefit from health dialogues with the school health nurse," *Health Education Journal*, vol. 66, no. 1, pp. 58–67, 2007.

[78] E. K. Clausson, *School health nursing—perceiving recording and improving schoolchildrens health [Ph.D. thesis]*, Nordic School of Public Health, Gothenburg, Sweden, 2008.

[79] I. K. Crombie, L. Irvine, L. Elliott, and H. Wallace, *Closing the Health Inequalities Gap: An International Perspective*, World Health Organization, Copenhagen, Denmark, 2005.

[80] M. Strand, C. Brown, T. P. Torgersen, and Ø. Giæver, *Setting the Political Agenda to Tackle Health Inequalities. Studies on Social and Economic Determinents of Population Health, No. 4*, World Health Organisation, Copenhagen, Denmark, 2009.

Planning for Serious Illness amongst Community-Dwelling Older Adults

Donna Goodridge

College of Nursing, University of Saskatchewan, Room 421 Ellis Hall, 103 Hospital Drive, Saskatoon, SK, Canada S7N 0W8

Correspondence should be addressed to Donna Goodridge; donna.goodridge@usask.ca

Academic Editor: Kaja Põlluste

Older adults have long been encouraged to maintain their autonomy by expressing their wishes for health care before they become too ill to meaningfully participate in decision making. This study explored the manner in which community-dwelling adults aged 55 and older plan for serious illness. An online survey was conducted within the province of Saskatchewan, Canada, with 283 adults ranging in age from 55 to 88 years. Planning for future medical care was important for the majority (78.4%) of respondents, although only 25.4% possessed a written advance care plan and 41.5% had designated a substitute decision maker. Sixty percent of respondents reported conversations about their treatment wishes; nearly half had discussed unacceptable states of health. Associations between key predictor variables and planning behaviors (discussions about treatment wishes or unacceptable states of health; designation of a substitute decision maker; preparation of a written advance care plan) were assessed using binary logistic regression. After controlling for all predictor variables, self-reported knowledge about advance care planning was the key variable significantly associated with all four planning behaviors. The efforts of nurses to educate older adults regarding the process of advance care planning can play an important role in enhancing autonomy.

1. Introduction

Given that almost three quarters of older adults lack decision-making capacity when urgent choices about life-sustaining treatment need to be made [1], older adults have long been encouraged by nurses and other health care providers to express their wishes for health care while they are healthy enough to meaningfully participate in treatment decision-making. Advance care planning has been recently promoted by the Centers for Disease Control and Prevention [2] as a process contributing to overall public health through its focus on supporting the individuals' health care choices and preventing unnecessary suffering. Widespread social marketing of advance care planning has made many excellent online and print resources available to the public [2–4].

Although advance care planning is now seen as an iterative process that includes the way in which people think about and communicate their values and preferences so that they may receive the health care they desire in the case of life-threatening illness [5], much of the extant research in this area has focused upon the completion of written advance care plans. Using a population-based approach, this study addressed the research question "How do community-dwelling adults aged 55 years and older plan for serious illness, either formally (e.g., by designating a substitute decision maker and preparing written advance care plans) or informally (e.g., by discussing states of health considered to be unacceptable to continue living or desired medical care in the event of serious illness)?" The overall objective of this study was to identify the associations between formal and informal planning for serious illness and key sociodemographic, health, and knowledge variables. Based on a review of current literature on advance care planning, it was hypothesized that sociodemographic variables (including age, gender, urban or rural location, education level, and income level), values (importance of planning for future care), and self-reported knowledge of advance care planning would be statistically significant predictors of behaviors relating to planning for serious illness.

It is estimated that between 18% and 36% of all American adults in the general public have completed an advance directive [6]. Rates of advance directive completion amongst distinct subpopulations, such as persons with terminal illnesses and older adults, have been reported to range from 15% to 84.9% [1, 7–13]. Completion of an advance directive is associated with a wide range of factors, including "older age, greater disease burden, type and acuity of condition, White race, higher socioeconomic status, knowledge about advance directives or end-of-life treatment options, a positive attitude toward end-of-life discussions, a long-standing relationship with a primary care physician, and whether the patient's primary care physician has an advance directive" [6].

While the clinical utility of advance directives has been rightfully questioned [14–20] and the uptake by intended consumers less than hoped in spite of widely available resources, support for the overall process of people considering and sharing key values and preferences for health care in the face of serious illness remains strong [5]. Social marketing campaigns have increasingly focused public attention on promoting dialogue, rather than completing forms, as a means of supporting the preferences and autonomy of individuals who may not be able to communicate his or her wishes for care in the future.

A number of studies have examined the extent to which discussions related to advance care planning are taking place, as well as the outcomes of these dialogues. Between 75% and 91% of participants over age 65 in the Canadian Study of Health and Aging [21] had considered who might make health decisions for them if they were unable to do this for themselves. The same study revealed that between 46% and 69% had discussed their preferences for end-of-life care with someone else. The benefits of having discussed preferences for future care were noted in a study of patients with advanced cancer by Wright and colleagues [22] and encompassed less aggressive medical care, including lower rates of ventilation (adjusted OR 0.26; 95% CI 0.08–0.83), resuscitation (adjusted OR 0.16 95% CI 0.03–0.80), ICU admission (adjusted OR 0.35; 95% CI 0.14–0.90), and earlier hospice admission (adjusted OR 3.37 95% CI 1.12–10.13), as well as better patient quality of life and improved bereavement adjustment. Discussions early in the trajectory of cancer have also recently been demonstrated to be associated with less aggressive treatment and greater use of hospice care [23].

Despite these positive outcomes, many people remain skeptical about the benefits of advance care planning, fuelled in part by society's denial of the inevitability of death [24, 25] and death's "sequestration" from mainstream society [26]. The choice *not* to engage in advance care planning is complex and highly individual but may include any one or more of the following reasons: believing that one's health is good and it is not necessary; believing that advance care planning is only for the terminally ill, elderly, or infirm; challenges discussing death; not being "ready"; lack of knowledge; difficulty completing the form; reluctance to broach the subject with the physician; fear of being a burden; incompatibility with cultural and spiritual traditions; preference to delegate treatment decision-making to family or others; lack of confidence that a written document would change the course of treatment received [15, 23, 27–30].

2. Materials and Methods

2.1. Study Setting, Population, and Design. This study was conducted in April, 2012, within the province of Saskatchewan, a province located in Western Canada with a population just over one million people [31]. One third of the province's population is considered rural, with the remainder divided between two urban centres.

The sample of 238 community dwelling older adults over the age 55 years represents a subgroup of the entire sample of 827 individuals obtained for a larger project, who were stratified by age, region, and sex to be representative of the population of the province. The entire sample was randomly selected from a pool of volunteers who had agreed to participate in online commercial market surveys (SaskWatch Research). Only data related to adults over age 55 years are presented in this analysis. This project received ethical approval from the University of Saskatchewan Behavioral Review Board. Participants provided consent for the data to be used in subsequent presentations and publications.

2.2. Description of Variables. The survey was comprised of structured, closed-ended items salient to planning for serious illness care. Demographic data included age; sex; personal income; education; residence (urban or rural). Respondents were asked to identify the number and type of health conditions with which they lived from a list of common illnesses, as well as to respond to the following question: "How important do you think it is to plan for medical care at the end-of-life? (not at all important, somewhat important, important, or very important)." Respondents were asked to indicate their level of knowledge about advance care planning and living wills on a three-point scale (not at all familiar; some basic understanding; fairly or very good understanding). Those who reported a written living will or advance directive were also asked to identify sources of help received with preparing this document (consultation with lawyer; consultation with lawyer and family; consultation with family; consultation with someone else; prepared by myself).

2.3. Data Analysis. Statistical analysis was completed using SPSS 19.0. Given that an age of 65 years has been recognized as the point at which many Canadians retire from paid employment, respondents were divided into two groups: those 65 and younger and those older than 65 years. Level of significance (σ) was set at 0.05. Comparisons between the groups were completed using the Kruskal-Wallis test (with multiple Mann-Whitney tests adjusted with Bonferroni corrections for post hoc analysis) and chi-square tests of proportion where appropriate. In order to determine the characteristics influencing outcome behaviors variables (discussions of unacceptable states of health; discussion of wishes for treatment, designation of a substitute decision maker; preparation of a written directive), binary logistic regression

TABLE 1: Demographic and health characteristics of the sample (by age group and overall).

	55–64 years ($N = 171$) %	≥65 years ($n = 112$) %	Overall ($N = 283$) %
Sex			
Male	45.6	47.3	47.3
Female	55.4	52.7	52.7
Education			
<or completed high school	20.1	14.4	17.9
Some post-secondary	52.1	55.0	53.2
Completed postsecondary	27.8	30.6	28.9
Annual personal income			
<\$60,000	23.4[†]	42.0[†]	30.7
\$60,000 or more	49.7[†]	28.6[†]	41.3
Refused	26.9	29.5	21.8
Residence			
Large urban	43.3	41.1	41.4
Other	56.7	58.9	58.6
Number of health conditions			
None	27.5[†]	10.7[†]	20.8
1–3 conditions	58.5	55.4	57.2
4 or more conditions	14.0[^]	33.9[^]	21.9

[†] $P < 0.05$ using the chi-square test for proportions with a Bonferonni correction.
[^] $P < 0.001$ using the chi-square test for proportions with a Bonferonni correction.

TABLE 2: Values, knowledge, and behaviors related to planning for the end of Life.

	55–64 years ($N = 171$) %	≥65 years ($n = 112$) %	Overall ($N = 283$) %
Importance of planning for future medical care			
Not at all or somewhat important	23.4	18.8	21.6
Important or very important	76.6	81.3	78.4
Importance of planning for own funeral			
Not at all or somewhat important	39.2	35.7	37.8
Important or very important	60.8	64.3	62.2
Familiarity with term "living will"			
Not at all familiar	7.0	6.3	6.7
Some basic understanding	32.7	30.4	31.8
Fairly or very good understanding	60.2	63.4	61.5
Familiarity with term "advance care plan"			
Not at all familiar	28.1	23.2	26.1
Some basic understanding	35.1	37.5	36.0
Fairly or very good understanding	36.8	39.3	37.6
Discussed unacceptable states of health	53.2	43.8	49.5
Discussed wishes for treatment	53.8[†]	69.6[†]	60.1
Designated a substitute decision-maker	34.5[†]	52.7[†]	41.7
Prepared written LW or ACP	20.5[†]	33.0[†]	25.4

[†] $P < 0.05$ using the chi-square test for proportions with a Bonferonni correction.

was conducted. The strength of association was measured by the odds ratio (OR) and 95% confidence interval (CI).

3. Results

Table 1 compares the demographic and health characteristics of the sample between respondents aged 55–64 years (younger group) and those who were 65 years and older (older group). Just over half (52.7%) of the 283 respondents were females. Respondents ranged in age from 55 to 88 years. The majority (82.1%) of all respondents had education beyond completion of high school. A higher proportion of the older group reported incomes of less than \$60,000 than the younger group, while the opposite was true for incomes above \$60,000. There were no differences between the age

TABLE 3: Adjusted[1] associations between respondent characteristics and serious illness planning behaviors.

	Discussed treatment wishes	Discussed unacceptable conditions	Designated substituted decision-maker	LW or ACP completed
	OR (95% CI)	OR (95% CI)	OR (95% CI)	OR (95% CI)
Sex				
Female	2.05[‡]	1.25	1.21	1.47
(ref: male)	(1.16–3.62)	(0.72–2.18)	(0.70–2.09)	(0.77–2.80)
Age				
≥65 years	1.75	1.23	2.30[‡]	1.86
(ref: <65 years)	(0.98–3.11)	(0.71–2.13)	(1.32–3.99)	(0.99–3.50)
Education				
Some postsecondary education	1.26	1.59	0.93	0.98
(ref: ≤high school)	(0.60–2.65)	(0.76–3.29)	(0.45–1.93)	(0.41–2.33)
Completed postsecondary	1.64	1.72	0.70	0.79
(ref: ≤high school)	(0.7–3.81)	(0.75–3.92)	(0.30–1.60)	(0.29–2.13)
Annual personal income				
≥$60,000 (ref: <$60,000)	0.62 (0.31–1.22)	0.84 (0.43–1.61)	1.04 (0.54–2.00)	0.56 (0.26–1.21)
Unspecified (ref: <$60,000)	0.59 (0.29–1.26)	0.82 (0.41–1.62)	0.87 (0.44–1.71)	0.86 (0.40–1.85)
Rural residence (ref: urban)	0.83 (0.48–1.42)	0.86 (0.51–1.45)	0.65 (0.38–1.09)	0.47[†] (0.25–0.86)
Health conditions				
1-2 conditions	1.14	0.81	1.06	1.05
(ref: 0 conditions)	(0.53–2.49)	(0.38–1.72)	(0.50–2.29)	(0.42–2.60)
3 or more conditions	1.20	1.30	0.96	0.85
(ref: 0 conditions)	(0.60–2.40)	(0.66–2.59)	(0.47–1.89)	(0.37–1.92)
Value				
Important to plan for care	1.67	1.24	2.32[†]	4.31[*]
(ref: not important)	(0.87–3.19)	(0.64–2.41)	(1.15–4.70)	(1.42–13.07)
Knowledge of ACP				
Understood term	3.45[^]	5.62[^]	2.49[‡]	9.87[^]
(ref: not familiar)	(1.87–6.34)	(2.90–10.92)	(1.87–6.34)	(2.90–33.50)

[1] Adjusted for each of the variables listed in the table.
[*] $P < 0.10$.
[†] $P < 0.05$.
[‡] $P < 0.01$.
[^] $P < 0.001$.

groups in location of residence. Participants residing outside of primary urban centres (populations >250,000) comprised 58.6% of the total sample. A significantly higher ($P < 0.001$) proportion of the older group reported four or more health conditions compared to the younger group, although the proportions were similar between the groups for those reporting one to three health conditions.

Table 2 compares the responses of the younger and older age groups in terms of values, knowledge, and behaviors related to planning for the end of life. The majority of respondents indicated they felt it was important or very important to plan for medical care in the event of serious illness (78.4%) and to plan for one's own funeral (62.2%). While 61.5% of respondents reported a good understanding

of the term "living will," substantially fewer indicated they had a good understanding of the term "advance care plan." Approximately half of all respondents had discussed states of health in which they would find it unacceptable to live with someone close to them in the past year. One-third of those aged 65 and older reported they had a written directive compared to 20.5% of adults below age 65. Respondents in the older group were significantly more likely ($P < 0.05$) to have discussed wishes for treatment, designated a substitute decision maker, and to have prepared either an advance care plan or living will.

Respondents without a written advance care plan were asked to identify reasons for not preparing this document. The majority (60.0%) indicated they had not considered this yet, while 21.2% suggested that their families would make decisions about future health care for them and 18.2% indicated that their families together with their physician would decide. Only one respondent reported that care decisions would be made by the physician.

For the 72 respondents who had prepared a written advance care plan, the most common source of assistance to prepare the document was a lawyer (50%). A third of respondents cited families as a source of assistance, while 22.2% indicated they had completed the plan by themselves. Few (4.2%) respondents had the assistance of a health care professional in writing the directive.

Table 3 displays the adjusted association between the outcome variables (discussions about treatment wishes or unacceptable states of health; designation of a substitute decision maker; preparation of a written advance care plan) and the hypothesized predictor variables. After adjustment for all the variables listed in Table 3, women were twice as likely as men (O.R. = 2.05, 95% CI 1.16–3.62) to have discussed treatment wishes but were similar to men in terms of reporting discussion regarding unacceptable conditions, designating a substitute decision maker, or completing a written advance care plan. Those over 65 years of age were significantly more likely than those between the ages of 55 and 65 to have designated a substitute decision maker (O.R. = 2.30, 95% CI 1.32–3.99). The older group was not more likely to have completed a written advance care plan, although this association approached significance ($P = 0.06$). Education, income, and the number of self-reported health conditions were not associated with any of the four planning behaviors under consideration. Respondents from rural areas were significantly less likely (O.R. = 0.47, 95% CI 0.25–0.86) than those from urban centres to have completed a written advance care plan. Those who believed it was important to plan for care were more than twice as likely to have designated a substitute decision maker (O.R. = 2.32, 95% CI 1.15–4.70) and more than four times as likely to have completed a written advance care plan (O.R. = 4.31, 95% CI 1.42–13.07). Respondents who reported a good understanding of advance care planning had a significantly greater likelihood of engaging in all planning behaviors: discussion of treatment wishes (O.R. = 3.45, 95% CI 1.87–6.34); discussion of states of health they would find unacceptable to live with (O.R. = 5.62, 95% CI 2.92–10.92); designating a substitute decision maker (O.R. = 2.49, 95% CI 1.87–6.34); completing a written advance care plan (O.R. = 9.87, 95% CI 2.90–33.50).

4. Discussion

The findings of this study demonstrate that neither formal nor informal planning for serious illness can yet be considered widespread amongst community-dwelling adults aged 55 and older. Formal planning for serious illness, in the form of designating substitute decision makers and preparing advance care plans, was reported by fewer than half of the respondents in this study. These proportions are similar to those reported in other studies [1, 7–13]. The proportion of respondents who engaged in informal planning for serious

illness, such as conversations about treatment preferences and unacceptable health conditions, was only marginally higher, at 50% and 60%.

In examining the demographic and health variables associated with planning behaviors, women were twice as likely as men to have discussed treatment wishes with someone close to them, but just as likely as men to have discussed unacceptable states of health, to have designated a substitute decision maker, or to have prepared a written advance care plan. Similar findings were reported by Garrett et al. [21], who reported women to be more likely to consider having a conversation about end-of-life wishes, but found no sex differences with respect to preparing an advance care plan.

In the adjusted model, there were no associations between age and informal planning behaviors. Older age proved significant only for the formal planning behavior of having designated a substitute decision maker, although the association between older age and having prepared an advance care plan approached significance ($P = 0.06$). Given the formal nature of both these activities and the fact that half of the advance care plans were completed with the assistance of lawyers, it may be that older adults are more willing to consider planning for serious illness under the umbrella of estate planning than health. Interestingly, the model found no associations between the number of health conditions reported by respondents and planning behaviors. It may be that an increasing number of health conditions are an expected sequela of the aging process and insufficient in and of themselves to trigger concern that planning for serious illness is warranted.

The Transtheoretical Model [23] is increasingly used to explain variability in personal "readiness" to engage in advance care planning [20, 30]. The reason most frequently cited by respondents in this study for not preparing an advance care plan was that they "had not considered it yet." Those individuals may have been in the "precontemplation" phase, described in the Transtheoretical Model, and were not ready to engage in formal planning behaviors. The decision to participate in planning for serious illness activities would, according to this model, mean that the "benefits" must outweigh the "costs" of the behavior perceived by the individual. The "costs" associated with the uncomfortable recognition and acceptance that one is personally vulnerable to poor health or death in the foreseeable future may have been such that respondents were not yet "ready" to engage in planning behaviors. If planning for serious illness is indeed a way to promote autonomy that is valued by older adults, it is worthwhile to further consider the factors that enhance readiness to participate in planning behaviors.

A significant proportion (21.6%) of respondents did not feel planning for future medical care to be important. Those who did not consider planning to be important were significantly less likely to have designated a substitute decision maker or have completed a written advance plan. While governments and health care providers continue to promulgate the benefits of planning for serious illness, it is important to bear in mind that a significant proportion of our patients may not share this value. Nurses who seek to educate patients about strategies to plan for future medical care must first take the time to appraise whether, in fact, a given individual believes these activities to be of value. Understanding the experiences that shape the individual's perspective on advance care planning is critical to a truly "patient-centred" approach.

Knowledge about advance care planning was consistently and independently associated with all types of planning for serious illness behaviors (discussions about treatment wishes or unacceptable states of health; designation of a substitute decision maker; preparation of a written advance care plan). The fact that respondents from rural areas, however, were only half as likely as those from urban areas to have an advance care plan suggests that access to information about planning for serious illness may, in fact, be a key driver for planning behavior. While the survey did not evaluate the access respondents had to education about advance care planning, access to health services is often limited in rural settings (CIHI). It is worthwhile to bear in mind, however, that the association between knowledge and behavior does not demonstrate causality, whereby more education about advance care planning leads directly to greater participation in planning. Individuals who were already receptive to the importance of planning for serious illness may have availed themselves of opportunities to educate themselves about this process. Nurses may play a significant role in identifying "teachable moments" and providing support and education to those who demonstrate an interest and willingness to learn more about ways to best plan for future serious illness. Tailoring interventions to the individual's level of readiness is referred to as "stage-matching" within the Transtheoretical Model [32].

5. Limitations

While this survey was representative of the population of the province in terms of sex and region, the sample did not include the entire population of the province. Stratification by socioeconomic status or additional variables was not possible, although level of education may reflect socioeconomic status to some extent. Random selection occurred from the pool of those individuals who had agreed to participate in online surveys conducted by SaskWatch Research, and thus selection bias may have been present. Verification that ACP or LW documents were completed was not possible.

6. Nursing Implications

Supporting the autonomy of older adults is a key concern of nursing practice. Education of the patients with respect to the process of advance care planning has been recognized as a public health issue in which nurses may make a significant contribution. As advocates for supporting the autonomy of older adults, however, nurses who engage in practice related to advance care planning must keep in mind that, for almost one quarter of respondents in this study, planning for serious illness was not considered important. That some individuals do not hold planning as a value is an important consideration when planning nursing interventions designed to educate and foster participation in advance care planning, highlighting the need to match interventions to levels of readiness.

Conflict of Interests

The author has no conflict of interests to declare.

References

[1] M. J. Silveira, S. Y. H. Kim, and K. M. Langa, "Advance directives and outcomes of surrogate decision making before death," *The New England Journal of Medicine*, vol. 362, no. 13, pp. 1211–1218, 2010.

[2] Centers for Disease Control and Prevention, "Give peace of mind: advance care planning," 2012, http://www.cdc.gov/aging/advancecareplanning/index.htm.

[3] The National Council for Palliative Care, University of Nottingham and NHS National End of Life Care Programme, "Planning for your future care," 2009, http://www.nhs.uk/Livewell/Endoflifecare/Documents/Planning_your_future_care%5B1%5D.pdf.

[4] Canadian Hospice and Palliative Care Association, "Speak up: start the conversation about end of life care," 2012, http://www.advancecareplanning.ca/community-organizations/download-the-speak-up-campaign-kit.aspx.

[5] M. E. Tinetti, "The retreat from advance care planning," *The Journal of the American Medical Association*, vol. 307, no. 9, pp. 915–916, 2012.

[6] US Department of Health and Human Services, "Advance directives and advance care planning," Report to Congress, 2008, http://aspe.hhs.gov/daltcp/reports/2008/ADCongRpt.htm#structure.htm#structure.

[7] L. C. Hanson, J. A. Tulsky, and M. Danis, "Can clinical interventions change care at the end of life?" *Annals of Internal Medicine*, vol. 126, no. 5, pp. 381–388, 1997.

[8] D. G. Larson and D. R. Tobin, "End-of-life conversations: evolving practice and theory," *Journal of the American Medical Association*, vol. 284, no. 12, pp. 1573–1578, 2000.

[9] M. D. Mezey, R. Leitman, E. L. Mitty, M. M. Bottrell, and G. C. Ramsey, "Why hospital patients do and do not execute an advance directive," *Nursing Outlook*, vol. 48, no. 4, pp. 165–171, 2000.

[10] G. Bravo, M. F. Dubois, and M. Pâquet, "Advance Directives for health care and research: prevalence and correlates," *Alzheimer Disease and Associated Disorders*, vol. 17, no. 4, pp. 215–222, 2003.

[11] L. G. Collins, S. M. Parks, and L. Winter, "The state of advance care planning: one decade after SUPPORT," *American Journal of Hospice and Palliative Medicine*, vol. 23, no. 5, pp. 378–384, 2006.

[12] P. Wu, K. A. Lorenz, and J. Chodosh, "Advance care planning among the oldest old," *Journal of Palliative Medicine*, vol. 11, no. 2, pp. 152–157, 2008.

[13] K. Meussen, L. Van den Block, M. Echteld et al., "Advance care planning in Belgium and the Netherlands: a nationwide retrospective study via sentinel networks of general practitioners," *Journal of Pain and Symptom Management*, vol. 42, no. 4, pp. 565–577, 2011.

[14] R. L. Sudore and T. R. Fried, "Redefining the "planning" in advance care planning: preparing for end-of-life decision

making," *Annals of Internal Medicine*, vol. 153, no. 4, pp. 256–261, 2010.

[15] A. Fagerlin and C. E. Schneider, "The failure of the living will," *Hastings Center Report*, vol. 34, no. 2, pp. 30–42, 2004.

[16] A. F. Connors Jr., N. V. Dawson, N. A. Desbiens et al., "A controlled trial to improve care for seriously ill hospitalized patients: the study to understand prognoses and preferences for outcomes and risks of treatments (SUPPORT)," *Journal of the American Medical Association*, vol. 274, no. 20, pp. 1591–1598, 1995.

[17] M. Danis, E. Mutran, J. M. Garrett et al., "A prospective study of the impact of patient preferences on life- sustaining treatment and hospital cost," *Critical Care Medicine*, vol. 24, no. 11, pp. 1811–1817, 1996.

[18] J. Teno, J. Lynn, N. Wenger et al., "Advance directives for seriously ill hospitalized patients: effectiveness with the patient self-determination act and the SUPPORT intervention," *Journal of the American Geriatrics Society*, vol. 45, no. 4, pp. 500–507, 1997.

[19] H. S. Perkins, "Controlling death: the false promise of advance directives," *Annals of Internal Medicine*, vol. 147, no. 1, pp. 51–57, 2007.

[20] R. L. Sudore, A. D. Schickedanz, C. S. Landefeld et al., "Engagement in multiple steps of the advance care planning process: a descriptive study of diverse older adults," *Journal of the American Geriatrics Society*, vol. 56, no. 6, pp. 1006–1013, 2008.

[21] D. D. Garrett, H. Tuokko, K. I. Stajduhar, J. Lindsay, and S. Buehler, "Planning for end-of-life care: findings from the canadian study of health and aging," *Canadian Journal on Aging*, vol. 27, no. 1, pp. 11–21, 2008.

[22] A. A. Wright, B. Zhang, A. Ray et al., "Associations between end-of-life discussions, patient mental health, medical care near death, and caregiver bereavement adjustment," *Journal of the American Medical Association*, vol. 300, no. 14, pp. 1665–1673, 2008.

[23] A. Clarke and J. Seymour, "'At the foot of a very long ladder': discussing the end of life with older people and informal caregivers," *Journal of Pain and Symptom Management*, vol. 40, no. 6, pp. 857–869, 2010.

[24] P. Aries, *Western Attitudes Towards Death*, Johns Hopkins University Press, Baltimore, Md, USA, 1974.

[25] E. Becker, *The Denial of Death*, Free Press, New York, NY, USA, 1973.

[26] A. Kellehear, "Are we a "death-denying" society? A sociological review," *Social Science and Medicine*, vol. 18, no. 9, pp. 713–721, 1984.

[27] J. A. Carrese, J. L. Mullaney, R. R. Faden, and T. E. Finucane, "Planning for death but not serious future illness: qualitative study of housebound elderly patients," *British Medical Journal*, vol. 325, no. 7356, pp. 125–127, 2002.

[28] L. C. Welch, J. M. Teno, and V. Mor, "End-of-life care in black and white: race matters for medical care of dying patients and their families," *Journal of the American Geriatrics Society*, vol. 53, no. 7, pp. 1145–1153, 2005.

[29] M. J. Johnstone and O. Kanitsaki, "Ethics and advance care planning in a culturally diverse society," *Journal of Transcultural Nursing*, vol. 20, no. 4, pp. 405–416, 2009.

[30] A. D. Schickedanz, D. Schillinger, C. S. Landefeld, S. J. Knight, B. A. Williams, and R. L. Sudore, "A clinical framework for improving the advance care planning process: start with

patients' self-identified barriers," *Journal of the American Geriatrics Society*, vol. 57, no. 1, pp. 31–39, 2009.

[31] Statistics Canada, Saskatchewan Population Report: Census of Canada, 2011, http://www.stats.gov.sk.ca/stats/pop/Censuspopulation2011.pdf.

[32] J. O. Prochaska, W. F. Velicer, J. L. Fava, J. S. Rossi, and J. Y. Tsoh, "Evaluating a population-based recruitment approach and a stage-based expert system intervention for smoking cessation," *Addictive Behaviors*, vol. 26, no. 4, pp. 583–602, 2001.

Permissions

The contributors of this book come from diverse backgrounds, making this book a truly international effort. This book will bring forth new frontiers with its revolutionizing research information and detailed analysis of the nascent developments around the world.

We would like to thank all the contributing authors for lending their expertise to make the book truly unique. They have played a crucial role in the development of this book. Without their invaluable contributions this book wouldn't have been possible. They have made vital efforts to compile up to date information on the varied aspects of this subject to make this book a valuable addition to the collection of many professionals and students.

This book was conceptualized with the vision of imparting up-to-date information and advanced data in this field. To ensure the same, a matchless editorial board was set up. Every individual on the board went through rigorous rounds of assessment to prove their worth. After which they invested a large part of their time researching and compiling the most relevant data for our readers. Conferences and sessions were held from time to time between the editorial board and the contributing authors to present the data in the most comprehensible form. The editorial team has worked tirelessly to provide valuable and valid information to help people across the globe.

Every chapter published in this book has been scrutinized by our experts. Their significance has been extensively debated. The topics covered herein carry significant findings which will fuel the growth of the discipline. They may even be implemented as practical applications or may be referred to as a beginning point for another development. Chapters in this book were first published by Hindawi Publishing Corporation; hereby published with permission under the Creative Commons Attribution License or equivalent.

The editorial board has been involved in producing this book since its inception. They have spent rigorous hours researching and exploring the diverse topics which have resulted in the successful publishing of this book. They have passed on their knowledge of decades through this book. To expedite this challenging task, the publisher supported the team at every step. A small team of assistant editors was also appointed to further simplify the editing procedure and attain best results for the readers.

Our editorial team has been hand-picked from every corner of the world. Their multi-ethnicity adds dynamic inputs to the discussions which result in innovative outcomes. These outcomes are then further discussed with the researchers and contributors who give their valuable feedback and opinion regarding the same. The feedback is then collaborated with the researches and they are edited in a comprehensive manner to aid the understanding of the subject.

Apart from the editorial board, the designing team has also invested a significant amount of their time in understanding the subject and creating the most relevant covers. They scrutinized every image to scout for the most suitable representation of the subject and create an appropriate cover for the book.

The publishing team has been involved in this book since its early stages. They were actively engaged in every process, be it collecting the data, connecting with the contributors or procuring relevant information. The team has been an ardent support to the editorial, designing and production team. Their endless efforts to recruit the best for this project, has resulted in the accomplishment of this book. They are a veteran in the field of academics and their pool of knowledge is as vast as their experience in printing. Their expertise and guidance has proved useful at every step. Their uncompromising quality standards have made this book an exceptional effort. Their encouragement from time to time has been an inspiration for everyone.

The publisher and the editorial board hope that this book will prove to be a valuable piece of knowledge for researchers, students, practitioners and scholars across the globe.

List of Contributors

Kristin Ownby, Renae Schumann, Linda Dune and David Kohne
The University of Texas Health Science Center School of Nursing at Houston, 6901 Bertner Avenue, Room 691, Houston, TX 77030, USA

Jane L. Phillips
School of Nursing, The University of Notre Dame Australia, The Cunningham Centre for Palliative Care, St Vincent's & Mater Health Sydney, 170 Darlinghurst Road, Sydney, NSW 2010, Australia

John X. Rolley
Cardiac Investigation Unit, St Vincent's Hospital, P.O. Box 2900, Fitzroy, VIC 3065, Australia

Patricia M. Davidson
Cardiovascular Nursing Research, St Vincent's Hospital and Centre for Cardiovascular and Chronic Care, Faculty of Nursing, Midwifery & Health, University of Technology Sydney, Broadway, NSW 2007, Australia

Elizabeth Kendall and Carolyn Ehrlich
Centre for National Research on Disability and Rehabilitation Medicine, Griffith Health Institute, Griffith University, Logan Campus, Meadowbrook, QLD 4131, Australia

Michele M. Foster
School of Social Work & Human Services, The University of Queensland, St. Lucia, QLD 4072, Australia

Wendy Chaboyer
NHMRC Centre of Research Excellence in Nursing Interventions for Hospitalised Patients, Research Centre for Clinical and Community Practice Innovation and Griffith Health Institute, Griffith University, Gold Coast Campus, Southport, QLD 4215, Australia

Janet E. Squires
Clinical Epidemiology Program, Ottawa Hospital Research Institute, Ottawa, ON, Canada K1H 8L6
School of Nursing, University of Ottawa, Ottawa, ON, Canada K1H 8M5

Alison M. Hutchinson
Cabrini-Deakin Centre for Nursing Research, School of Nursing and Midwifery, Deakin University and Cabrini Health, Melbourne, VIC 3KM, Australia

Anne-Marie Bostrom
Division of Nursing, Department of Neurobiology, Care Sciences and Society, Karolinska Institute, 14183 Huddinge, Sweden
Department of Geriatric Medicine, Danderyd Hospital, 18287 Danderyd, Sweden

Kelly Deis, Greta G. Cummings and Carole A. Estabrooks
Faculty of Nursing, University of Alberta, Edmonton, AB, Canada T6G 1C9

Peter G. Norton
Department of Family Medicine, University of Calgary, Calgary, AB, Canada T2M 0H5

Stephanie K. Daniels
Research Service Line, Department of Communication Sciences and Disorders, Michael E. DeBakey VA Medical Center and
University of Houston, 2002 Holcombe Boulevard, Houston, TX 77030, USA

Jane A. Anderson
Health Services Research and Development Center of Excellence, Department of Neurology, Michael E. DeBakey VA Medical Center and Baylor College of Medicine, 2002 Holcombe Boulevard, Houston, TX 77030, USA

Nancy J. Petersen
Health Services Research and Development Center of Excellence, Department of Medicine, Michael E. DeBakey VA Medical Center and Baylor College of Medicine, 2002 Holcombe Boulevard, Houston, TX 77030, USA

Christina Purpora
School of Nursing and Health Professions, University of San Francisco, 2130 Fulton Street, San Francisco, CA 94117, USA

Mary A. Blegen
Department of Community Health Systems, School of Nursing, University of California, San Francisco, Koret Way, P.O. Box 0608, San Francisco, CA 94143, USA

Leah L. Shever
Nursing Research, Quality, and Innovation, University of Michigan Health System, 300 North Ingalls, Room NI 5A07, Ann Arbor, MI 48109-5446, USA

Marita G. Titler
University of Michigan School of Nursing and University of Michigan Health System, 400 North Ingalls, Suite 4170, Ann Arbor, MI 48109-5482, USA

Aleda M. H. Chen
Assistant Professor of Pharmacy Practice, School of Pharmacy, Cedarville University, 251 N. Main Street, Cedarville, OH 45314, USA

Karen S. Yehle
School of Nursing, Purdue University, 502 N. University Street, JNSN 238, West Lafayette, IN 47907, USA
Center on Aging and the Life Course, Purdue University, West Lafayette, IN 47907, USA
Regenstrief Center for Healthcare Engineering, Purdue University, West Lafayette, IN 47907, USA

Nancy M. Albert
Office of Research & Innovation, Nursing Institute and CNS, Kaufman Center for Heart Failure, Heart and Vascular Institute,

Kenneth F. Ferraro
Center on Aging and the Life Course, Purdue University, West Lafayette, IN 47907, USA
Distinguished Professor of Sociology, Purdue University, Bill and Sally Hanley Hall, 1202 W. State Street, West Lafayette, IN 47907, USA

Kimberly S. Plake
Center on Aging and the Life Course, Purdue University, West Lafayette, IN 47907, USA
Regenstrief Center for Healthcare Engineering, Purdue University, West Lafayette, IN 47907, USA
Pharmacy Practice, College of Pharmacy, Purdue University, Heine Pharmacy Building, 575 Stadium Mall Drive, West Lafayette, IN 47907, USA

Holly L. Mason and Matthew M. Murawski
Pharmacy Administration, College of Pharmacy, Purdue University, Heine Pharmacy Building, 575 Stadium Mall Drive, West Lafayette, IN 47907, USA

Weihua Zhang
Nell Hodgson Woodruff School of Nursing, Emory University, 1520 Clifton Road, Atlanta, GA 30322-4207, USA

Betty S. Lane
Clayton State University, 2000 Clayton State Boulevard, Morrow, GA 30260-0285, USA

Mary E. McNally
Faculty of Dentistry, Dalhousie University, P.O. Box 15000, Halifax, NS, Canada B3H 4R2
Atlantic Health Promotion Research Centre, Dalhousie University, P.O. Box 15000, Halifax, NS, Canada B3H 4R2

Ruth Martin-Misener
School of Nursing, Faculty of Health Professions, Dalhousie University, P.O. Box 15000, Halifax, NS, Canada B3H 4R2

Christopher C. L. Wyatt
Faculty of Dentistry, University of British Columbia, 2329 West Mall, Vancouver, BC, Canada V6T 1Z4

Karen P. McNeil and Sandra J. Crowell
Atlantic Health Promotion Research Centre, Dalhousie University, P.O. Box 15000, Halifax, NS, Canada B3H 4R2

Debora C. Matthews
Faculty of Dentistry, Dalhousie University, P.O. Box 15000, Halifax, NS, Canada B3H 4R2

Joanne B. Clovis
School of Dental Hygiene, Faculty of Dentistry, Dalhousie University, P.O. Box 15000, Halifax, NS, Canada B3H 4R2

Khaldoun M. Aldiabat
School of Nursing, University of Northern British Columbia, 3333 University Way, Prince George, BC, Canada V2N 4Z9

Michael Clinton
Rafic Hariri School of Nursing, American University of Beirut, Riad El-Solh, Beirut 1107 2020, Lebanon

Rita A. Jablonski
School of Nursing, The Pennsylvania State University, 201 Health and Human Development East, University Park, PA 16802, USA

Nop T. Ratanasiripong and Kathleen T. Chai
School of Nursing, California State University, Dominguez Hills, CA 90747, USA

Marianne Frilund
°Abo Akademi University, Vaasa, Finland
Novia University of Applied Sciences, Vaasa, Finland

Lisbeth Fagerström
°Abo Akademi University, Vaasa, Finland
Buskerud University College, Drammen, Norway

Katie Eriksson
Department of Caring Science, °Abo Akademi University, Vaasa, Finland
Helsinki Hospital District of Helsinki and Uusimaa, Finland

Patrik Eklund
Department of Computing Science, Ume°a University, Ume°a, Sweden

Anthony James Roberson
Capstone College of Nursing, The University of AL, Tuscaloosa, Alabama 35487-0358, USA

Diane K. Kjervik
Health Care Environments Division, School of Nursing, University of North Carolina at Chapel Hill, 528 Carrington Hall, Chapel Hill, NC 27599-7460, USA

Sandra P. Small
School of Nursing, Memorial University of Newfoundland, St. John's, NL, Canada A1B 3V6

Kaysi Eastlick Kushner and Anne Neufeld
Faculty of Nursing, University of Alberta, 11405 87 Avenue, Edmonton, AB, Canada T6G 1C9

Heather Pierce
Faculty of Nursing, Midwifery and Health, University of Technology, Sydney, P.O. Box 123, Broadway, NSW 2007, Australia

Caroline S. E. Homer
Centre for Midwifery, Child and Family Health, Faculty of Nursing, Midwifery and Health, University of Technology, Sydney, P.O. Box 123, Broadway, NSW 2007, Australia

Hannah G. Dahlen
Family and Community Health Research Group, School of Nursing and Midwifery, University of Western Sydney, Locked Bag 1797 Penrith, NSW 2751, Australia

Jenny King
Pelvic Floor Unit, Department of Women's and Children's Health, Westmead Hospital, P.O. Box 533, Wentworthville, NSW 2145, Australia

Dana Tschannen
Division of Nursing Business and Health Systems, School of Nursing, University of Michigan, 400 N Ingalls, Room 4152, Ann Arbor, MI 48109-5482, USA

Eunjoo Lee
College of Nursing, Kyungpook National University, Daegu 702-701, Republic of Korea

Tomoko Nishida
Department of Nursing, Sugiyama Jogakuen University, 17-3 Hoshigaoka-Motomachi, Chikusa-Ku, Nagoya 464-8662, Japan

Eriko Ando
Division of Health, Bureau of Health and Welfare, 1-1 Sannomaru 3-Chome, Naka-Ku, Nagoya 460-8508, Japan

Hisataka Sakakibara
Department of Nursing, Nagoya University Graduate School of Medicine, 1-1-20 Daiko-Minami, Higashi-Ku, Nagoya 461-8673, Japan

Agneta Breitholtz
Department of Neurobiology, Care Sciences and Society (NVS), Karolinska Institutet, 141 83 Huddinge, Sweden
School of Health, Care and Social Welfare, M¨alardalen University, P.O. Box 883, 721 23 V¨aster°as, Sweden

Ingrid Snellman
School of Health, Care and Social Welfare, M¨alardalen University, P.O. Box 325, 631 05 Eskilstuna, Sweden

Ingegerd Fagerberg
Department of Neurobiology, Care Sciences and Society (NVS), Karolinska Institutet, 141 83 Huddinge, Sweden
Department of Health Care Sciences, Ersta Sk¨ondal University College, P.O. Box 11189, 100 61 Stockholm, Sweden

Morgan Heinzelmann and Jessica Gill
National Institute of Nursing Research, National Institutes of Health, Bethesda, MD 20814, USA

Michelle R. Frazelle
School of Nursing, Virginia Commonwealth University, 1100 East Leigh Street, Richmond, VA 23298-0567, USA

Cindy L. Munro
School of Nursing, Virginia Commonwealth University, 1100 East Leigh Street, Richmond, VA 23298-0567, USA
School of Nursing, University of South Florida, 12901 Bruce B Downs Boulevard, Tampa, FL 33612, USA

Anne Clancy
Department of Health and SocialWork, School of Nursing, Harstad University College, 9480 Harstad, Norway
University of Tromsø, 9019 Tromso, Norway

Patricia Leahy-Warren, Mary Rose Day and Helen Mulcahy
School of Nursing & Midwifery, Brookfield Health Sciences Complex University College Cork, Cork, Ireland

Donna Goodridge
College of Nursing, University of Saskatchewan, Room 421 Ellis Hall, 103 Hospital Drive, Saskatoon, SK, Canada S7N 0W8

CPSIA information can be obtained
at www.ICGtesting.com
Printed in the USA
BVOW07*0630130617

486758BV00007B/2076/P

9 781632 422958